Praise for *The Autoimmune Fix*

"The hero who has contributed so much to the field of non-celiac gluten sensitivity and celiac disease now shines a light on a mysterious epidemic that is still in the shadows for many: autoimmune disease. Dr. O'Bryan very elegantly connects the dots between environmental triggers such as food and how they can affect the very immune system that's supposed to protect us. *The Autoimmune Fix* doesn't pull any punches. It unflinchingly identifies the foods that put you at risk for future autoimmune disease, foods you might love, foods you might think nothing about eating daily, but it also gives you actual detailed recipes and protocols that will have you eating and living your way to health. Dr. O'Bryan also talks about predictive autoimmunity, one of my favorite subjects. With autoimmunity, you have two choices: Wait until millions are suffering from full-blown autoimmune disorders, then put them on a lifetime of immune suppressants and biologics as well as years of suffering. Or, you can use predictive antibodies to detect autoimmunity in the early stages of the disease and then take steps to halt or even reverse the course of the incipient autoimmune disorder. *The Autoimmune Fix* wisely tells us to take the latter, more proactive choice, and to paraphrase what Dr. O'Bryan says in his book: It's not the doctors you see, the drugs you take, or the surgeries and therapies you undergo; what will impact your health, ultimately, are the choices you make in your life—and getting this book is one of those choices."

—*Aristo Vojdani, PhD, MSc, CLS, CEO, Immunosciences Lab, Inc., and author of* Neuroimmunity *and* The Brain-Gut Connection

"We are so thrilled to support Dr. O'Bryan's work *The Autoimmune Fix*, a book whose time has come. Medicine is evolving and there is a new paradigm for preventing and reversing autoimmune disease, one that is empowering and surprisingly simple to implement. So thankful for this step-by-step manual out in the world to make it easy for anyone to take control of their health."

—*James Maskell, founder and CEO, Evolution of Medicine*

"Dr. Tom O'Bryan is a pioneer in the field of clinical autoimmunity. His explanations of extremely sophisticated mechanisms into everyday language help all of us to understand the path out of autoimmunity and into health. He's been holding the line for patients who have been misdiagnosed and has helped countless people over the years. If you're not feeling right, there's a chance you may be suffering from this hidden cause. This book is a must-read!"

—*Pedram Shojai, OMD, founder, Well.org and* New York Times *bestselling author,* The Urban Monk

"Dr. O'Bryan, does not just 'get' the zeitgeist of immune dysfunction as a primary driver of major degenerative illness, he helps to define it! A great narrative underpinned with relevant research served up with practical solutions—ingest this, then switch your eating habits to those recommended; they will both have a profound effect on your health and life."

—Dr. Michael Ash DO, ND, BSc, RNT,
managing director & head of research and development, Nutri-Link, Ltd.

"I have admired and been informed by Dr. Tom O'Bryan's perspective and approach to the topic of autoimmune disease for many years. In *The Autoimmune Fix* he brings his broad knowledge, with careful consideration of the scientific evidence, directly to those suffering from autoimmunity and those wishing to avoid that fate. He does not just ring the alarm bell, but provides proactive solutions to dealing with this epidemic sweeping through western industrialized society. When it comes to understanding this modern autoimmunity epidemic it doesn't get any better than this."

—David M. Brady, ND, CCN, DACBN, VP health sciences and director, Human Nutrition Institute, University of Bridgeport, and author of The Fibro Fix

"Dr. O'Bryan's understanding of the physiopathology of autoimmune disease is second to none. His ability to translate complex research findings into practical, applicable recommendations that can be individualized to suit each patient's case is admirable. Because of his ability to make complexity accessible, translational, and applicable, I recommend every nutrition practitioner to read Dr. O'Bryan's book."

—Miguel Toribio-Mateas MSc (Clin NeuroSc) BSc (Hons) NutMed ABAAHP FBANT CNCH Reg., chairman of the British Association for Applied Nutrition and Nutritional Therapy

"We all know that an ounce of prevention is worth a pound of cure. Well, when you read this book and implement the author's advice you will be stacking the weights in your favor, helping yourself enjoy a healthier, longer life. Why? Because Dr. Tom O'Bryan has written a different kind of book here. He describes how you can prevent auto-immunity from occurring in the first place. Fortune favors the prepared mind; now you have this book in your hand, don't let it go."

—Antony Haynes, nutritional therapist, functional medicine practitioner, author, lecturer, and head of Technical Services, Nutri-Link, Ltd.

"This is a fascinatingly detailed book about the outcome of autoimmunity —its causes, mechanisms, and effects on the body. It tells you what to eat, and more importantly, what not to eat, if you want to remain healthy, keep doing your marathon running and not be subject to the diseases caused by our affluent Westernized lifestyle and junk foods, and to which most of us still fall prey. Read it and be enlightened! Warmly recommended for those worried about their bodies—and brains."

—Michael N. Marsh, professor, Wolfson College, University of Oxford

"Dr. O'Bryan's information is always cutting edge and he is a brilliant clinician and author. His new book *The Autoimmune Fix* should be read by anyone suffering from autoimmunity. The information contained in the book can be life changing."

—*Datis Kharrazian, DHSc, DC, FACN, CNS,*
associate clinical professor, Loma Linda University School of Medicine

"During the past two decades, no single person has contributed more to the understanding and importance of recognizing the negative effects that gluten has played in human health than Dr. Tom O'Bryan. The hundreds of seminars, lectures, and conferences where Dr. O'Bryan has presented this breakthrough information to literally thousands of physicians are proven true by the results these physicians have experienced as they applied this knowledge to tens of thousands of their patients.

Dr. O'Bryan's new book *The Autoimmune Fix* will prove to become an essential tool to help assist the growing number of individuals whose health and lives are being impacted by the exposure to gluten on their immune system and quality of life. It is with gratitude and pride that I wish to offer my encouragement for everyone to get a copy of Dr. O'Bryan's book as well as to each physician to also get a personal copy of this book and one for their waiting room as well."

—*Tom Schembari, president, NuMedica Advancing Nutrition*

"When new health information is identified, it can sometimes take a long time before doctors actually implement this information in their treatment protocols. I have had the privilege of working with Dr. Tom O'Bryan for more than a decade and admire his passion and commitment to pushing new health information to the forefront, supporting it with his own research and clinical experience, particularly to help other clinicians and patients identify possible triggers of autoimmune disease. The sooner these triggers are identified in a person, the higher the chance of arresting or reversing the disease development. Dr. O'Bryan does a splendid job of explaining this difficult topic. You will be grateful you've read this."

—*Jean Bellin, president, Cyrex Laboratories and past president, Metagenics Nutrition*

"As a doctor and brain scientist, I understand that autoimmune diseases pose one of the greatest threats to our bodies and our minds. Not only do they damage our organs, but they erode self-esteem and can be difficult to identify and treat. In this book, Tom O'Bryan offers a sensitive and comprehensive account of autoimmune disease, all at once engaging us in both the reasons they occur and what we can do about them. With the vast amount of information available, it's important to know where to look when you or a loved one needs help. Look no further! With the combination of the highest scientific integrity and the ease of understanding, this book is a gem, worth getting and guarding, for it is bound to be regarded as a classic of its time."

—*Srini Pillay, MD, assistant professor, Harvard Medical School,*
and award-winning author of Life Unlocked

"Dr. Tom O'Bryan's new book *The Autoimmune Fix* takes his readers down his path to health enlightenment, which is a much deeper understanding of the underlying cause of disease and poor health. Dr. O'Bryan clearly lays out why individuals with certain genetic predispositions will react to certain foods, which will trigger inflammation that will lead to intestinal permeability and the start of a process which, if not checked, will trigger poor health, autoimmune diseases, or worse. More importantly, Dr. O'Bryan lays out how to avoid all this and regain your health using his two phases of transition, which are described in this book in great detail and also include very helpful Transition Protocol Recipes to be used during his two phases of transition.

"I believe that anyone interested in living a healthier and longer life should read *The Autoimmune Fix*, including all doctors and health care practitioners, as it will lead all to a much greater understanding of health and disease."

— *Scott Adams, founder, Celiac.com*

"In my opinion, everyone should read this book. My colleague Dr. Tom O'Bryan has been researching the serious progressive effects of the autoimmune spectrum for decades. He has gained incredible insights into its causes, effects, and how to vanquish the symptoms. This book contains his lifetime work. The concept of the autoimmune illness is complex to get your head around. However, Dr. O'Bryan expertly explains it to us step by step so you can understand why your body is steadily deteriorating and how to reverse this downward spiral. It is a progressive inflammatory state in your body that provokes your immune system to respond and attack itself. He explains this in easy-to-read detail so that parents can understand the implications for their children. He tells us that it is the quantity and quality of our food that is important. He reveals that the stand-out culprits are gluten, dairy, and sugar. Read this book and follow the steps to dampen down the fire of reactivity that can rage through your body."

— *Rodney Ford, MD, MBBS, FRACP, pediatric gastroenterologist and allergist and author of* The Gluten Syndrome *and* Gluten: ZERO Global

HOW TO STOP THE HIDDEN
AUTOIMMUNE DAMAGE
THAT KEEPS YOU SICK, FAT, AND TIRED
BEFORE IT TURNS INTO DISEASE

The Autoimmune Fix

TOM O'BRYAN, DC, CCN, DACBN

——————— FOREWORD BY ———————

NEW YORK TIMES BESTSELLING AUTHOR MARK HYMAN, MD

RODALE

RODALE *wellness*

Live happy. Be healthy. Get inspired.

Sign up today to get exclusive access to our authors,
exclusive bonuses, and the most authoritative, useful, and cutting-edge
information on health, wellness, fitness, and living your life to the fullest.

Visit us online at RodaleWellness.com
Join us at RodaleWellness.com/Join

© 2016 by Dr. Tom O'Bryan

All rights reserved. No part of this publication may be reproduced or transmitted in
any form or by any means, electronic or mechanical, including photocopying,
recording, or any other information storage and retrieval system, without the written
permission of the publisher.

Rodale books may be purchased for business or promotional use or for special sales.
For information, please write to:
Special Markets Department, Rodale Inc., 733 Third Avenue, New York, NY 10017

Printed in the United States of America

Rodale Inc. makes every effort to use acid-free ♾, recycled paper ♻.

Graphic on page 6 from *The New England Journal of Medicine*,
Melissa R. Arbuckle, Micah T. McClain, Mark V. Rubertone, et al.,
"Development of Autoantibodies before the Clinical Onset of Systemic Lupus
Erythematosus," vol. no. 349, Copyright © 2003 Massachusetts Medical Society.
Reprinted with permission from Massachusetts Medical Society.

Book design by Joanna Williams

Library of Congress Cataloging-in-Publication Data is on file with the publisher.
ISBN   978-1-62336-700-8   hardcover

Distributed to the trade by Macmillan

2 4 6 8 10 9 7 5 3 1   hardcover

☘ RODALE.

Follow us @RodaleBooks on

We inspire health, healing, happiness, and love in the world.
Starting with you.

TO KELLY, JASON, AND MIA
LOVE YOU FROM EVERYWHERE

CONTENTS

FOREWORD

The number of people in the United States with chronic conditions is rapidly rising. It is predicted that by the year 2030 close to half of the entire population will be diagnosed with some form of chronic disease. This has many implications. First, it means that more people are getting sicker earlier in life. Second, it's predicted that by 2044 the cost to Medicare and Medicaid to treat these chronic conditions will be more than all of the taxes collected by our government. What's more, the most common chronic conditions are grouped as autoimmune diseases, in which the body—in an effort to protect itself—is attacking instead.

How are we as a community going to deal with this? The answer is that health doesn't happen in the doctor's office. Health happens where we live, in our kitchens where we cook, and where we eat. I strongly believe that the fork is the most powerful tool we have to transform our health, and I know that my friend and colleague, Dr. Tom O'Bryan, agrees.

Today we know that the foods most of us were taught to enjoy our entire lives, and many of us still eat every day, are actually making us sick. These foods include wheat products as well as sugar, dairy, and commercially processed fats. Once you can understand this fact, you're going to change your relationship with the foods you're eating, and you're going to feel better. This book provides that lesson.

The traditional medical community is partly to blame for the health problems millions of us are facing. When we suggested that the answer to fighting obesity was a low-fat diet, we told our patients to eat whole grain pasta and bread and margarine. Yet over the years, we found, in fact, that our advice was wrong, because the exact opposite happened. Low-fat eating wasn't the cure for the obesity epidemic; it was a primary cause. I call the result *diabesity*.

Now we know that eating foods high in the right fats makes you thin. Sugar makes you fat. And flour products, which the body converts into sugar, are one of the biggest triggers of the diabesity epidemic.

The way in which we grind flour and the way in which it's grown produce wheat with a much higher starch content compared to what our ancestors ate. The average whole wheat bread has more sugar content than sugar. If you have two slices of whole wheat bread, you're going to raise your blood sugar more than if you ate a candy bar. In this book, you'll learn that not only does this increase in blood sugar lead to obesity, it creates the silent killer of inflammation, which is at the root cause of most chronic illnesses doctors treat every day.

So if you think "I'm having whole wheat bread, that's a good thing. It's healthy," Dr. O'Bryan is here to clear up the confusion. Most food industry companies are adding whole grains to their products to make them sound healthy just as we had *low fat* assigned to food labels 10, 20, 30 years ago. Dr. O'Bryan is going to teach you how to get them out of your diet. The truth is, any kind of gluten-containing flour product is a problem for the majority of people.

Over the years, I've seen more than 15,000 patients at the UltraWellness Center in Lenox, Massachusetts. There is nobody who comes into my office, not one single person, who doesn't get a gluten sensitivity test. Anybody who has any chronic illness or any of its symptoms is considered "gluten guilty" until proven otherwise.

If you are one of the many millions of people who know that they don't feel quite right, but don't know exactly why, this book is for you. The information you're about to read takes you outside of the traditional health-care system that is not providing the answers that you are looking for. Instead, you'll learn how to implement strategies to change your everyday behaviors, so that you can begin to feel better, lose the weight you want, and regain your energy.

This exciting new book may be your first introduction to the world of functional medicine. Dr. O'Bryan and I, as well as thousands of doctors and health practitioners around the world, believe that functional medicine is the future of medicine. It seeks to identify and address the root causes of disease and views the body as one integrated system, not a collection of independent organs divided up by medical specialties. Functional medicine practitioners are specifically trained to treat the whole system, not just the symptoms. In this way, we can address the underlying causes of disease, often with the least invasive means possible. This line of thinking brings us back full circle, to your fork.

By choosing the right foods and avoiding the wrong ones, you can break your addictions to sugar and carbs, lower inflammation, and take back your health. You'll also learn how to accurately diagnose the underlying problems that are pushing you further along the path to poor health, or what Dr. O'Bryan refers to as the autoimmune spectrum.

Tom and I went through our original functional medicine training together, almost 20 years ago. He is without a doubt part of the solution to the current health crisis, as he teaches thousands of health practitioners across the globe every year about the autoimmune spectrum. His gluten-free lifestyle and life story provide the best examples for the rest of us to follow. Adapting his suggestions, you too will become part of our community, get to better health, and improve your quality of life.

—Mark Hyman, MD, director of the Cleveland Clinic Center for Functional Medicine, chairman of the Institute for Functional Medicine, and *New York Times* bestselling author of *The Blood Sugar Solution, The Blood Sugar Solution 10-Day Detox Diet Cookbook,* and *Eat Fat, Get Thin*

Acknowledgments

This book is an accumulation of my 30+ years of study. It began with my mentors, and it is my honor to acknowledge them. Dr. George Goodheart taught me "body language never lies" and to always ask the question "Why is the body doing what it is doing?" Dr. Jeffrey Bland taught me how to investigate "the why" and keep the larger perspective in mind. Dr. Aristo Vojdani whose life's work gives us the tools to measure the immune system. And Dr. Leonard Faye, whose common sense approach taught me how the body is a completely interconnected and integrated masterpiece.

My grandparents, Bepe and Assunta Ceschini, came to the United States through Ellis Island in 1922 at the ages of 24 and 22. They came with very little money, did not speak English, arrived without a specific destination, and simply wanted a better life for themselves and their future family. Their courage has always been my foundation when times get tough.

My parents, Thom and Nellie, who gave all they had so their children would have more opportunity. My sister Karen's tireless patience allows me to be my best self. My brother Dennis has an authenticity that is a model to us all. And to Marzi, my confidante, whose untiring support feeds my body and soul.

TheDr.com is the momentum for carrying out my message. My heartfelt thanks goes to the entire team that keeps the wheels greased and the machine running: Karen Cortis, Michelle Ross, Kris Blakeman, Lynn Douglas, Laura Danaher, Melissa Mersch, Gena Stokes, Maria Michelle, and Erin Crutcher. Mary Agnes and Tommy Antonopoulos and the entire team at viralintegrity.com have been my biggest cheerleaders and are responsible for disseminating my internet and social media content. They tune the frequency of my message to carry it out to the world.

When I met the Rodale publishing team, I knew I had come home. It was 35 years ago that Rodale's publication *Prevention* magazine and Dr. Jonathan Wright's case studies demonstrated that health care could be rational and effective. Thank you, Rodale! Today I am blessed to work with Rodale Books. My editor Marisa Vigilante and her assistant Isabelle Hughes have been integral to this book's success.

My publishing team has been extraordinary. My agents Celeste Fine and John Maas, whose patience and guidance have been exemplary. Thank you for providing the road map for every aspect of this book's journey. Tom Malterre's camaraderie and support is only second to the depth of his knowledge on the topics in this book. Thank you, Alissa Segersten, creator of the wonderful recipes in this book; I would sit at your table in total bliss every day. Pamela Liflander, whose editorial support allowed my ideas to flow freely and created an order for this body of knowledge. This was no easy task. Thank you, Pam!

My ongoing thanks to my patients, who share their stories, come for help, trust my guidance, and celebrate their results. And lastly, I also want to thank you, the reader, for taking a chance and investing your time and dollars into reading this book. My prayer is that you find guidance to a healthier future for yourself and the next generation.

INTRODUCTION

As millions of people desperately seek solutions to an epidemic of mysterious and debilitating health issues, I'm going to show you that the underlying cause of many of these diseases is related to your immune system: the mechanism in your body that is designed to protect you yet is so overwhelmed it is unintentionally doing you a whole lot of harm.

When the body attacks itself and causes organ and tissue damage, we call the disorder *autoimmunity*. A person can go a lifetime with the earliest symptoms of autoimmunity—which can include joint pain, weight gain, brain fog, gut imbalances, depression, mood disorders, and fatigue— without ever receiving a diagnosis of a disease. Instead, you're told by doctors or well-meaning family and friends that "you're fine, it's just stress," even though your inner voice may be telling you that something's wrong. The doctors who evaluate these symptoms are well intentioned, but because nothing shows up as a crisis on a blood test, you might have received generic advice, like "lose weight," "get more sleep," "eat cleaner," or "reduce your stress." Or worse, you might walk out of the doctor's office with a prescription for antianxiety medications to help you "calm down." It's no wonder we lose hope as our conditions worsen, mystified as to what could possibly be wrong with our health. After all, our doctors said we're healthy.

The truth, and what I'd like to share with you in this book, is that autoimmunity occurs on a spectrum. You don't wake up with diabetes one day—it develops slowly, almost imperceptibly, over time. You don't wake up with Alzheimer's disease either—it's a decades-long process with many steps of progression over the years. Scientists now know that for autoimmune diseases, including diabetes and Alzheimer's, the process starts as early as your twenties or thirties, with multiple steps of declining health along the way. In the case of Alzheimer's, it might begin with brain fog, then forgetfulness, confusion, memory loss, and, eventually, dementia. For diabetes, the spectrum might begin with food cravings, then blood sugar imbalances (hypoglycemia), next metabolic syndrome with weight gain, then followed by neuropathies (numbness and tingling that come and go), and finally a diagnosis of diabetes with a high risk of heart disease.

Aside from our discomfort, the largest problem we face is that a medical diagnosis can occur only *after* there is significant tissue damage. By then, the fix is severe: a lifetime of medications and an uphill battle to reverse disease. While science has been making clear advances in the treatment of many of the 80-plus autoimmune diseases, wouldn't you like to know, sooner rather than later, if autoimmunity is causing your symptoms?

The stakes are high: Currently, in the United States, the number one cause of morbidity and mortality—meaning getting sick and eventually dying of some disease—is your immune system trying to protect you. Doctors and researchers have known for decades that the primary cause of getting sick and dying in the world is cardiovascular disease, with cancer being second and autoimmune diseases (as a whole) third. However, there is a paradigm shift occurring in understanding the development of heart disease and cancer. What was originally perceived as a lipid (fats)–storage disease of the arterial wall, atherosclerosis is now recognized as a chronic inflammatory disease. From this perspective, and with the knowledge that the only system of the body addressing inflammation is your immune system, we now believe that the immune system triggers are the number one mechanism behind getting sick and dying.[1]

I should know. Autoimmunity and gluten sensitivity, one of the most common mechanisms for launching the immune system into action, have been my world for the past 25 years. I've educated hundreds of thousands of members of the general public, and tens of thousands of doctors, nurses, and nutritionists across the globe, about how food selection, digestion, nutrition, and autoimmunity affect overall health. What's more, my own health story, as well as what my family has experienced, exemplifies the drama of the autoimmune spectrum.

MY JOURNEY

I was not one of those men who always knew that they wanted to be a doctor or who were motivated to become one because of a firsthand experience with chronic illness. In fact, I always thought I was a healthy kid. Growing up on the streets of Detroit, I had a passion for martial arts. In my early twenties, I was introduced to aikido, a form of martial arts that has been called moving Zen. This practice resonated in my soul—the premise of removing resistance and redirecting powerful energy and letting the body flow.

Even though I'm now known the world over for my work on autoimmunity and gluten sensitivity, believe it or not, in my early twenties I was a baker in an organic restaurant in Ann Arbor, Michigan. Ironically, I used to bake the best bread. People would come from miles around for my unleavened whole grain, organic bread. I'd bake 48 loaves a day of this fabulous, really good bread by hand. I was so hungry all the time when I was younger: I remember that I would often take the bread out of the oven, slice off an end piece, spread peanut butter over it, then drizzle honey on it and lay sliced bananas on top. I thought I was being so healthy: It was whole wheat bread and organic peanut butter and honey. The bananas were natural. Honey is natural, and certainly better than processed sugar. Yet feeding that one hunger craving was probably the worst thing I could have been doing for my health: I was eating a blood sugar time bomb. I was hungry and tired all the time because of my own chronic low blood sugar, but this snack was flooding my body with the equivalent of four Snickers bars. I'd feel great for a while, but the unavoidable crash would happen about an hour later, and I'd be exhausted all over again. Do you ever notice that you're tired and yawning about an hour after your last big meal? This spike and crash create the typical roller-coaster ride that many of us notice. I was just trying to live the healthiest life I could, so I kept eating my organic whole wheat bread, not recognizing the damage it was causing.

At the same time, being a long-haired "back to nature" hippie in Ann Arbor in 1970, I had a circle of friends who started reading articles about food and nutrition in *Prevention* magazine. I remember noticing the articles by Jonathan Wright, MD, from the University of Michigan, which is where I was studying. His point of view was my first introduction to health care, even though I was more interested in pursuing martial arts at the time.

After graduation, I decided to follow my passion to learn as much as I could about aikido, this gentle martial art. I moved to Japan and lived in a martial arts school as a *deshi*, honing my craft and cleaning the toilets for the grand master. Physically, I never felt better. My energy and endurance were up, and I was experiencing a full and joyous life. It's just occurring to me now in writing this book that one of the reasons I was so clearheaded and performed so well physically was that my diet was primarily rice, which doesn't have the toxic gluten proteins found in wheat; I had left my Western diet behind. Yet after a while, I was aching to get back to the United States. I had met my future wife before I went, and I missed her. So I came back and we were married within 6 months.

My wife suffered from back pain that stemmed from an accident when she was 12. The pain would flare up so severely that she would have to be hospitalized in traction for a week at a time. While I was searching for a new career and trying to find a way to relieve her pain, I met Dr. Harold Swanson, an 84-year-old chiropractor. When I first went to his office, I had to carry my wife in. Yet when he was finished, she could walk out. There was something about Dr. Swanson and the energy of chiropractic that reminded me of aikido, which translates from the Japanese to mean "get out of the way and allow the energy to flow." That same theory is the premise of chiropractic: that the body can heal itself by freeing its energy flow. The link between the two disciplines was remarkable, so I decided to become a chiropractor.

It took me a while to notice that I wasn't feeling well once I started back on my regular eating routine. I was at my physical peak after training with elite aikido practitioners; I was excited about getting married and thinking about what was in store in my future. Looking back, now I know I was running on adrenaline. Had I not been in the greatest shape of my life, I would have felt symptoms sooner.

In 1978, we moved to Chicago so I could study at the National University of Health Sciences, the most research-oriented chiropractic school. During my first weekend, I attended a seminar by Kirpal Singh, MD, a visiting scholar from Los Angeles, whose lecture on electroacupuncture literally changed my expectations of what a doctor could discern. He shared an anecdote of a 42-year-old woman that I remember verbatim to this day.

The woman had come to see him because she had just been diagnosed with adult-onset diabetes. After his initial examination, he told her, "I believe that when you were a young child, you had a virus, and it almost killed you. The virus settled into your pancreas, causing inflammation and upsetting your hormone balance to the point where you developed hypoglycemia. You've had hypoglycemia for the last 35 years. Now it just progressed into type 2 diabetes."

Dr. Singh recalled that the woman was shocked and said, "Doctor, you're right. I did have hypoglycemia for many, many years, but I never was sick as a child."

He calmly replied, "Yes, you were. If your mother is alive, call and ask her."

The woman called right from his office, and he recounted the conversation: "Hi Mom. I'm in a doctor's office. Everything is fine, but he just told me that I must have been deathly sick as a child. Was I really?"

Her mother replied, "Honey, it's true. You were so little, and our doctor was out of town. We tried everything because you had a really high fever, including putting ice packs on your feet. We didn't realize it at the time, but you almost died."

When I heard the story in its entirety, I just sat there, amazed. How did he know?

The next weekend, Sheldon Deal, DC, a former Mr. Arizona bodybuilder, came to lecture. Dr. Deal's talk was given in a hotel just off campus, and the stage featured a working color TV without volume. He opened his briefcase and took out a magnet about the size of today's smartphones, held it up, and walked over to the television. The picture on the television went upside down. When he walked away from it, the picture went right side up. Walked to it, it went upside down. He said, "That's what electromagnetic energy does to your nervous system." Back in 1978, people were first starting to wear electronic watches. It was the new big thing, and people were concerned. Today, the batteries in cell phones or Bluetooth devices are of even greater concern and might be contributing to inflammation in the brain and the development of brain tumors.[2] This information made me realize that our environmental exposures can have a silent but profound impact on our health.

Just like the previous weekend, I sat there in awe. This was certainly not the status quo of any medical education with which I was familiar. I was fired up to learn all that I could. I realized that chiropractic care meant so much more than manipulating bones and muscles. It also focused on diet, nutrition, environment, and what was later to be organized as the principles of functional medicine.

During my last year of study, my wife and I were trying to start a family, but we were having difficulty conceiving. I picked up the phone and called the seven most famous holistic doctors I'd heard of, and every one of them graciously took the time and gave me their advice. Each expert contributed one piece of information that helped me solve the puzzle, including something radical: going gluten-free. So I put a program together based on all of their recommendations, and in 6 weeks we were pregnant. One of the critical components that we addressed was gluten and dairy sensitivities, and we both began to change our diet. I started running again, and my marathon times were better than ever, but I never connected my increased performance to my new diet.

Good friends of ours quickly asked if I would help them get pregnant. They, too, had been through artificial insemination, and nothing had worked. In 3 months, a second woman was pregnant! I was ecstatic to see that I could help people who were suffering from hormone imbalances and infertility, and I couldn't wait to open my practice. I decided to focus my practice on treating couples with hormone imbalances and infertility.

When I graduated in 1980, I opened my practice, having already lined up 33 women as potential patients. I created a comprehensive, holistic approach to health care. I also took on leadership roles. I was at one point the president of the Illinois Chiropractic Society, and I was also responsible for initiating massage as a reimbursable therapy: In the early 1980s, I formalized the claim submission process by carefully documenting and standardizing the therapeutic value of massage for musculoskeletal concerns.

As my practice grew, I realized that patient after patient had food sensitivities that I could spot by putting them on a gluten-free diet. In fact, many of the women I saw with hormonal imbalances had a problem with gluten, manifesting as either PMS, infertility, amenorrhea, or unexplained miscarriages. We tested each of the women for celiac disease, and the results usually came back negative. This was a problem, because at that time, celiac was the only accepted disease linked to a wheat allergy or sensitivity. But the patients' bodies never lied: Their issues resolved or made significant improvements when they would follow my advice to avoid wheat completely. Back then, science had no accepted way of confirming this, but I knew what I saw: Hundreds of my patients were responding favorably to a gluten-free diet. This realization, and the subsequent treatment protocol I developed, got me into the world of treating gluten sensitivity with or without celiac disease.

Meanwhile, my own health was suffering, and I didn't even know it. At 40, I was a long-distance runner, still trim and with a nicely performing body. Then I was diagnosed with a cataract, which is very unusual for a healthy, 40-ish man. I took a few days to research the problem and found out that high lead levels can be a trigger for cataracts, but who has high lead levels in this day and age? I was certain it wasn't me, but I did the tests anyway. Wouldn't you know, I had the highest levels of lead poisoning of any of the hundreds of people I had ever tested. I reviewed my timeline, as life experiences often shed light on a problem, and I remembered that during the first 8 years of my life, my family lived in Detroit, just across the river from Ford's largest assembly plant. In the 1950s, there weren't pollution controls like there are now, and the air was highly toxic. Just think about the toxic water problems in Flint, Michigan, today.

Once I got the lead out of my system by following a protocol that included infrared saunas and the right nutrition that acted as a magnet to pull the lead out, I went back to running marathons and triathlons. Although I had a healthy lifestyle and ate good-quality foods, every once in a while I would feel like I needed more calories because my blood sugar would get low from exercising so aggressively. I knew the fix: I'd eat half a dozen apple-cinnamon doughnuts on the way to do a 15-mile run. After all, I'd burn it all off with the 2-plus hours of running. Nothing wrong with that kind of logic, right?

Then I had myself tested, using a protocol similar to the one you'll learn about in this book, and the results came back and astounded me: three different elevated levels of antibodies that would affect my brain function over time. I had elevated antibodies to myelin basic protein, which is the mechanism for developing multiple sclerosis. I had elevated antibodies to cerebellar peptides, linked to a loss of balance and brain processing speed. And I had elevated antibodies to ganglioside, which shrinks your brain and causes cognitive decline and dementias. This test clearly showed that I, too, was on the autoimmune spectrum.

Let me be clear: I had all three elevated antibodies, and I was eating well and doing triathlons at the same time. On the outside, no one would ever say I was infirm. I felt like a pretty healthy guy. I didn't have any symptoms, but you don't argue with elevated antibodies. These test results were not something you can wish away or take an aspirin for in response. So I cleaned up my act and went *completely* gluten- and dairy-free and applied the right nutritional protocol that would support my immune system so that I could heal. About 2 years later, I repeated the tests. The elevated antibodies were all gone; the antibodies were down to normal range.

My observations were not fully validated until 2001, when my friend David Perlmutter, MD, was lecturing. He presented a study of 10 men whose migraines were so debilitating they had been receiving workers' compensation for an average of 8 years. During the lecture, I started to think about the children in those families and how stressful their home environment must have been, constantly hearing, "Be quiet, *shhh, shhh,* Dad's got a headache." These families would have gone through their life savings and their retirement accounts just trying to survive. It turned out that all 10 men with unrelenting migraines had gluten sensitivity and *not celiac disease.* When the author of the study put them on a gluten-free diet, 7 out of 10 never had a headache again. Two got partial relief. The tenth one refused the diet. The MRIs of all 10 patients showed lesions on their brains, which were caused by inflammation that began with gluten sensitivity.

The pieces of the autoimmune story were beginning to come together. I realized then that millions of people were suffering from undiagnosed or, worse, poorly diagnosed autoimmune conditions causing tissue damage (like lesions on the brain) that would begin causing symptoms and eventually a disease diagnosis. I decided to focus my attention on nutrition education and the new world of functional medicine, a term first coined in the 1980s by one of my mentors, Jeffrey Bland, PhD. I wanted to spread my findings to a wider audience: that gluten sensitivity by itself was a tremendous problem, regardless of a confirmed celiac disease diagnosis. My work, and the work of others in functional medicine, also confirmed that if you have a sensitivity to gluten, or other food or environmental triggers, it can manifest as inflammation that can occur in *any* tissue of the body. We had found the trigger—the "gasoline on the fire"—that began the cascade of symptoms leading to autoimmune diseases. By this point, I was living entirely gluten-, dairy-, and sugar-free. At 52, I was feeling great, and my triathlete performances were competitive with the 30-year-old bracket.

I gave my first large lecture in 2004 to the International and American Academy of Clinical Nutritionists, and I haven't stopped speaking to this day. My lectures continue to be received as an "OMG" moment for most in the audience: No matter where in the world I'm speaking, the average well-intentioned doctor or other health practitioner simply does not understand the extent to which the lifestyle choices we make, including the foods we eat and the environment we create, can so severely affect our health.

This message hit home once again when my 80-year-old mother was found by her friends, sitting in a chair at home, conscious but completely incoherent. In the emergency room, the doctors diagnosed her with toxic metabolic encephalopathy—big Scrabble words that refer to a neurological disorder that includes hallucinations and irrational conversations, caused by toxicity in the bloodstream called *sepsis* (what I refer to as crud in the blood). By the time I got there, the attending doctor advised me that there was nothing I could do besides make my mother comfortable and watch her go; his own mother was suffering from the same thing. But I wasn't willing to accept that diagnosis. By that time, I had been practicing functional medicine for 20 years, and I knew that symptoms like my mother's were rarely the problem but rather a signal from the body of some other underlying issue. I realized that even though I knew so much about gluten sensitivity, I had never tested my mom. When I ordered the tests, we learned that my mother had celiac disease that had never been diagnosed. Her body's autoimmune response—exacerbated by the malabsorption, malnutrition, and dehydration that often accompany celiac in elderly patients—was causing the symptoms of toxic metabolic encephalopathy. I took her home from the hospital and put her on a gluten-free, dairy-free, sugar-free diet and increased her water intake to 3 liters of water a day. Within weeks, she was not only feeling better, she was demanding to get back behind the wheel of her car.

On one side of the autoimmune spectrum was my mother, who at 80 was diagnosed with celiac disease only because she had one really bad day. Over the course of her life, I don't remember her ever complaining about her health, but now I'm sure there were plenty of days when she must have been uncomfortable. Celiac, like any other autoimmune disease, doesn't come on overnight. Meanwhile, I'm sitting at the other end of the spectrum: Even though I was much younger and appeared healthy, I also had disease that could have caused devastating illness had it not been addressed. For both of us, lifestyle changes were the first step to healing.

WHAT'S IN IT FOR YOU?

Now it's my turn to help you. If you have stomach cramps, bloating, constipation, occasional headaches, or acne, and if you're fatigued even though you're drinking coffee all day, I'm here to tell you that's not normal. You don't have to live this way. These annoying symptoms, let alone the more immobilizing symptoms, are a message from your body saying "something's not right here." In this book, you'll learn how to listen to the messages your body is delivering, and you'll be able to discern them because you will fully understand the most overlooked mechanism that's directly affecting your health.

The good news is that it is not difficult to make changes in your lifestyle that will set the stage to transform your life and your health in just 3 weeks. The goal is to lower inflammation: the reason why you are feeling forgetful, sick, fat, or tired. Addressing these symptoms alone will not work, which is why you are frustrated. Instead, we're going to find what's causing the inflammation that's creating these symptoms.

Gluten (the family of proteins in wheat), dairy, and sugar are the most common triggers that set up the entire mechanism of inflammation and autoimmunity. There are others, but the clinical world of functional medicine considers those to be "the big three." Toxic chemicals and heavy metals found in the environment—like the lead I was carrying around—are also notorious initiators of the autoimmune mechanism. When you stop "throwing gasoline on the fire" by getting rid of these main food groups that cause inflammation and trigger autoimmunity, your body begins to cool down and reduce inflammation. Best of all, the science is clear: You then can arrest and eventually reverse the damage of many autoimmune diseases.

I'm not promising a panacea that will cure every possible disease in 3 weeks, but my program will put you on the right track. Following this plan will create an undeniable difference in how good you feel. Your sleep will improve, your energy will increase, and you'll finally be able to get rid of the extra weight you're carrying without having to starve yourself.

In fact, some of the symptoms that have often been holding you back for years will begin to fade away. Addressing inflammation is the primary reason why scientists, researchers, and doctors can share so many successful case studies in medical journals, and why you may have heard seemingly unbelievable testimonials about reversing attention-deficit/hyperactivity disorder (ADHD), acne in teenagers, depression in adults, severe crippling arthritis, tumors in the eye (yes, that's right), rheumatoid arthritis, psoriasis, lupus . . . the list goes on and on. Once the "emergency brake" of inflammation that has been holding their bodies back is released by addressing the foods that contribute to the immune system's response, people do get better. That's why I feel confident in saying that no matter what your current health issues, you will begin to transition into good health by following the program.

This book provides everything you'll need to understand the autoimmune mechanism, see how it's manifesting in your body, recognize where it began, and address the problem so that you can move forward and experience optimal health. Autoimmunity is a maze. I will show you the pathway out. What's more, you'll be so excited to have your health and vitality back that staying with the program becomes second nature.

STOP ACCEPTING MEDIOCRE HEALTH

Whenever I lecture on reversing autoimmunity, I start by asking my audience, "How many in the room are healthy?" Usually, almost everybody raises a hand. Then I ask, "How many in the room believe they have optimal physical, mental, and social well-being, and not merely the absence of disease and infirmity?" This statement is the definition of the word *health* in *Dorland's Illustrated Medical Dictionary*. At this point, the hands go down, except for 1 person out of 300. I smile and say to her, "Way to go. High-five to you." The truth is, we think we're healthy, and we're not. We accept mediocrity in our health and in our lives.

In this book, I am inciting a revolution, a revolution against mediocrity. There are two statistics that put my mission in perspective. First, the US health-care system is the most expensive in the world but reports consistently show that it grossly underperforms relative to other highly industrialized countries. Worse, according to the *New England Journal of Medicine*, we have finally crossed the line where for the first time in the history of the human species, our offspring will have a shorter projected life span than their parents. Our children are going to get sick earlier, get diagnosed with disease earlier, and die earlier than their parents from completely preventable diseases like diabetes, obesity, cardiovascular disease, and Alzheimer's disease. More kids are diagnosed with diabetes, ADHD, autism, and pediatric juvenile idiopathic arthritis than ever before. This is simply unacceptable.

The mediocre health care that we accept is producing a world where our children will die at an earlier age than us. Here's an example: When I went through my medical education, we were taught that adult-onset type 2 diabetes was going to be an upcoming epidemic. Now we don't call it adult-onset diabetes because so many children share the same condition. It's just type 2 diabetes—one of the greatest threats to health in the industrialized world. And the predictions were correct: The "upcoming epidemic" is here, now.

The outlook for adults isn't much better. We have collectively bought into the crazy notion that the aches, pains, and fatigue that limit us are due to the "fact" that we are getting older or are under a lot of stress. We listen to the ridiculous commercials on television about drugs that can make us happy again if we would only overlook the warnings that they might cause cancer, blindness, brain deterioration, or death. We block out the warning messages and accept the happy visuals. But your life, especially as you age, doesn't have to be a downward spiral of depression and poor health. Instead, you'll learn the science that explains why you haven't been experiencing optimal health, and you'll find out what you can do about it right now. You'll also learn why your nagging symptoms occur where they do.

Imagine that the human body is a chain of interconnected organs and systems. Whenever you pull on a chain, it will always break at the weakest link. Wherever your weak link is in your body, that's where inflammation will impact, causing symptoms. This weak link might be why you have a vague sense of not feeling well. Perhaps it's weight. Perhaps it's memory. Perhaps it's your thyroid. Perhaps it's your joints or your hormones. The weak link in your chain is where, or how, you will experience illness. You might have been associating these symptoms with getting older, but the reality is that age has very little to do with your sense of well-being.

Identifying this weak link gives us a window of opportunity to address the associated problem at the earliest possible moment. This investigation is the researcher's field of *predictive autoimmunity*; functional medicine is the clinician's field of what to do about it. Knowing what may be in store might be the motivation you need to take a good look at your family history as well as your current lifestyle and see what is out of balance. Then we can work together so that you can begin to feel good again.

We must stop going blindly forward thinking we're "fine." We have to wake up and learn how to take care of our bodies. As you start uncovering the story of autoimmunity, you'll learn more about yourself than you ever thought possible. Then you can take this information to your doctors, and instead of treating or stabilizing your symptoms—or worse, being told yet again that there is nothing wrong—you can finally address your total health in the most sustainable way. Most of our researchers today are looking for ways to suppress the immune response. I believe the first step is, once again, to stop throwing gasoline on the fire. Then you have a better chance of putting the fire out.

We can have a totally different status quo in terms of our collective health. However, unless we can address the mechanisms that send our immune system into attack mode, we will continue to age prematurely and develop diseases earlier in life. To do nothing to control the autoimmune response means that even if you have the genes to be vibrant and dynamic in your nineties, you're not likely to get there.

Don't take my word for it: The proof is in the research. The immune system is one of the areas that have sparked the most research and new findings in medicine over the past 25 years. In fact, according to Yehuda Shoenfeld, MD (the godfather of predictive autoimmunity, and someone you will hear about in this book), if you review the Nobel Prizes of the last 20 to 25 years, most of them were given in recognition of revelations about the immune system.

Yet it takes an average of 17 years for research findings to work their way down to your local doctors.[3] The problem is that you don't have 17 years to waste. Unless your doctors are completely up to date with the medical research, they may not be fully aware of what cutting-edge science now knows about the immune system. And it's very likely that unless they went to school in the past 10 years, this information was not addressed in their medical training. That's why this book is so critical to your health: because your doctor, even with the best of intentions, may not be treating you based on the most current science.

This book will introduce you to some of the thousands of studies done at the finest institutions and published in the most prestigious journals. The science clearly shows that modifying your eating habits to avoid the foods that trigger an immune response doesn't mean you are following a fad diet. It's the only way to address the inflammation in your body so that you can heal.

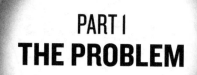

PART I
THE PROBLEM

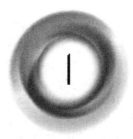

THE SPECTRUM OF AUTOIMMUNITY

In this chapter, we're going to talk about where disease comes from. Here's a question for you: Do think that you wake up one morning with a disease like diabetes or Alzheimer's or an extra 30 pounds? No. Scientists tell us these are results from decades-long processes that develop in a step-by-step sequence. But if you gain the big-picture view of the disease sequence, it becomes clear that there is a way to "nip it in the bud"—or, as scientists say, arrest the development of autoimmune disease—and stay healthy longer and with a shorter period of disability at the end of life.

My work in the world of celiac disease and wheat sensitivity has made me one of the leading experts in this field. Because celiac disease is the one autoimmune disease that has clearly been mapped—what makes you vulnerable (genetics), what's the trigger (gluten in wheat, rye, and barley), and what's the "last straw" before it begins (intestinal permeability)—it is a good model to study. I'm going to refer to it throughout this chapter, as well as the rest of the book, as a classic example of the *autoimmune spectrum.*

A spectrum is used to classify an idea or object in terms of its position on a scale between two extreme or opposite points. The spectrum of autoimmunity is a progressive state of disease that runs from vibrant health at one end to degenerative disease at the other. In between lies a broad range of varied but related stages that build on each other, usually moving in the direction of more disease. This is how we suffer from autoimmune damage long before we're diagnosed with autoimmune disease and long before the first symptoms occur. Again, on one end of the spectrum, there are no obvious symptoms: This is referred to as *benign autoimmunity*. On the other end is a well-defined health problem: disease or clinical illness. The in-between area of the spectrum holds the *disease process* (the accumulation of damage), which is referred to as *pathogenic autoimmunity*. The benefit of understanding this spectrum is so we can consciously shift our direction away from disease and back to vibrant health. That is the purpose of this book.

This health deterioration can be measured in terms of its intensity by the level of antibodies. When there is a slight elevation of antibodies, some people may have noticeable symptoms, while others with tremendously high levels of antibodies may have no symptoms at all. Yet both types of people are on the spectrum, and they will progress along the spectrum until they are diagnosed with a chronic or deadly disease. This is why it does not matter whether you notice symptoms or not: If you have elevated antibodies, they are fueling tissue degeneration.

Whenever we are exposed to any environmental trigger (such as gluten, peanuts, mold . . .), our immune system is activated to protect us. This is happening 24/7, and it's designed to work in the background so we don't notice it. This is referred to as *normal immunity*: You feel nothing. If the level of insult (the amount of exposure) increases, you might experience some kind of mild irritation, like a runny nose, sore muscles, or brain fog. If the level of exposure continues to increase, the immune system has to respond more aggressively, which begins the inflammatory cascade. Excess inflammation beyond the normal range will cause cellular damage. Continued cellular damage will cause tissue damage. Continued tissue damage will cause organ inflammation. Continued organ inflammation will increase the intensity of symptoms, and you develop elevated antibodies to that organ. Continued elevated antibodies to an organ leads to organ damage. Now you have symptoms that can be identified as an autoimmune disease.

This mechanism is the primary pathway in the development of autoimmune disease, opposite.

In 2003, Melissa Arbuckle, MD, PhD, and her colleagues published a landmark study in the *New England Journal of Medicine* that chronicled the autoimmune disease spectrum. Dr. Arbuckle investigated the

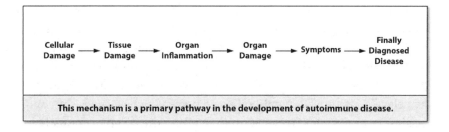

Cellular Damage → Tissue Damage → Organ Inflammation → Organ Damage → Symptoms → Finally Diagnosed Disease

This mechanism is a primary pathway in the development of autoimmune disease.

patient history of 130 veterans in the VA hospital system who had been diagnosed with lupus, a classic autoimmune disease that affects skin, joints, and organs.[1] During their years of active duty, all servicemen and women have their blood drawn many times. Luckily for Dr. Arbuckle's team, the US government has been freezing and saving blood samples since 1978. She asked for permission to examine frozen blood samples taken when the current lupus patients were healthy and serving in the Armed Forces.

Her study showed that every single veteran who had a positive diagnosis of lupus had markers for seven different elevated antibodies that caused lupus in their bloodwork years before they had any symptoms. The level of antibodies increased every year until they reached a plateau, at which point the organ damage was severe enough for symptoms to appear. This stage is called *early pathogenic autoimmunity*. By the time the patients reached this plateau, they were sick enough to see a doctor.

As time went by, more cells were attacked, inflammation increased, and symptoms became worse. Finally, when the symptoms were no longer tolerable, the servicemen and -women went to the doctor and were diagnosed with lupus. Yet each of the men and women in the study were on the autoimmune spectrum for lupus at least 5 years earlier. We can't feel when antibodies are killing off our cells in the earlier stages, so there is nothing to alert us to tissue damage until it progresses to the point where clinical illness is apparent.

If this were you, when would you want to know that you were on the spectrum of autoimmunity? Would you wait until you had enough organ damage to have noticeable symptoms, or would you try to catch disease before there is so much damage that the symptoms demand medical attention?

In the graph below, look at the seven different antibodies that can cause lupus. When the study participants first noticed symptoms of lupus, we see that just over 18 percent of those eventually diagnosed with lupus, technically referred to as systemic lupus erythematosus (SLE), had elevated anti-Sm antibodies 5 years beforehand; 28 percent had elevated anti-dsDNA antibodies; 48 percent had elevated ANA antibodies; 56 percent had elevated anti-La antibodies; 59 percent had elevated anti-Ro antibodies; and 64 percent had elevated aPL antibodies.

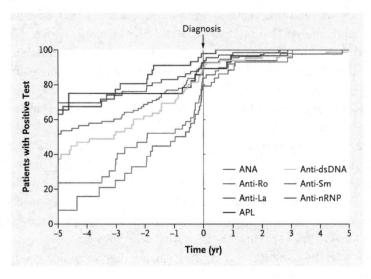

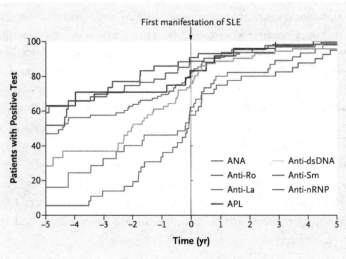

Similarly, when patients received the diagnosis of SLE, we see in the bottom graph that all seven antibodies were elevated more than 5 years beforehand. This is a critical concept to understand: The antibodies are elevated, thus damaging targeted tissue, years before there are noticeable symptoms or a diagnosis is made.

The severity of the symptoms depends on how long you have been on the autoimmune disease spectrum and how much tissue damage has accrued. The "gift" of having symptoms is that it will force you to take notice and do something to address a problem. It is the window of opportunity to do something about these often seemingly unconnected symptoms *before* there is so much tissue damage one gets a disease. Your recurring symptoms like fatigue, bloating, lack of energy, and memory lapses, or seemingly unrelated symptoms that come out of nowhere, might be messengers from your immune system letting you know that something's out of balance.

Yet let's be clear: Symptoms are not the first manifestation of a problem; they're the last straw when your body cannot compensate further. While your body has been working very hard compensating for your tissue damage and trying to maintain balance, its abilities to "adapt" by compensating to maintain balance (a process known as *allostasis*) are worn out. Now the accumulating damage begins producing symptoms. Once that ball starts rolling, unless you stop it, the problem only gets bigger and bigger.

Oddly, chronic health conditions are almost accepted as normal parts of life: fatigue, pain, depression, obesity, insomnia, anxiety, headaches, and many more. These symptoms may be common, but they are not normal. The difference is huge: *Common* means a lot of people have it; *normal* means "that's the way it's supposed to be." The "common" symptoms (being sick, fat, tired, and forgetful) should not be accepted as "normal," and knowing this should be empowering enough for all of us to say to our doctors, "Wait a minute, is what I'm experiencing common or normal?" The truth is, no one should have to live with symptoms, no one should accept them, and no one should ignore them.

The worst thing that you can do is neglect your symptoms or habitually take pain relievers to deal with them. While there's nothing wrong with occasionlly taking aspirin, ibuprofen, or other nonsteroidal anti-inflammatories (referred to as NSAIDs), or even prescription pain relievers every once in a while, when you are taking them regularly, you've exposed yourself to a new problem. Up to 65 percent of people who take NSAIDs for 6 months or longer develop inflammation in the intestines, which can lead to arthritis in any joint in your body.[2] The NSAIDs can cause a secondary autoimmune reaction that I call *collateral damage*, which you'll learn about later.

The second problem with relying on pain relievers is that you never address the underlying issue that is causing the pain. Imagine that you are driving a car and a light appears on your dashboard. Would you pull over and reach underneath the dashboard, look for the wire that's connected to the warning light, cut the wire, and then head back on the road and continue driving? My guess is no. We know better than that—our cars won't last long and might put us in danger if we ignore the warning light. Do you think your body is any different? Yet we do something similar to our bodies when we take pain relievers without looking for the underlying trigger for the pain.

Neglecting or suppressing symptoms allows the underlying imbalance to continue causing more tissue damage. While it's perfectly normal and expected to want to feel better right away, we need to address the mechanism causing the discomfort or the degeneration will continue to the point where medications will no longer address the symptoms. For example, while antibiotics can effectively treat acne, they bring only short-term relief and don't address the root cause of the problem. What's more, taking them comes with many long-term consequences, such as damage to bones, scarring, and autoimmune hepatitis.[3]

LOOK AT BLOODWORK CAREFULLY

When your doctor reviews results of a blood test with you, and there is an *H* or *L* next to a blood marker, signifying high or low, and the doctor tells you that your results "are normal," ask the doctor this question: "Doctor, is it common or is it normal?" This one question will possibly open up a line of communication as to why this number is high or low, because it is certainly not normal.

If you want vibrant health, you have to decipher what your body is trying to tell you. The truth is, the body's language never lies; we just have to learn how to understand what our body is saying. That's the whole goal of this book: to teach you how to listen to your body and ask it the right questions. Once you understand the basics of how your immune system gets activated to protect you from perceived threats, and learn its language, you can find the trigger or root cause of your symptoms and identify which offending invader put you on the autoimmune spectrum. Next, you can identify where you are on the spectrum, which opens a window of opportunity to address the underlying mechanism years before enough tissue damage has accrued, symptoms begin, and a diagnosable disease has occurred. Then you can reverse the trend and roll back the ball to optimal health through simple lifestyle changes.

KNOW YOUR IMMUNE SYSTEM

The vast majority of us are moving toward the dangerous, far end of the autoimmune spectrum as a consequence of our immune system trying to protect us from the increased exposures of a toxic environment. The goal is to move all of us toward the other end of the spectrum, back to normal immunity. The first step is to get the big picture of how the immune system works.

Your immune system acts like the armed forces—it's there to protect you and is composed of different branches that work together. There is a metaphorical army, navy, air force, marines, and coast guard (which are referred to by doctors as the antibodies IgA, IgG, IgE, IgM, and IgD, but more on that later), each of which has a distinct role that protects us and allows us to survive and thrive on the planet.

There are actually four different immune systems in the body, and each can produce the five types of autoimmune responses listed above. The largest one is found in the gastrointestinal tract (the gut), where 70 to 85 percent of your immunity resides. There is another immune system in the liver called the Kupffer cells. The third comprises the white blood cells found in the bloodstream. Finally, there's one in the brain made of glia cells.

Each of these systems operates separately, but all follow the same owner's manual and communicate with each other. Each immune system is constructed of at least two arms: the cellular, or *innate immune system*, which acts as the protective handguns firing chemical bullets, and the humoral, or *adaptive immune system*, which is the heavy artillery that's called in when you need backup.

When faced with an invader, whether it is made of cancer cells, bacteria, viruses, parasites, offensive dietary proteins and peptides, or even chemicals such as medications, the innate/cellular arms produce *cytokines*, the biochemical bullets I refer to as the first responders. These cytokines recognize and then destroy whatever they consider threatening. A number of different types of cytokines are produced, and the immune system determines which one to launch depending on the threat. For example, we support the immune system through vaccinations, and we receive separate immunizations for measles and mumps; each time, we are targeting a different cytokine. If the cellular arms' defensive strategy cannot get the job done, the immune system calls up the "big guns." This is when the humoral/adaptive immune system kicks in, and its soldiers launch targeted missiles called *antibodies*.

This complex biological system works 24/7, and its limited arsenal is all we have to protect our internal health from the outside world. The immune system has to work very hard in today's world, and it can become overtaxed easily. Sometimes, offending invaders slip through the cracks and trigger (1) infections or (2) the nagging symptoms that you may be putting up with that do not progress into a diagnosable infection. Either response can progress into major diseases. This is particularly true for children and the elderly, as the immune system takes time to fully mature and often wears down as we get older.

A second problem is that our bodies today are exactly the same as those of our ancestors who lived thousands of years ago, yet the threats we are exposed to today are completely different. As my good friend Mark Houston, MD, a vascular biologist (a specialist in blood vessels), says, "The human body has a limited number of response systems available to respond to an unlimited number of insults." Our ancestors required immune protection against only a few viruses and a handful of bugs—parasites, worms, and bacteria. Their immune system was designed to identify and destroy them. Our immune system today is exactly the same, yet the threats to our health now include the same handful of parasites, worms, bugs, and bacteria as well as "an unlimited number of insults"—including superbugs (bacteria that have become resistant to antibiotics); hybridized and genetically modified foods; tens of thousands of toxic chemicals, including herbicides and pesticides; and heavy metals like lead, mercury, and cadmium—as a result of the modernization of society. It's been said, for example, that the Roman civilization ended with the building of poisonous lead-lined aqueducts because human immune systems are not designed to fight lead. The point is, our bodies continue to respond to all of these and many more offending agents (which, together, are called *antigens*) as if we're fighting a bug, parasite, bacteria, or virus. That's it. That's all we have as our protective response system.

ELEVATED ANTIBODIES ARE THE IMMUNE SYSTEM'S BAZOOKA STRATEGY

When the innate immune system cannot get rid of the offending invader by creating inflammation, the adaptive immune system is called in to fight the battle with antibodies, the trained assassins that go after a specific target. Anywhere the antibodies find an invader, they fire their missiles. If you've ever received blood test results with the words "elevated levels of antibodies," or an *H* next to the antibody marker, this refers to the fact that the big guns are working overtime to contain a perceived threat, and whether or not you have any symptoms, the tissue damage from those antibodies is accruing.

Each one of the big guns releases its own brand of antibodies: IgA, IgG, IgE, IgM, and IgD. IgM is the first antibody produced when a threat is suspected and the big guns are called in. If it can't neutralize the threat completely, the other antibodies are produced, and they take over the task. If you ate something that your sensors register as a threat, IgA is the follow-up response launched from the epithelial surfaces (the lining of your intestines, lungs, and blood vessels). IgG is a systemic response activated when an offending agent enters the blood. We know that IgD exists, but we still are unclear as to its function.

If an IgE response is activated, IgE stimulates the release of histamine molecules that can be life threatening when excessive, such as with allergies to food, like peanuts, or exposure to certain venoms, like bee stings. If you or someone in your family has been diagnosed with allergies, you may already be familiar with the test that simulates an

IgE response—that's the skin prick test that confirms if you have an allergy. However, it is not the only test that confirms a sensitivity to an offending food.

If you tell your doctor that every time your child eats a lot of cheese he ends up with a nose full of mucus, she will send you to an allergist who will perform an IgE test for a dairy allergy. If the test comes back negative, should your child still eat cheese? An allergist might say it's safe to eat cheese because there is no IgE allergy response present. However, there are other branches of the armed forces in your body to check. Antibody tests (IgA, IgG, IgM) might prove that while your child does not have a dairy IgE allergy, there could be a response from a different armed force. It may not be the air force (IgE), but it could be the army (IgG), or the marines (IgA).

Is a skin prick test comprehensive in determining a food sensitivity? No, it is not. It's a very good test, but it highlights only one of a number of ways your immune system would respond to an offending food. If your doctor doesn't take a more comprehensive approach, your child may continue exposure to dairy, which will continue to make him feel sick.

Your brain may direct the immune system to create someone in charge (a general) whose job is to make sure you are protected for the rest of your life from that offending food. For example, you may have General Gluten, who instructs the immune system to create antibodies against gluten and keep the ability to reproduce them for the rest of your life. These generals are called *memory B cells,* and their job is to protect you from future exposures to the toxic things that your immune system has already recognized as a problem. For example, back when you were a child, you probably received a measles vaccination. If I were to do a blood test on you right now, I would likely see that you do not have antibodies to measles because you haven't been recently exposed to them. But when you first had the vaccine that contained a small amount of measles virus, your blood test would have told a different story.

Now remember, your immune system is the armed forces, and it has many generals sitting around with nothing to do. Once you received the measles vaccination, the body was faced with an invader, and it got into gear. The brain responds with instructions, "General, you're now called General Measles, take care of this." General Measles builds an assembly line that starts producing antibody soldiers trained to go after measles, and each one is carrying very powerful bazookas. These antibodies fire their missiles as they travel through the bloodstream, looking for and destroying measles wherever they can find it.

When the measles bugs introduced from the vaccination are gone, General Measles says, "Turn off the assembly line; I don't need any more soldiers right now." But because General Measles is a memory B cell, if you are ever exposed to measles again, all General Measles has to do is flip the switch to get the assembly line up and running; he doesn't have to rebuild it. That's the purpose of a booster shot: It turns the assembly line back on. It just takes a couple of days after being activated by a booster to create enough measles antibodies, or any other antibodies, to protect you. That's why if you travel to a place like Africa, you need vaccinations months in advance for yellow fever and dengue fever—the potential bugs that you may be exposed to on your trip. But if you go back to Africa 15 years later, you just need a booster shot 2 weeks before you go. You do not have to build the assembly line again. The booster shot will wake up General Yellow Fever, or General Dengue Fever, and they will turn on the assembly line so you have antibodies in your bloodstream ready to protect you.

Antibodies that have been produced to protect you from yellow fever or dengue fever—or gluten or dairy—are circulating in the bloodstream looking for the bugs or foods they have been trained to attack. After the offending bug or food has been destroyed by the antibodies, it takes a month or two to turn off the assembly line. The already-produced antibodies in your bloodstream have a life span of 2 to 3 months. Thus, high levels of antibodies keep circulating in the bloodstream, working, attacking, and sometimes causing collateral damage long after an exposure (like gluten). This process can continue for as long as 3 to 5 months.

This means that it takes only one exposure to activate a specific general, and you'll have this protective response continuing long after. If you're ever exposed to yellow fever, or a little gluten, the protective mechanism is reactivated, the antibody load goes up, and your immune system is in full force protecting you. This is why you can't have "just a little" when it comes to gluten or other foods you may be sensitive to. For example, in a landmark study published in the *Lancet* in 2001, celiac patients were followed for more than 20 years, and their eating patterns were recorded. It was found that those patients who ate gluten once per month, even if they didn't feel bad, suffered tremendous consequences. Here's the exact quote: "Non-adherence to the GFD [gluten-free diet], defined as eating gluten once per month, increased the relative risk of death sixfold."[4] Seems like a high price to pay for an occasional cupcake.

When your immune system continues making elevated levels of antibodies, it's a pretty serious thing in the big picture, even though many doctors ignore it if you have no other symptoms. For example, if you had elevated levels of antibodies to your thyroid, most doctors would consider it an incidental finding if you don't have noticeable thyroid symptoms. Yet it's not incidental at all: It's a message from your immune system that you have a problem. Elevated antibodies are a signal that the immune system is working with its last option to respond to a perceived threat before the development of disease. Elevated levels of antibodies to your own tissue cause inflammation and tissue damage. Period. You won't feel the damage that's accruing when you have elevated levels of antibodies until your immune system kills off so much tissue that symptoms emerge.

Elevated antibodies can also occur when our innate immune system (the "first responders") becomes depleted and ineffective. Our immune system gets worn out just by monitoring the way we live our hectic lives.[5] We are traveling on the highway of life and our transmission is screaming in low gear, but we're not moving as fast as we want to even though we are stressing the engine and the transmission. Some doctors might advise you to slow down if you seem stressed or burned out, but I don't believe that option is realistic in today's society. To me, it's a cop-out when doctors tell people to "cut the stress out of your life" or "slow down." We cannot cut down on our demands, whether they are taking care of the kids, dealing with rush-hour traffic, or keeping our A game at work. We're simply not going to slow down in life. Nobody's going to slow down, and frankly, you shouldn't have to.

Instead, I'm going to teach you how you can shift into drive so you're going much faster with less effort. Then we can cruise through life without a screaming transmission, burn less fuel, and support our immune system. I believe it's our birthright to live a life of passion—we just should not have to burn out our bodies to do this. Part of my personal creed and where I find my joy comes from George Bernard Shaw:

The Being used for a purpose recognized by your Self
as a mighty one.

The Being a force of nature, instead of a selfish, feverish clod
of ailments and grievances complaining the world will not
devote itself to making you happy.

Learning to shift gears is pretty simple, and you'll learn exactly how in this book. When you eat foods that your immune system responds to as a problem, you create metabolic stress that will manifest at your weak link. Instead, by eating power foods, you can reduce this unnecessary stress. You'll learn in this book to stop eating the exact foods that make you sick, fat, tired, or forgetful. By doing so, your body can perform at the level you want it to perform.

INFLAMMATION IS THE IMMUNE SYSTEM'S FORTRESS STRATEGY

Inflammation is the natural response of the immune system to a threat. When the immune system produces cytokines and antibodies, these responders attack the offending invader in a process that both destroys the invader and creates a barrier between your body and the infection, injury, or stress. This barrier or fortress strategy increases bloodflow and sends immune-enhancing white blood cells and antibodies to the areas of the body or brain that require healing. In some instances, like when you get a small cut on your hand, this barrier creates heat and tenderness that you can see and feel: You may notice tenderness, redness, and swelling. But in other cases, inflammation is internal and not so obvious: There is still tenderness, redness, and swelling, but you just can't feel it—like atherosclerosis, which progresses to heart disease. This is considered to be a "sleeper" condition; you don't know it's happening. If you didn't go looking for this type of inflammation with highly sensitive blood tests, you wouldn't even know it's there. Understanding that there are two types of inflammation is very important, as it is the basis of your ability to identify "what's cookin" in your body while there's still time to reverse the damage.

Inflammation is the primary tool in our immune system's arsenal that keeps you healthy. This is critical to remember, because inflammation gets a bad rap. The truth is, inflammation is not bad for you. *Excessive* inflammation is bad for you. Once the offending invader is destroyed and the damage to your body is repaired (like when the cut on your finger heals), the inflammation barrier is removed. However, inflammation usually continues if the threat remains. This might occur when the ammunition in your inflammatory response wasn't powerful enough to vanquish the invader, or when we continue to expose ourselves, such as in the case of unknown food sensitivities, when we keep eating the wrong foods, throwing gasoline on the fire.

When inflammation gets out of control, you might notice subtle symptoms and think perhaps that maybe you're "getting older." At first, you might notice you have gained a few pounds or are a little more tired than usual. Perhaps you've gained 3 pounds in the last year and your pants are tighter. But if you multiplied that weight gain by 10 years, now you're up a pant size or two and have developed a spare tire around your midsection. The type of body fat found on your midsection is called *adipose fat*, and it produces 17 different hormones, 15 of which fuel even more inflammation. Adipose body fat usually develops from following the wrong lifestyle habits and can lead to weight gain and systemic inflammation throughout the body. A simple screening test to identify if you are carrying dangerous levels of adipose fat is known as a *body composition analysis*.

Ongoing, chronic inflammation is linked directly to tissue damage that accumulates and eventually triggers dysfunction. The cascade of excessive inflammation is the initiator of a degenerative process leading to weight gain, fatigue, depression, chronic pain, anxiety, insomnia, and autoimmune diseases. Practically every degenerative disease is linked to excessive inflammation, including cancer, heart disease, diabetes, lupus, multiple sclerosis, Parkinson's, and Alzheimer's. Scientists have now shown that atherosclerosis (the plugging up of your pipes causing cardiovascular disease) and cancer have autoimmune components in their initiating and fueling stages. In total, autoimmunity is estimated to affect one in five American women, and one in seven men.

INFLAMMATION AND THE WEAK LINK
IN YOUR CHAIN

Where inflammation first presents as symptoms is the weak link in your chain. This location is determined by your genetics, your antecedents (how you have lived your life so far), and your environmental exposures. Symptoms on the autoimmune spectrum can be expressed in many ways, depending on where the weak link in the chain of your overall health lies. For example, if someone has a gluten sensitivity, it may manifest as compromised brain function, such as headaches, memory loss, or seizures. In the next person, the same sensitivity may manifest as constipation. In the next person, it may manifest as liver disease.

Excess inflammation pulls on your chain, and wherever the weak link in your health chain is, that's where tissue damage will occur. If it's your thyroid, you may notice that you are more chilled or have trouble losing weight. If it's your liver, you may find that alcohol has a stronger effect on you than it did before. If you are a woman, you might have more PMS. If it's your brain, you may forget simple things, like where you've left your keys, or have trouble with your memory in general. If it's your muscles, you may notice that you are not as strong as you used to be or you have more trouble walking up stairs.

It may take you a number of visits, or even a number of doctors, before you get the right diagnosis. For example, individuals with celiac disease typically require an average of five doctors and 11 years of symptoms before they receive the correct clinical diagnosis of celiac disease. By the time your symptoms are disrupting your daily life, the tissue damage of inflammation has been accruing for years. *Years.* These symptoms could eventually send you to a doctor, who may focus on treating the symptoms of inflammation (the joint pain, the headaches, the high blood sugar, etc.) but is less likely to address the root cause. Whatever is pulling on your chain may never be addressed, and the excess inflammation is likely to cause another problem at your next weakest link. In medicine, that's called a *comorbidity.*

For example, the measurement of successful pharmaceutical treatment of diabetes is a blood marker called hemoglobin A1C. The standard approach is to increase the dosage of medication until hemoglobin A1C levels come into the normal range. If you follow your doctor's advice and take your medications to the point where your blood sugar is stable, your lab results will look acceptable (you'll have normal hemo-globin A1C), but the medication itself may be putting you at a high risk of comorbidities, like mental deterioration or fatal heart attacks, because the underlying mechanism of inflammation that actually caused the increase in blood sugar is not addressed with this medication. The inflammation is still causing tissue damage to your blood vessels and brain. I'm sorry I have to be the one to tell you, but people with type 2 diabetes have a shorter life span, earlier onset of cardiovascular disease, and more brain deterioration (cognitive decline) than the general popu-lation—and that's when you follow your doctor's instructions and take your medicine that stabilizes only the symptom you initially presented with (excess blood sugar). According to a 2011 meta-analysis (a study summarizing many studies) of the use of medications to treat diabetes that appeared in the *New England Journal of Medicine,* researchers found that as compared with standard therapy, an increase in dosage medica-tions to get hemoglobin A1C down to an acceptable range reduced 5-year nonfatal heart attacks by 21 percent. That sounds pretty good, doesn't it? But you have to read the entire study to find out that it also increases 5-year mortality (death) by more than 19 percent.[6]

I fully support taking medications that treat symptoms, but we also must treat the underlying inflammation causing the disease. Thou-sands of clinicians have found that by including an anti-inflammatory approach to health care, like the one you'll learn about in this book, you can arrest and even in some cases reverse degenerative diseases such as diabetes and other autoimmune diseases.

EXCESS OXIDATIVE STRESS PRODUCES INFLAMMATION GONE WILD

Within every cell are tiny powerhouses called *mitochondria.* As oxygen is taken into the body, the mitochondria use it to create the energy we need to keep the body functioning. During this process, part of the "exhaust" creates extra oxygen molecules called *free radicals.* These free radicals can damage the outer walls of our cells, and when enough damage accrues, it affects the function of tissues and organs, and then symptoms begin to show up. Usually, free radicals are neutralized by antioxidant vitamins and polyphenols that act like sponges, sopping up the free radicals.

We get these vitamins from eating colorful fruits and vegetables—that's why I recommend eating different-colored vegetables every day in Chapter 7. Every color contains a different family of vitamins, polyphenols, and antioxidants that are great for you.

However, if our diet is lacking in antioxidants, or we're overexposed to antigens, free radicals can pile up and create oxidative stress, which damages any cell in your body. It just depends where the weak link is in your chain. Oxidative stress is a primary mechanism of inflammation production and the resulting cellular damage, which progresses into tissue damage. When enough tissue damage has occurred, organ dysfunction begins and eventually progresses into organ disease. This is the point when you usually get a diagnosis.

Did you know that every time you fly you are exposed to excessive radiation from solar flares, which increases your oxidative stress load? For example, when solar flares are at their strongest, you may be exposed to the equivalent of seven chest x-rays' worth of radiation during a single flight from New York to Los Angeles. This is important, because radiation causes oxidative stress. Excessive exposure is a major contributor to why female flight attendants have one of the highest incidences of hormone imbalances and pregnancy complications of any profession and why pilots have one of the highest incidents of leukemia and lymphoma of any profession.[7] These people are sitting in an aluminum box, being exposed to radiation causing excess oxidative stress every day. I recommend to all my flight attendant/pilot patients that they take five times the amount of antioxidant vitamins that everyone else needs. They need lots of sponges to soak up the free radicals that cause the oxidative stress.

Another way to think about oxidative stress is an example I learned from my mentor, Jeffrey Bland, PhD, the cofounder of functional medicine. He taught me that it takes 976,000 mousetraps lying side by side to fill a football field. If you cock each mousetrap and load it with a Ping-Pong ball, the football field will look entirely white—all you see are the balls. If you walked along the sidelines and threw one additional Ping-Pong ball onto the field, it would hit a mousetrap that would launch its own ball: *Pop!* Now there are two balls in the air, the one you threw out and the one in the mousetrap that just popped. These two balls hit two more mousetraps: *Pop, pop!* Now there are four Ping-Pong balls in the air—*Pop!*—then eight, then sixteen, and so on: *Pop, pop, pop, pop, pop, pop,*

pop, pop. You've created a cascade reaction of launching balls that continues long after the first one was thrown.

Just as in this example, after the initial irritant causes inflammation, the oxidative stress increases exponentially, as if it had a life of its own. You've crossed the threshold of what your antioxidant load—your fire extinguishers—can put out. If you keep throwing gasoline on a fire, creating more inflammation (by eating foods that you are sensitive to, for example), oxidative stress will continue to fuel further inflammation, which then leads to more tissue damage, dysfunction, and eventually disease.

Here's an example of how simple food selection can reduce the damage of excessive oxidative stress. According to a 2004 meta-analysis reported in the *British Medical Journal,* you can reduce your risk of cardiovascular disease by 75 percent, increase total life expectancy by 6.6 years, and increase life expectancy free from cardiovascular disease by 9 years when you put a healthy, antioxidant-rich eating plan together (so you get more sponges to soak up the free radicals and reduce oxidative stress). The beneficial foods to eat daily include cold-water fish, dark chocolate (yes, you read that right, daily dark chocolate), garlic, almonds, red wine, and just under a pound of fruits and vegetables.[8] Remember, that's *every day.* It's not enough to simply eat a 1-pound bag of carrots, though, so go for diversity. Eat some carrots and some broccoli and some purple cabbage and some tomatoes or red peppers to get all the different types of antioxidants.

We'll follow Samantha's story throughout the book, starting on page 22, so you can see how each of the different components causing the autoimmune spectrum affected her. Unfortunately, this part of her story is just the beginning.

IDENTIFYING AUTOIMMUNE DISEASES

There are more than 80 autoimmune diseases, and many more autoimmune conditions. The difference between a disease and a condition is clear. *Conditions* are the result of dysfunction. Autoimmune *disease* occurs when the dysfunction has progressed to organ damage. If you are producing antibodies to your own tissue, each one of those antibodies represents a different condition. For example, there are seven antibodies present for lupus, and each one represents a different mechanism contributing to the dysfunction. That's why there are many different organs or tissues that can be affected when you have lupus.

The National Institutes of Health tells us that while many autoimmune diseases are rare, collectively they affect approximately 8 percent of the United States population—24 million people,[9] more than those affected by either cancer (9 million) or heart disease (22 million). Yet according to Dr. Jeffrey Bland, the number is probably much higher, as this calculation reflects only those who are correctly diagnosed. Better estimates suggest that more than 72 million people in the United States, or approximately 22 percent of the population, have an autoimmune disease. Remember, in total, autoimmunity is estimated to affect one in five American women, and one in seven men. You might be one of them.

People who are on the autoimmune spectrum commonly have more than one condition. For example, more than 20 percent of children with celiac disease already have mild cardiac dysfunction:[10] Their celiac is at one end of the spectrum with a confirmed diagnosis, but their heart disease is all the way at the early end of the spectrum, without symptoms yet. This means that if you have an autoimmune condition, you probably still have other weak links in your chain, and wherever they are, they will become activated unless you stop the cascade of inflammation.

The most common are:

- Alopecia (hair loss)
- Alzheimer's disease
- Amyotrophic lateral sclerosis (ALS, also known as Lou Gehrig's disease)
- Diabetes
- Inflammatory bowel diseases (Crohn's and colitis)
- Multiple sclerosis
- Nephropathies (kidney diseases)
- Neuropathies (brain and nervous system diseases)
- Osteoarthritis
- Parkinson's disease
- Psoriasis
- Rheumatoid arthritis
- Thyroid disease

MEET SAMANTHA

My patient, colleague, and good friend Samantha had one of the worst cases of lupus ever seen at the world-renowned lupus research center at UCLA Rheumatology. No exaggeration, Samantha died twice on the ER table. As a result of the necessary aggressive chemotherapy and steroid therapy, she lost 8 inches in height due to the severe osteoporosis causing multiple fractures in her midback. Samantha has finally come out of her nightmare both dynamic and healthy. However, her story is a warning to all of us about the importance of not only listening to what your body is trying to tell you but also acting on that message.

Fifteen years before she was diagnosed with lupus, Samantha was told that constipation for 2 weeks at a time was "normal." As early as age 7, she remembers having severe ear infections, difficulty catching her breath, and extreme fatigue. When Samantha's mom would suggest that they leave the house to run an errand, Samantha was typically reluctant because she was always tired and just didn't feel well. However, she'd psych herself up and go, even though she had constant stomach cramps, fatigue, and muscle weakness.

The intensity of the pain, the earaches, the allergies, and the fatigue would fluctuate, and life went on. Samantha remembers that as a child and through her teenage years, she never felt well after she ate, but she assumed that her queasiness was normal. During her teen years, she had uncontrollable acne. Her regular physician put her on birth control pills by the time she was 13 to control heavy menstruation, and when that didn't clear up her skin, her dermatologist prescribed isotretinoin (Accutane). Unfortunately, the Accutane made her feel depressed, and it didn't reverse the acne.

Throughout her teen years, Samantha's motto was "I'm just going to push through feeling bad; it's no big deal. My doctor tells me that I'm a healthy kid. I'm going to party. I'm going to have fun. I want to enjoy my life." So she tried to lead a normal teenage life even though she felt lousy. At 20 years old and 5 foot 11, Samantha was as active as she could be; she played tennis and danced ballet, until she started having cramps in her calf during her last weeks as a sophomore in college. One morning, she got up early, and as she stood up, she fell flat on her face. Samantha noticed her leg was swollen. She went to her nurse practitioner, who took her off the Accutane, which is known to cause leg cramps. Just to hedge her bet, the NP sent Samantha to the hospital to get an ultrasound on her leg.

Samantha was extremely fortunate that the ultrasound found a blood clot in her leg, which meant that she had to start taking blood thinners. Within 2 weeks, the blood clot in her calf broke off and traveled into her lung, causing a pulmonary embolism. This is a serious condition and can be life threatening. The embolism was thought to have been caused by antiphospholipid syndrome (Hughes syndrome), a disorder characterized by an increased tendency to form abnormal blood clots that can lead to strokes and unexplained miscarriages. This was the first autoimmune disease Samantha was diagnosed with. Her specialized hematologist at USC Medical Center told her, "If you're not on Coumadin [warfarin, a blood thinner] the rest of your life, you're going to get another blood clot, and you're going to die."

At that point, Samantha went to a chiropractor who specialized exclusively in spinal care. Again, Samantha was lucky: The chiropractor recognized that she needed more help beyond his expertise. He suggested that Samantha see his own chiropractor, who specialized in functional medicine.

Samantha's experience is classic. She was on the autoimmune spectrum very early in life, but no one thought to look for it. As early as age 3 she was having severe ear infections. Then by age 7 she had stomach pains, the constipation, and the toxicity that developed from it. All of these symptoms were a huge red flag that something was going on with her immune system, contributing to creating the environment where recurring ear infections take place. She followed traditional medicine's advice, but it never addressed the cause of her symptoms. So it's no surprise that even when she took the drugs like birth control, Accutane, allergy meds, and inhalers that the doctor suggested, nothing really resolved her symptoms. Her parents did the best they could, and her positive attitude kept her going, but eventually Samantha's pile of symptoms caught up with her and created an even bigger health problem.

A more comprehensive list, created by the American Autoimmune Related Diseases Association,[11] includes the following. I'm showing you this list in its entirety so you can see how many different diseases are actually on the autoimmune spectrum.

1. Acute disseminated encephalomyelitis (ADEM)
2. Acute necrotizing encephalopathy
3. Addison's disease
4. Agammaglobulinemia
5. Alopecia areata
6. Amyloidosis
7. Ankylosing spondylitis
8. Anti-GBM/anti-TBM nephritis
9. Antiphospholipid syndrome (APS)
10. Autoimmune angioedema
11. Autoimmune aplastic anemia
12. Autoimmune dysautonomia
13. Autoimmune hepatitis
14. Autoimmune hyperlipidemia
15. Autoimmune immunodeficiency
16. Autoimmune inner ear disease (AIED)
17. Autoimmune myocarditis
18. Autoimmune oophoritis
19. Autoimmune pancreatitis
20. Autoimmune retinopathy
21. Autoimmune thrombocytopenic purpura (ATP)
22. Autoimmune thyroid disease
23. Autoimmune urticaria
24. Axonal and neuronal neuropathies
25. Balo disease
26. Behçet's disease
27. Bullous pemphigoid
28. Cardiomyopathy
29. Castleman disease
30. Celiac disease
31. Chagas disease
32. Chronic fatigue syndrome
33. Chronic inflammatory demyelinating polyneuropathy (CIDP)
34. Chronic recurrent multifocal osteomyelitis (CRMO)
35. Churg-Strauss syndrome
36. Cicatricial pemphigoid/ benign mucous pemphigoid
37. Cogan's syndrome
38. Cold agglutinin disease
39. Congenital heart block
40. Coxsackie myocarditis

41. CREST syndrome
42. Crohn's disease
43. Demyelinating neuropathies
44. Dermatitis herpetiformis
45. Dermatomyositis
46. Devic's disease (neuromyelitis optica)
47. Discoid lupus erythematosus
48. Dressler's syndrome
49. Endometriosis
50. Eosinophilic esophagitis
51. Eosinophilic fasciitis
52. Erythema nodosum
53. Essential mixed cryoglobulinemia
54. Evans syndrome
55. Experimental allergic encephalomyelitis
56. Fibromyalgia
57. Fibrosing alveolitis
58. Giant cell arteritis (temporal arteritis)
59. Giant cell myocarditis
60. Glomerulonephritis
61. Goodpasture syndrome
62. Granulomatosis with polyangiitis (GPA)
63. Graves' disease
64. Guillain-Barré syndrome
65. Hashimoto's encephalitis
66. Hashimoto's thyroiditis
67. Hemolytic anemia
68. Henoch-Schönlein purpura
69. Herpes gestationis
70. Hypogammaglobulinemia
71. Idiopathic pulmonary fibrosis
72. Idiopathic thrombocytopenic purpura (ITP)
73. IgA nephropathy
74. IgG4-related sclerosing disease
75. Immunoregulatory lipoproteins
76. Inclusion body myositis
77. Interstitial cystitis
78. Juvenile arthritis
79. Juvenile diabetes (type 1 diabetes)
80. Juvenile myositis
81. Kawasaki disease
82. Lambert-Eaton syndrome
83. Leukocytoclastic vasculitis
84. Lichen planus
85. Lichen sclerosus
86. Ligneous conjunctivitis
87. Linear IgA disease (LAD)
88. Lupus (SLE)
89. Lyme disease, chronic
90. Ménière's disease
91. Microscopic polyangiitis
92. Mixed connective tissue disease (MCTD)
93. Mooren's ulcer

94. Mucha-Habermann disease
95. Multiple sclerosis
96. Myasthenia gravis
97. Myositis
98. Narcolepsy
99. Neuromyelitis optica (Devic's syndrome)
100. Neutropenia
101. Ocular cicatricial pemphigoid
102. Optic neuritis
103. Palindromic rheumatism
104. PANDAS (pediatric autoimmune neuropsychiatric disorders associated with streptococcal infections)
105. Paraneoplastic cerebellar degeneration
106. Paroxysmal nocturnal hemoglobinuria (PNH)
107. Parry-Romberg syndrome
108. Parsonage-Turner syndrome
109. Pars planitis (peripheral uveitis)
110. Pemphigus
111. Peripheral neuropathy
112. Perivenous encephalomyelitis
113. Pernicious anemia
114. POEMS syndrome
115. Polyarteritis nodosa
116. Polyglandular syndromes (type I, II, and III autoimmune)
117. Polymyalgia rheumatica
118. Polymyositis
119. Postmyocardial infarction syndrome
120. Postpericardiotomy syndrome
121. Primary biliary cirrhosis
122. Primary sclerosing cholangitis
123. Progesterone dermatitis
124. Psoriasis
125. Psoriatic arthritis
126. Pure red cell aplasia
127. Pyoderma gangrenosum
128. Raynaud's phenomenon
129. Reactive arthritis
130. Reflex sympathetic dystrophy
131. Reiter's syndrome
132. Relapsing polychondritis
133. Restless legs syndrome
134. Retroperitoneal fibrosis
135. Rheumatic fever
136. Rheumatoid arthritis
137. Sarcoidosis
138. Schmidt syndrome
139. Scleritis
140. Scleroderma
141. Sjögren's syndrome
142. Sperm and testicular autoimmunity
143. Stiff person syndrome

144. Subacute bacterial endocarditis (SBE)
145. Susac's syndrome
146. Sympathetic ophthalmia
147. Takayasu's arteritis
148. Temporal arteritis/giant cell arteritis
149. Thrombotic thrombocytopenic purpura (TTP)
150. Tolosa-Hunt syndrome
151. Transverse myelitis
152. Type 1 diabetes
153. Ulcerative colitis
154. Undifferentiated connective tissue disease (UCTD)
155. Uveitis
156. Vasculitis
157. Vesiculobullous dermatosis
158. Vitiligo
159. Wegener's granulomatosis/ granulomatosis with polyangiitis (GPA)

A FOCUS ON CELIAC DISEASE AND NON-CELIAC WHEAT SENSITIVITY

Celiac disease is the most researched autoimmune disease, and it is the only one for which the environmental trigger has been identified (gluten in wheat, rye, or barley). It is a chronic autoimmune reaction to gluten where autoantibodies are produced that attack the intestines and other tissues. The intestines are a tube that is about 20 to 25 feet long. The inside of the tube is lined with *microvilli* (page 28) that look just like shag carpeting. Each of the microvilli absorbs different nutrients. Celiac disease happens when these microvilli wear down due to exposure to gluten, and you are left with a flat surface, much like Berber carpet, and therefore your intestine can no longer absorb nutrients properly. You end up malnourished, regardless of how many nutrients you're actually consuming. People with celiac disease often feel sick, fatigued, and depressed and may complain of brain fog. The University of Chicago Celiac Disease Center has identified more than 300 symptoms and conditions that are potentially related. In Chapter 4, you'll take a simple quiz to find out if the symptoms you are experiencing are related to celiac or non-celiac gluten sensitivity.

Treatment for celiac disease involves following a strict gluten-free diet for life. This disease teaches us that if you can identify the environmental trigger and eliminate it, you may eventually stop the process of

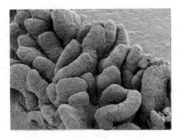

The microvilli in our intestines look like shag carpeting. We absorb all of our nutrients through each shag.

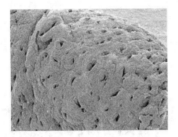

When the microvilli wear down, the shag disappear, and you're left with ' berber' or flat carpet.

Reprinted with permission from Macmillan Publishers Ltd: *The American Journal of Gastroentology*, 2004.

the autoimmune attack. However, if you reintroduce gluten, the accelerated "wearing down" will return.

Gluten sensitivity, on the other hand, is a separate gluten reaction that is primarily caused by the innate immune branch. The most significant difference between a gluten sensitivity and celiac disease is that a gluten sensitivity does not wear down the microvilli. There will be, however, just as much or more inflammation with gluten sensitivity as there is with celiac disease. As a matter of fact, the most recent studies show a higher incidence of people on the autoimmune spectrum with gluten sensitivity than with celiac disease. People with gluten sensitivity develop the same types of symptoms as people with celiac disease when exposed to gluten, including anxiety, headaches, brain fog, chronic fatigue, weight gain, depression, and a loss of well-being. These symptoms are part of the autoimmune spectrum and, if left untreated, will progress to the same damaging diseases we've been talking about:

obesity, dementia, diabetes, heart disease, and so on. Many more people have non-celiac gluten sensitivity than celiac disease, and they do just as well when following a gluten-free diet.

The importance of differentiating between celiac disease and a gluten sensitivity was first apparent in a study reported in 2009 in the prestigious *Journal of the American Medical Association* (*JAMA*). This study looked at 351,000 biopsies of intestinal linings. The researchers identified a total of 46,121 patients on the celiac spectrum: 29,096 with celiac disease and 17,025 with earlier stages of celiac development before their shags had been completely worn down. However, there were another 13,000 people in the study who did not have worn-down shags and did not have positive bloodwork, yet they had gluten sensitivity and inflammation.[12] This is the largest study connecting gluten sensitivity with mortality ever published. Celiacs had a 39 percent increased risk of early mortality. People with inflammation from a gluten sensitivity had a 72 percent increased risk of early mortality. The group that experienced the most dangerous risk of early mortality displayed only malabsorption symptoms (osteoporosis, anemia, fatigue). Fully understanding your risk regarding gluten sensitivities of any kind is a critical step that few doctors realize or will investigate. But I'm telling you these truths because you need to know how important it is to listen to your body and take your health seriously.

Irritable bowel syndrome (IBS) accounts for more visits to gastroenterologists (20 percent) than any other complaint. The frequency of non-celiac gluten sensitivity is highlighted in a 2014 article in the *American Journal of Gastroenterology*.[13] The study showed that the frequency of IBS with accompanying celiac disease is about 1 percent. But the frequency of irritable bowel disease with accompanying non-celiac gluten sensitivity is 30 percent. The remaining 70 percent of IBS patients do not have an identified gluten sensitivity. Yet when the majority of people with IBS follow a gluten-free diet, the symptoms disappear. Unfortunately, most gastroenterologists have not incorporated the results of these studies into their practice.

Most people refer to a reaction to gluten without a confirmed celiac diagnosis as a gluten sensitivity, but a better description is wheat sensitivity. While celiac disease is an immune reaction to the poorly digested proteins found in wheat, rye, and barley, a non-celiac sensitivity to wheat can be the response to any of the many components of wheat. It could be the entire molecule of wheat, not just the gluten proteins. It could be the lectins in wheat called wheat germ agglutinins, which are widely known to trigger the formation of blood clots. It could be a sensitivity to a family of carbohydrates in wheat known as FODMAPs, a component most directly attributed to gassiness, bloating, constipation, and diarrhea. Or it could be a reaction to the family of chemicals in wheat called benzodiazepines (yes, wheat includes these compounds found in prescription anxiety drugs, which is one reason why many people find carbs comforting). Therefore, we refer to non-celiac wheat sensitivity (NCWS) as the umbrella term, and gluten sensitivity would fall under that umbrella.

Interestingly, the premier neurologist in the world specializing in the impact of gluten sensitivity on the brain, with or without celiac disease, is Marios Hadjivassiliou, MD, who believes that gluten sensitivity is associated with autoimmune disease and that celiac is just one manifestation of it. He has proven that gluten sensitivity in and of itself is a systemic autoimmune disease. Dr. Hadjivassiliou is a consultant neurologist at Sheffield Teaching Hospitals NHS Foundation Trust, the world's first clinic to specialize in the neurological manifestations of gluten-related disorders, with or without celiac disease. Dr. Hadjivassiliou conducted extensive research into gluten ataxia (when one loses the ability to walk easily), having first described the condition in the 1990s after seeing a number of patients with unexplained balance and coordination problems. The majority of these patients did not have celiac disease but did have gluten sensitivity.

In 2015, in a study released from three of the government-certified gluten-related disorder centers in Italy, non-celiac wheat sensitivity was identified as causing autoimmune diseases at least as frequently, and in some cases more frequently, as celiac disease. Hashimoto's thyroid disease was the most frequent one identified. Additionally and even more startling, elevated antibodies to a common whole-body trigger (antinuclear antibodies, or ANA antibodies, that may manifest as lupus, rheumatoid arthritis, Sjögren's syndrome, scleroderma, or polymyositis) were double in NCWS patients compared to that in celiacs.[14]

This finding suggests that non-celiac wheat sensitivity is not an individual autoimmune disease listed alongside rheumatoid arthritis or psoriasis, but rather it's the initiator to many systemic autoimmune diseases. This does not mean that everyone with a systemic autoimmune disease has a sensitivity to gluten, but it does show the very high correlation. Gluten sensitivities can manifest in many different ways and can be just as severe, if not more so, than celiac disease. If your exposure continues, you may likely progress further along the autoimmune spectrum, and your condition might change from just a gluten sensitivity to a full-fledged autoimmune disease.

While this might not happen every time someone has elevated antibodies to gluten, in this recent study, the ANA antibodies were elevated 24 percent of the time in celiacs and 46 percent of the time in people with NCWS (yes, you read that right; almost double). This means the elevated antibodies traveling in the bloodstream can be destroying tissue wherever your weak link is (brain, kidney, liver, thyroid, etc.) if you have NCWS. If you've been diagnosed with celiac disease, you are 10 times more likely to have other autoimmune diseases than someone who doesn't have celiac disease.[15] Today we are beginning to see that with non-celiac wheat sensitivity, you are just as likely, or more likely, to get other autoimmune conditions than the general population. Clearly, NCWS is the big kahuna. Celiac disease is just one important manifestation of a sensitivity to wheat.

The same study showed that 50 to 55 percent of those with NCWS carry the gene we thought was "the celiac gene," which 93 to 100 percent of those with celiac disease carry (DQ2 or DQ8). Does this suggest that those genes are in fact related to many more wheat sensitivities outside of celiac disease? We haven't yet followed NCWS as a contributor to every autoimmune disease. With more than 300 conditions identified with celiac, could those 300 conditions also be correlated to NCWS? Only time and research will tell us. But we now know for sure that a sensitivity to wheat, whether it is a sensitivity to the gluten proteins, to the lectins, or to any other component of wheat, can wreak havoc anywhere in your body, with an end result of increased risk of developing an autoimmune disease.

It's important to clarify the difference between fad diets and the prevalence of gluten-related disorders and celiac disease. Fad diets come and go. They are highly promoted methods for losing weight in a less-than-sustainable way. However, wheat sensitivities, among other

GLUTEN MAY AFFECT ANYTHING

According to the University of Chicago Celiac Disease Center, more than 300 different conditions may be associated with a sensitivity to gluten. Any of these may be the reason you are feeling sick, fat, forgetful, or tired.

Here's an example of how a gluten sensitivity will cause osteoporosis. If you have Berber carpet in your intestinal lining due to celiac disease, you can't absorb calcium, and you are at risk for developing osteoporosis. I'm not saying that everyone with osteoporosis has celiac disease, but what I do know is that many do, and those who do have celiac will not get the intended benefits of standard osteoporosis medications, such as alendronic acid (Fosamax). Other scientists agree. In one study in the *Archives of Internal Medicine,* it was reported that "the prevalence of celiac disease in osteoporosis is high enough to justify a recommendation for blood screening of all patients with osteoporosis for celiac disease."[16] The reason this testing would benefit those with osteoporosis is that a bisphosphonate drug like Fosamax, which will help increase bone development, does not stop the calcium and other nutrient malabsorption related to celiac disease. Fosamax stimulates the laying down of new bone matrix, the scaffolding inside the bones, but if you're not absorbing calcium, magnesium, vitamin K, strontium, and boron, the scaffolding isn't supporting anything. You're building new bone out of balsa wood instead of oak. No wonder why postmenopausal women with osteoporosis who take Fosamax have just as many fractures as the women who don't take Fosamax: The medication isn't treating their nutrient deficiencies.

food sensitivities, are real medical conditions and can put you on the autoimmune spectrum. So while it might be trendy to be gluten-free, that's not my intention. I want you to be gluten aware—to find out if your immune system has a problem with these foods.

WHAT'S NEXT

There is a triad of factors required for the development of the autoimmune spectrum. In the next chapter, we'll review the three main factors that have been identified in the development of autoimmune disease. These factors include the genes (the deck of cards you've been dealt in life, over which you have more influence than you think, as you'll learn), environmental exposures (with gluten being the most common), and intestinal permeability (the leaky gut).

> To download my article, "The Conundrum of Gluten Sensitivity and Autoimmunity—Why Tests Are Often Wrong," and a bonus guide, "The Hidden Sources of Gluten," go to GlutenAndAutoimmunity.com.

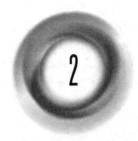

CULPRITS AND CAUSES

GENETICS, EXPOSURE, AND INTESTINAL PERMEABILITY

While inflammation is the mechanism behind practically all degenerative diseases, what stokes the flames that fuel the fire? Why does inflammation cause disease? We don't develop disease simply by eating gluten or dairy or any other food that we are sensitive to; we develop disease from damage caused by excessive inflammation. Remember, inflammation is not bad for you in and of itself. It's the mechanism by which our body protects us from invaders. *Excessive* inflammation is bad for you.

For inflammation to continue to a chronic state, have a life of its own (*pop, pop, pop*), and cause autoimmunity, three distinct factors must be present: a genetic susceptibility, environmental triggers, and a loss of intestinal barrier function. All three have been shown to be necessary to develop the majority of autoimmune diseases. If you take just one of the three out of the picture, your body can begin to heal.

In this chapter, you'll learn how to identify these three factors and determine if they affect you. Then, the rest of the book will show you how to modify and hopefully eliminate the factors you can control. By doing so, you'll be able to reset your immune response and arrest the development of the autoimmune process.[1]

One of the unrecognized but critical contributors to chronic inflammation is known as *molecular mimicry*. Understanding how this mechanism works will help you see how even the smallest toxic exposure can have wide-ranging and long-term negative effects on your health.

MOVING TARGETS: MOLECULAR MIMICRY

There are two types of antibodies you need to know about: antibodies to toxins and antibodies to your own tissue. We learned about the antibodies to toxins in Chapter 1. The second type of antibodies are called *autoantibodies*: antibodies that are produced against your own tissue.

The body experiences some cellular damage every day, just in the course of life, from aging cells to the hormones we produce or the chemicals we're exposed to. In fact, we generate a whole new body's worth of cells every 7 years. Some of those cells turn over quickly: The inside lining of your gut turns over every 3 to 7 days. Other cells, like your bones, turn over much slower. The body then has to get rid of the old and damaged cells to make room for new cells to develop.

One of the ways it accomplishes this cellular replenishment is with autoantibodies. Every day, the immune system is supposed to create the exact right number of autoantibodies to get rid of specific damaged cells. There's a different autoantibody for lung cells, adrenal cells, myelin sheath cells, other brain cells, thyroid cells, etc. The ongoing process can be measured with a blood test, and when everything is working correctly, your autoantibodies are recorded as a *normal reference range*. This means that your autoantibodies are being produced at the correct rate—referred to as *benign autoimmunity*. You're perfectly healthy.

Now, back to the antibodies that protect your body from toxic exposures. When you are exposed to a toxin (food, mold, stress, hormones, bugs, etc.), the inflammatory cycle begins by activating the innate immune system (the first responders), but if the exposure is greater than it can manage, your adaptive immune system (the big guns) takes over. These antibodies to toxins are powerful but not as precise as autoantibodies. Imagine a biochemical "terminator" wildly firing a machine gun out the window of a moving car. He might get the bad guys, but he's creating lots of broken glass and debris. This debris is a mix of your damaged cells as well as the remnant bits and pieces of the offending invaders your immune system was working so hard at destroying. I call this the *collateral damage* of the immune response.

Collateral damage can be a mess of epic proportion, creating inflammation, oxidative stress, and damaged tissue. When organ tissue has been damaged, the organ affected by the collateral damage becomes dysfunctional. This causes inflammation, which causes tissue damage, which causes organ damage, which then begins producing noticeable symptoms. For example, when you start having tissue damage in your thyroid, the thyroid will dysfunction, resulting in symptoms like cold hands and feet (do you wear socks to bed?), the inability to lose weight, or waking up in the morning and wishing you had 20 more minutes in bed. Eventually, you'll have fatigue that is immobilizing enough that it will send you to a doctor. Most doctors will check thyroid hormone levels and, if the results are normal, will chalk up your fatigue to stress. They should also have checked your thyroid antibody levels.

Now I'm going to tell you something that most doctors were not taught in medical school. Ready? *The antibodies we produce to protect us from toxins can easily mistake and destroy other molecules that look very similar to toxins.* Infectious agents, foods, or bacteria may confuse the body's immune system because they are structurally similar to human tissue.[2] Wow. I'm including a reference—one of many that I have—so you can read the science yourself or show it to your doctor.

To simplify things, let's call the amino acid structure of gluten A-A-B-C-D. Each of the letters represents different amino acids. When gluten molecules enter the bloodstream, your immune system starts making gluten antibodies A-A-B-C-D. These antibodies travel through the bloodstream, looking for A-A-B-C-D, firing missiles wherever it finds A-A-B-C-D. The problem is that the surface of your brain, or the part of your thyroid facing the bloodstream, also contains a structure similar to gluten's A-A-B-C-D. The antibodies produced to attack gluten may attack anything that looks like A-A-B-C-D, whether it's in your brain or your thyroid, or any other tissue where your weak link resides. This mechanism is called molecular mimicry, and when it happens, it is a primary mechanism by which the autoimmune cascade begins from gluten. Molecular mimicry increases inflammation in the tissue, eventually damaging the tissue, and, if continued unchecked, will damage the organ. The body now starts to produce autoantibodies to get rid of the damaged organ cells. That's not a problem, unless the antibodies to toxins continue to be produced as a result of frequent exposure. If so, they'll continually damage the organs, resulting in autoantibodies to get rid of the damaged organ cells until eventually the production of the autoantibodies is self-perpetuating. Now not only have you developed symptoms, but you've initiated the autoimmune mechanism.

The A-A-B-C-D amino acid chain is a common building block for most of our tissues. Molecular mimicry to A-A-B-C-D can occur anywhere in the body, from your kidneys to your gall bladder, muscles, bones, brain, heart, even in the conjunctiva of your eye. That's why the symptoms of gluten sensitivity can manifest anywhere, because the immune system is mistakenly attacking its own tissue in its attempt to get rid of gluten. Where the tissue becomes the most damaged is determined by the weak link in your health chain, which is determined by your genetics and your antecedents, or how you've lived your life. These are two of the three necessary factors for the presentation of autoimmune disease.

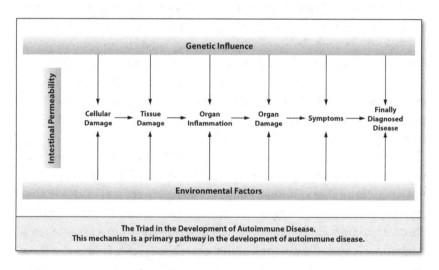

The Triad in the Development of Autoimmune Disease.
This mechanism is a primary pathway in the development of autoimmune disease.

FACTOR I: GENETICS

It's quite unlikely that you are the only person in your family who is on the autoimmune spectrum or has progressed to the point of having enough tissue damage that there are symptoms, perhaps even a diagnosed disease. My guess is that someone you are related to is also on the autoimmune spectrum; he or she may just be at a different point. Also, that person's symptoms or conditions might be entirely different from yours. The reason I'm so confident is that the first factor necessary for excessive inflammation to create autoimmunity is your genetics.

Your genetic code affects your health in many different ways. The first is the most direct: the ability for your immune system to misinterpret antigens via molecular mimicry, leading to elevated antibodies and the destruction of your tissue.

The particular way your system attacks its own tissue also depends on your unique genetic predisposition; that is, where the weak link in your chain occurs. Your family's history of autoimmune diseases might look like a straight line: Your father and grandfather both had heart disease. Or it might look more like a scattergram: Your father had heart disease, your sister had a miscarriage, and a brother had a stroke. Both instances reflect a genetic susceptibility to autoimmune disease. The only difference is that in the scattergram model, the weak link in the chain was not as clear, at least at first. But when you test properly, as we'll outline in Chapter 5, you'll see that all three are possible symptoms of the disease antiphospholipid syndrome.

The reason why everyone in your family is not on the autoimmune spectrum is because of two things—genetics and what are called antecedents (how you've lived your life so far, including diet choices, toxin exposures, stress, etc.). While you might share the same gene pool, one person's genes might be expressed and the other's not, depending on how you lived your life.

If you are genetically predisposed to a certain autoimmune disease, you are vulnerable to developing heightened antibody levels for that tissue or organ. For example, you might develop food allergies if your genes are skewed to produce excessive IgE antibodies. For other people, chronic inflammation can lead to either stroke, heart disease, diabetes, Alzheimer's, or cancer, because they each have genes that make them susceptible to these specific conditions. Still others may develop acne or other skin conditions. Yet it's important to remember that genes rarely cause disease. Your genes may say, "This is the weak link in your chain. If you pull at the chain too hard with excessive inflammation, this is where the chain is going to break." Disease appears when you put stress on the chain, which will break at your weak link. If you have the genes for susceptibility to celiac disease, you're highly vulnerable to celiac if the other elements necessary for it present themselves: The environmental trigger that sets it off (gluten) is activated, and there is intestinal permeability. Without the other two modulators, it's very unlikely that you will develop celiac disease, even if it's part of your genetic code. These two modulators affect your *epigenetics*. Epigenetics is the study of the distinct way that your environment and lifestyle affect the expression of your genes.

Epigenetics (now there's a good Scrabble word) is a huge, complicated topic, but the bottom-line explanation is that it is what happens in the environment around your genes, not the genes themselves, that determines your state of health or disease.

Here's an example. When you're trying to answer the question "Is coffee good for you?" the answer isn't black or white. There's a lot of conflicting science out there. Some studies show coffee is beneficial, and other studies show coffee is bad and puts you at greater risk of heart attacks. Well, how can that be? Here's the answer: It depends on your genes.

There's a gene we all have called CYP1A2. It helps us break down toxic chemicals we're exposed to. It comes in two types, 1A and 1F. We all inherit one of the two versions of this gene from our parents—it's the deck of cards we were dealt in life. If you have the 1A version, your risk of having a heart attack before the age of 50 that is associated with drinking coffee is as follows:

Less than 1 cup per day = no increased risk.

1 cup per day = 61% reduced risk.

2 to 3 cups per day = 65% reduced risk.

4 cups per day = 19% reduced risk.

You, and all other 1As out there, would benefit from drinking 1 to 3 cups of coffee a day.

But if you have the 1F version of this same gene, your risk of having a heart attack before the age of 50 associated with drinking coffee is as follows:

Less than 1 cup per day = no increased risk.

1 cup per day = 112% increased risk.

2 to 3 cups per day = 143% increased risk.

4 cups per day = 307% increased risk.

As the Soup Nazi would say, "No coffee for you."

The epigenetic factor involved in this scenario is the coffee. The coffee is the trigger. If you have the 1F version of the CYP1A2 gene and you are not exposed to coffee (the environmental trigger), there is no evidence that you are at risk for a heart attack before the age of 50.[3] Your genes are your genes—they don't determine that you'll get the disease, they just determine the weak links in your chain. Pull on the chain (drinking coffee if you're a CYP1A2[1F]) and you run the risk of the chain breaking (a heart attack before the age of 50).

Epigenetics teaches us that while genes influence our health, they are not our destiny. Studies of twins give us a great example for how this works. If you were to take identical twins and keep them in the same environment, they would continue to look identical as they got older. But if you change their environments, including feeding them different foods and experiencing different stresses and different lifestyles, the twins will actually look different, and their health will be different. These differences are caused by whether or not a certain genetic expression was activated, depending on those external factors. Even if you have genes for autoimmunity that put you at risk, those genes will not necessarily translate into disease.

For example, many people with genes for celiac disease or non-celiac wheat sensitivity may lead their entire lives without ever developing the symptoms of these diseases. For some people, the symptoms are immediately apparent, within the first year of life. Others will develop symptoms later on. Some people are able to eat gluten-filled foods for many years and stay symptom-free, until they switch from tolerance and a state of health to a loss of oral tolerance, activating the genes, and producing antibodies (now they're on the spectrum), leading to the developing of disease. Researchers have discovered that the frequency of confirmed celiac disease has doubled every 15 years. It was 1 in 500 in the 1970s, 1 in 250 in the 1980s, and 1 out of 100 in the 2000s.[4]

This is really great news because it shows that we can control our own health. If we understand the mechanism by which a disease develops, it gives us the opportunity to reverse engineer the direction we're going and move toward a higher level of health. In the last paragraph of his excellent book *Genetic Engineering*, Jeffrey Bland, PhD, says it all:

> Throughout your life, the most profound influences on your health, vitality, and function are not the doctors you have visited or the drugs, surgery, or other therapy you've undertaken. The

most profound influences are the cumulative effects of the decisions you make about your diet and lifestyle, and how those decisions affect the expression of your genes.

It's how you live your life that decides what genes get turned on and whether you're vibrantly healthy or terribly sick, or anything in between. Testing will confirm if you carry the gene and determine where your weak link is.

While we can't change our genes, we can address the two other factors of the autoimmunity triad: intestinal permeability and environmental exposures. Even if you have a genetic predisposition to autoimmunity, you can keep inflammation under control by making the right lifestyle choices. You'll see these explained in greater detail when we get to the Transition Protocol in Chapter 6. Genetics and environmental exposures have to work together to create the mechanism that pushes you forward on the autoimmune spectrum.

FACTOR 2: ENVIRONMENTAL EXPOSURES

The second component in the triad development of autoimmune disease is crossing the threshold of an environmental exposure—the straw that breaks the camel's back, so to speak. When the introduction of any antigen exceeds the limit of our bodies' ability to say, "Oh, that's kind of an undesirable, but it's no big deal," when we cross that threshold of exposure, then the foods or toxins that we are exposed to will cause excessive inflammation, which then causes joint pain, weight gain, brain fog, exhaustion, and so many other reactions. These antigens begin the cycle of autoimmunity, because it is in response to them that the armed forces we discussed in Chapter 1 are called out to protect you.

The signs that your body is being exposed to unhealthy antigens in the form of offending foods, molds, pesticides, preservatives, or additives include fatigue, difficulty concentrating, achiness, and muscle twitches, as well as rashes, bloating, chronic colds, or skin infections. High-sugar foods, processed dairy, and wheat can be just as toxic to the body as environmental pollutants. In this way, your current diet may literally be making you sick.

Your body can launch an immune response to foods, causing either a *food allergy* or a *food sensitivity*. Food allergens are associated with systemic inflammation and can cause a rash, hives, stuffy nose, watery eyes, vomiting, choking, coughing, asthma, or external inflammation (swollen hands, feet, or lips). In extreme cases, you can develop internal inflammation that can lead to *anaphylaxis*, a deadly condition where the throat closes and air cannot pass through to the lungs. The most common food allergies in the United States include wheat, dairy, corn, peanuts, soy, shellfish, strawberries, and eggs.

Food sensitivities may look completely different from an allergic reaction, yet they are just as difficult to deal with—they both cause excessive inflammation. A food sensitivity is often marked by a delayed reaction: The body may not respond to the problematic food for up to 72 hours after the food is consumed. This means that your reaction to a food you eat today may occur immediately or as late as 3 days later. The reaction can be anywhere from mild stomach cramps to an immobilizing migraine headache and everything in between.

People commonly develop sensitivities to the same foods that cause allergic reactions. Gluten, dairy, and sugar are generally the most common food sensitivities, although you can develop a food sensitivity to almost any type of food. The longer a person goes without recognizing a food sensitivity and continues to eat the food, accumulating excessive inflammation with the resulting tissue damage eventually causing organ damage, the more likely he or she will develop an autoimmune disease. Unfortunately, until now, the testing has been less than complete, so many people do not know they have a sensitivity to gluten. This is why people who have a sensitivity to gluten but are still eating it are 10 times more likely to have other autoimmune diseases like rheumatoid arthritis or Hashimoto's thyroiditis.[5]

However, once the food causing the problems can be identified and avoided, the immune system can begin to recover and the body starts healing. I have seen firsthand the profound changes that can occur with a patient's health once the person removes the offending foods from the diet. From infertility to rheumatoid arthritis to psoriasis to juvenile inflammatory arthritis to migraines to seizures, there is no condition that may not be helped by removing offending foods, thus calming down an inflammatory cascade.

Gluten Is Not Bad for You; Bad Gluten Is Bad for You

Gluten is a family of proteins found in many grains. The family of gluten proteins includes wheat, rye, barley, rice, corn, quinoa, and more. It is the family of toxic gluten proteins found in wheat, rye, and barley that no human can digest completely. In the chart below, the Triticeae family of grains are the toxic gluten-containing grains. The rest are safe to eat unless you have a sensitivity to them. For example, we know that 44 percent of people with celiac disease have a sensitivity to corn.[6]

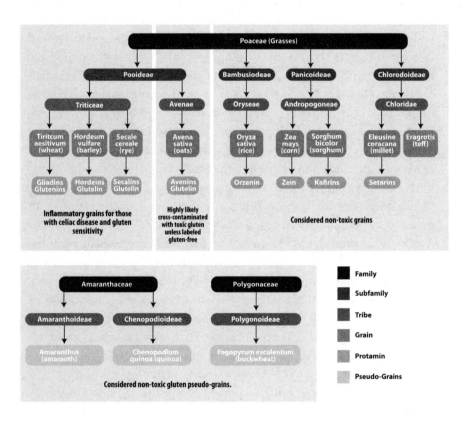

The USDA, FDA, Academy of Nutrition and Dietetics, American Heart Association, and American Diabetes Association all agree we should have a diet dominated by grains. In fact, 50 percent of all human calories worldwide now come from the grains wheat, corn, and rice. I disagree with this recommendation. My colleagues Mark Hyman, MD, David Perlmutter, MD, William Davis, MD, Jeffrey Bland, PhD, Deanna Minich, PhD, Sara Gottfried, MD, and tens of thousands of clinicians around the world also strongly disagree with this emphasis on grains as the primary source of calories. I personally believe that grains are good for most people, in moderation, but excess grain consumption is a strong contributor to the obesity and diabetes epidemics occurring in our world today.

Now let me be clear about wheat. Wheat has saved millions of lives. If there is a famine in Africa and we ship boatloads of wheat there, we save millions of lives. However, because no human has the enzymes to fully digest the proteins of wheat, rye, and barley, these grains will cause inflammation and intestinal permeability every time they are eaten. My friend and colleague Alessio Fasano, MD, conducted research at Harvard University and recently published a paper that showed that gluten in wheat causes intestinal permeability in every human. His team studied four populations: recently diagnosed celiacs (thus recently eating gluten), celiac patients in remission (who haven't eaten gluten in at least 12 months), non-celiac gluten sensitivity patients, and patients with no sensitivity to gluten. In his conclusion, Dr. Fasano states, "Increased intestinal permeability after gliadin exposure (a piece of poorly digested gluten) occurs in all individuals."[7]

Our body produces enzymes that act like scissors, which are meant to cut proteins into individual amino acids, just like a string of pearls. Gluten's strange molecular composition makes this process difficult. The sequence of the amino acids that make up gluten isn't recognized by the scissors as it attempts to break up the gluten and instead, the best the scissors can do is break off indigestible clumps. This means that for humans, gluten has absolutely no nutritional value: We eat it and excrete it. You can go a life-time without eating gluten and have no adverse side effects.

The consequence of gluten's poor digestibility may be absolutely nothing. The vast majority of people eat gluten without digesting it and are symptom-free. Yet some people have consequences leading to symptoms because they possess the first factor: genetic susceptibility. For them, they now have two factors in place: the genetics that reject gluten, plus the exposure to it. For those people, gluten is highly irritating to both the gut and the immune system. For many people with gluten sensitivity, the brain seems to be particularly vulnerable, causing memory lapses, poor attention, difficulty concentrating, fatigue, and more.

MEET MOLLY

Molly was 3 years old when her parents noticed that she had a tumor in her right eye (A). Her medical history revealed a premature cessation of breastfeeding, intolerance to baby foods, and abdominal distention. By the time she was 2, Molly had recurrent ear infections that were treated with antibiotics. Her weight and height percentiles were way below normal compared to her age group.

Molly's tumor was diagnosed as Kaposi's sarcoma, which often occurs with HIV patients, yet Molly's HIV antibody test was negative. However, her blood tests showed that she had high antibodies to gluten; a positive endoscopy for celiac disease confirmed that her microvilli (the shags) were worn down. The ophthalmologists recommended a biopsy on Molly's eye to test the tumor to determine its cause, but Molly's parents were nervous: She had a negative reaction to general anesthesia during her previous endoscopy. They asked if they could wait a few weeks. In the meantime, they started Molly on a gluten-free diet.

Two weeks later, she returned to the ophthalmologists. The tumor in her eye was smaller (B). After Molly followed a gluten-free diet for 2 full months, the tumor disappeared completely (C).

The ophthalmologists were startled by this unusual response. When they published this case study, they stated, "In conclusion, we present a very unusual conjunctival tumor in a patient with celiac disease that showed complete regression by a gluten-free diet. Prompt regression of the conjunctival lesion during gluten-free diet suggests a possible relationship to celiac disease and an autoimmune process."

Obviously, the weak link in the chain for this little girl was her eye. This was likely her genetic vulnerability, and the environmental trigger was the gluten she was eating. How a gluten sensitivity will manifest for you is determined by your genetics (the weak link in your chain) and your environmental triggers.

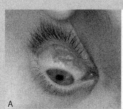
A
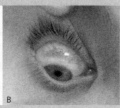
B
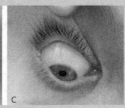
C

The problem with gluten seems to be getting worse, and you may have noticed the large number of food manufacturers who have jumped on the gluten-free bandwagon. In truth, the gluten content in grains has increased over the years. During the process of "improving" the commercial applications of wheat, the US agricultural industry over the last 50 years has increased its gluten content through hybridization. That makes the digestibility of today's grains much more difficult than the grains you may have grown up eating. So while some see eating gluten-free as a trend or fad diet, for those with a gluten sensitivity, it's absolutely imperative to eat gluten-free all the time.

A doctor can perform a variety of different blood tests to confirm a gluten sensitivity, and a positive diagnosis of celiac disease requires an endoscopy. However, you can test yourself for a gluten sensitivity by following my elimination diet. It's designed to determine if an unsuspecting food is actually causing problems for you. In the next 3 weeks, you will eliminate all gluten foods and assess how you feel. Then you can reintroduce gluten and see if you have a reaction. If you do, you'll know that you have a gluten sensitivity.

The Trouble with Sugar

We all know that sugar is loaded into sodas, desserts, and treats, but you might not realize that it has found its way into almost every meal we eat. Sugar has become one of the two primary food additives—the other is salt—used to enhance the taste of all processed foods. What's more, natural sugars are the basic building blocks of all carbohydrates, including grains, fruits, and vegetables.

The sugar that we add to our foods can be made from a variety of plants that produce it as a way to store energy, just like we store energy as body fat. Some 120 million tons of refined sugar is produced yearly, 70 percent from sugarcane and 30 percent from sugar beets.

Sugar itself is not bad for you, but bad sugar is bad for you. There are few health benefits and even less nutritional value to processed sugar. Sugar in its most natural state, sugarcane, actually has some nutritional value. In developing countries, children chew on sugarcane every day and don't get cavities. But in the United States, children who eat lots of sugar-laden sweets end up with lots of cavities. When children chew on sugarcane, they are exposed to the entire plant and ingest many other vitamins, minerals, polyphenols, and antioxidants as well as sucrose, the chemical extract of table sugar. Our children, on the other hand, are snacking on highly refined sugar in its most potent state. Sugar beets contain hemoglobin, the protein best known for carrying oxygen in the bloodstream in humans. Yet when sugar beets go through a multistage refining process, there is no hemoglobin left in the product. Don't be fooled by brown sugar or "sugar in the raw" as a healthy alternative: It's just refined sugar with caramel color or molasses added.

If you are a "sugar junkie," you may have already recognized that every time your body craves sugar, you may need a little more of it to get that feeling of satisfaction. The reason sugar is so much more addictive than eating naturally sweet fruits is because it's highly concentrated. I enjoy gluten-free poppy-seed pastries, and I allow myself one every 3 to 4 months, but if I were to extract the active ingredient in poppy seeds that contributes to enjoying the taste so much, I'd be eating pure heroin. One of my favorite television shows, *MythBusters*, once proved that eating just two poppy-seed bagels is enough to test positive for morphine, which is a by-product of heroin, which is made from poppy plants. White table sugar is the same kind of end-stage extract of sugarcane or sugar beets as heroin is to poppy seeds, and just as addictive and lethal.

Eating excess processed sugar, defined as eating more than your body can fully digest, is a primary fuel that increases systemic inflammation. In Chapter 1, I described how we have some inflammation in our body all the time, simply from the immune process getting rid of old and damaged cells. Sugar is one of the 10 most inflammatory foods in any quantity, and eating excess amounts of sugar is like throwing gasoline on a fire: It turns a manageable campfire into a roaring blaze. A diet high in refined sugar is also considered to be the primary trigger in the development of obesity.

Overexposure to sugar suppresses your immune system, making it inefficient, especially when it has to fight off infections. Sugar will suppress white blood cells for about 10 minutes after it's consumed.[8] So, for example, if you eat lots of sugar when you have a cold, your recovery will take days longer.

We've all heard that eating too much sugar is a trigger in developing diabetes. We now know there are three types of diabetes. Type 1 diabetes has always been known to be an autoimmune disease, and it occurs when antibodies have destroyed enough cells of the pancreas so that it is unable to produce enough insulin. Type 2 diabetes is related to years of excessive intake of sugar, wearing out our sugar-regulating system. People with type 2 diabetes do not need extra insulin: What they need are medications that help get the insulin from the bloodstream into their cells. This is called *insulin resistance,* which is an autoimmune mechanism. We now know that type 2 diabetes has a very strong autoimmune component. Insulin resistance is associated with a unique profile of IgG antibodies, which are associated with increased inflammation that produces excessive *visceral adipose tissue* (VAT). VAT is the spare tire you may be carrying around your waist—it's the result of another autoimmune mechanism. In 2005, researchers found a third form of diabetes called type 3. This is an insulin resistance in the brain causing dementia. Researchers are now connecting type 3 diabetes with Alzheimer's disease. In the last two scenarios, excess sugar exposure wears out the brain's and body's ability to manage insulin levels. You have plenty of insulin; it's just not being used properly.

Of the many complications of excess sugar, here are some of the physiological impacts for developing autoimmune disease that relate to both an increase in inflammation negatively affecting the immune system.

- Sugar upsets the mineral relationships in your body. It causes chromium and copper deficiencies and interferes with absorption of calcium and magnesium. These minerals, particularly chromium, are essential in the production of antibodies.[9]

- Sugar feeds cancer cells and has been connected with the development of cancer of the breast, ovaries, prostate, rectum, pancreas, biliary tract, lung, gallbladder, and stomach. The drain on antibody production to deal with these cancers depletes our immune function.[10]

- Sugar can cause many problems with the gastrointestinal tract, including an acidic digestive tract, indigestion, malabsorption in patients with functional bowel disease, and increased risk of the autoimmune diseases Crohn's disease and ulcerative colitis.[11]

- Sugar can cause premature aging. More antibodies are necessary to get rid of aging cells.[12]

- Sugar can cause autoimmune diseases such as arthritis, asthma, and multiple sclerosis.[13]
- Sugar can cause a decrease in your insulin sensitivity, thereby causing abnormally high insulin levels and eventual diabetes, which is often an autoimmune disease.[14]
- Sugar can lower your vitamin E levels, which can initiate the autoimmune process.[15]
- High sugar intake increases advanced glycation end products (AGEs: sugar molecules attaching to and thereby damaging proteins in the body).[16]
- Sugar causes food allergies.[17]
- Sugar can cause toxemia during pregnancy and can contribute to eczema in children.[18]
- Sugar can cause atherosclerosis and cardiovascular disease.[19]
- Sugar can impair the structure of your DNA.[20]
- Sugar can change the structure of protein and cause a permanent alteration in the way the proteins act in your body.[21]
- Sugar can make your skin age by changing the structure of collagen.[22]
- Sugar can cause emphysema.[23]
- Sugar lowers the ability of enzymes to function.[24]
- Sugar intake is higher in people with Parkinson's disease.[25]
- Sugar can increase kidney size and produce pathological changes in the kidney, such as the formation of kidney stones.[26]
- Sugar can damage your pancreas and compromise the lining of your capillaries.[27]
- Sugar can cause headaches, including migraines.[28]
- Sugar can increase your risk of gout.[29]
- Sugar can increase your risk of Alzheimer's disease.[30]
- Diets high in sugar will increase free radicals and oxidative stress.[31]
- Sugar adversely affects urinary electrolyte composition.[32]
- Sugar can slow down the ability of your adrenal glands to function.[33]

- Sugar has the potential for inducing abnormal metabolic processes in a normal healthy individual and for promoting chronic degenerative diseases.[34]
- High sugar intake can cause epileptic seizures.[35]
- Sugar causes high blood pressure in obese people.[36]
- Sugar may induce cell death.[37]
- Sugar can cause gum disease.[38]

When you eat a high-sugar meal, you'll initially feel a burst of energy as your blood sugar levels rise in your bloodstream. If it's the type of sugar that pours into the bloodstream too quickly, and the body cannot adapt quickly enough, your blood sugar will rise, peak, and begin to nose-dive. When this happens, you may feel tired, irritable, or unfocused or experience brain fog.

One of the goals of my program is to get you off this sugar roller coaster. Without processed sugar, your brain and body can have a chance to recalibrate. You may find that many of your emotional problems, including anxiousness, depression, and irritability, may dissipate during the 3-week phase of the Transition Protocol. Once you begin the 3-week program, you will be avoiding all forms of processed sugar and learning how to balance your total sugar intake throughout the day. While you might have heard that people feel irritable when they're first adjusting to a low-sugar diet, I want to assure you that I've taken this into consideration, and the program you'll be following is more complete than others that are simply "low carb." On my program, we will focus on maintaining blood sugar levels at a steady rate throughout the day, which is why you won't have an adverse reaction.

Although sugar substitutes don't add calories to your diet, they can cause tremendous problems over the long term and are just as dangerous as eating excessive processed sugar. For example, the artificial sweeteners aspartame (found in NutraSweet and Equal), saccharin (found in Sweet'N Low), and sucralose (found in Splenda) all raise blood sugar levels significantly higher than does refined sugar.[39] The mechanism by which this occurs is that these noncaloric artificial sweeteners alter the bacteria in the gut. We'll talk more about the gut and gut bacteria in Chapter 3, but know now that this increase in blood sugar levels leads not only to diabetes but to excessive weight gain.[40]

One way to monitor your sugar intake is by consulting a glycemic index (see page 52), which quantifies how fast a particular food will raise your blood sugar. Pure glucose is used as the base number for the index and is given a value of 100; all other carbohydrates are given values relative to glucose depending on how fast they get into your blood—the lower the index, the longer it takes and the more stable your blood sugar remains. The higher the index, the more likely you'll feel the roller coaster of blood sugar peaks and drops.

Foods that have a high index (greater than 60) include ice cream, breads, all other white flour products, white potatoes, bananas, raisins, potato chips, alcoholic beverages, and white rice. In fact, according to Dr. William Davis, the bestselling author of *Wheat Belly*, the glycemic index of wheat products is among the highest of all foods. Low glycemic index foods (under 45) are considered more nutritious. It's no surprise that they include most fruits, vegetables, and legumes.

The glycemic index can definitely help you make better food choices, and it points out several discrepancies of so-called healthy options. For example, just one slice of whole wheat bread is considered high on the glycemic index, coming in at 69; it's actually higher than a Snickers bar, which has a glycemic index of only 41, thanks to the peanuts in this candy bar.

The only drawback of the glycemic index is that it is limited to helping you calculate one meal at a time. My friend and bestselling author JJ Virgin points out in her book *JJ Virgin's Sugar Impact Diet* that the combined effect of all the sugar you take in during the day is much more important to know, compared to the glycemic index of any one food. Even seemingly small amounts of sugar from different foods over the course of the day can add up and have a huge impact on your health. She recommends, as I do, that you remove processed sugar from your diet. For example, champagne balsamic vinaigrette is really sweet even though it sounds healthy. If you have been putting that on your salad, you've been adding a high glycemic index sugar to an otherwise healthy meal. That may not be a problem by itself because it's not a large volume of sugar, but if you are also eating a dinner roll, and then have a plate of pasta, and share a dessert because you're trying to be healthy, the impact of the total sugar intake can be overwhelming to your blood sugar regulating system. This is the mechanism that eventually causes insulin resistance. So while none of these choices were horrible on their own, when combined, they can strongly affect your health.

(continued on page 54)

GLYCEMIC INDEX

Cereals		Snacks	
All-Bran	51	Chocolate bar	49
Bran Buds + psyllium	45	Corn chips	72
Bran flakes	74	Croissant	67
Cheerios	74	Doughnut	76
Corn Chex	83	Graham crackers	74
Cornflakes	83	Jelly beans	80
Cream of Wheat	66	Life Savers	70
Frosted Flakes	55	Oatmeal cookie	57
Grape-Nuts	67	Pizza, cheese & tomato	60
Life	66	Pizza Hut, supreme	33
Muesli, natural	54	Popcorn, light microwave	55
Nutri-Grain	56	Potato chips	66
Oatmeal, old fashioned	48	Pound cake	54
Puffed wheat	67	Power bars	58
Raisin bran	73	Saltine crackers	74
Rice Chex	89	Shortbread cookies	64
Shredded wheat	67	Snickers bar	41
Special K	54	Soup, green pea	83
Total	76	Strawberry jam	51
Apple	38	Wheat Thins	67
Apricots	57	Crackers	
Banana	56	Graham	74
Cantaloupe	65	Rice cakes	80
Cherries	22	Rye	68
Dates	103	Soda	72
Grapefruit	25	Wheat Thins	67
Grapes	46	Cereal Grains	
Kiwifruit	52	Barley	25
Mango	55	Basmati white rice	58
Orange	43	Bulgur	48
Papaya	58	Cornmeal	68
Peach	42	Couscous	65
Pear	58	Millet	71
Pineapple	66	Sugars	
Plums	39	Fructose	22
Prunes	15	Honey	62
Raisins	64	Maltose	105
Watermelon	72	Table sugar	64

Pasta		Beans	
Cheese tortellini	50	Baked	44
Fettucine	32	Black beans, boiled	30
Linguine	50	Butter, boiled	33
Macaroni	46	Cannellini beans	31
Spaghetti, 5 min boiled	33	Chickpeas, boiled	34
Spaghetti, 15 min	44	Kidney, boiled	29
Spaghetti, protein enriched	28	Kidney, canned	52
Vermicelli	35	Lentils, green, brown	30
Soups/Vegetables		Lima, boiled	32
Beets, canned	64	Navy beans	38
Black bean soup	64	Pinto, boiled	39
Carrots, fresh, boiled	49	Red lentils, boiled	24
Corn, sweet	56	Soy, boiled	16
French fries	75	**Breads/Muffins**	
Green pea soup	66	Apple muffin	44
Green peas, frozen	47	Bagel, plain	72
Lima beans, frozen	32	Baguette, French	95
Parsnips	97	Blueberry muffin	59
Peas, fresh, boiled	48	Croissant	67
Potato, red, baked	93	Dark rye	76
Potato, sweet	52	Hamburger bun	61
Potato, white, boiled	63	Oat and raisin muffin	54
Potato, white, mashed	70	Pita	57
Split pea soup with ham	66	Pizza, cheese	60
Tomato soup	38	Pumpernickel	49
Yam	54	Rye	64
Milk Products		Sourdough	54
Chocolate	35	Wheat	68
Custard	43	White	70
Ice cream, vanilla	60	**Drinks**	
Ice milk, vanilla	50	Apple juice	40
Skim milk	32	Colas	65
Soy milk	31	Gatorade	78
Tofu frozen dessert	115	Grapefruit juice	48
Whole milk	30	Orange juice	46
Yogurt, fruit	36	Pineapple juice	46
Yogurt, plain	14		

If you've been diagnosed with diabetes, you already know that you have a problem processing excess sugars. But if you are on the autoimmune spectrum, you might not realize how much sugar is affecting your health. One way to test this is with the homeostasis model assessment (HOMA), a blood test that is sensitive to blood sugar imbalances long before you develop diabetes or other blood sugar problems. You can also chalk up the extra 5 to 10 pounds that you are carrying around your midsection to excess sugar consumption. While this is not the only cause, sugar is a likely culprit. If your urine smells sweet, it's another indication that you are taking in too much sugar.

Dairy Is Difficult

Most dairy products you'll find in a supermarket are highly refined. To prolong the shelf life of milk products, two things are done: pasteurization and homogenization. Pasteurization is a process of heating the milk to very high temperatures to kill off bacteria. But during the process, milk enzymes and vitamins are destroyed. This is one reason why commercial yogurts are unlikely to have the amount of good bacteria that's labeled on the container: Bacteria cannot thrive in pasteurized milk. The homogenization process gives milk its creamy consistency. It changes the size and shape of milk fat, making it more likely to enter the bloodstream and create inflammation in the body. The smaller molecules of milk fat also bind to arterial walls. The body then protects the area by producing a layer of cholesterol, which is linked to heart disease.

Many large-scale dairy farms in the United States inject hormones into milking cows, including rBGH (genetically engineered bovine growth hormone), which is used to enhance milk production. In Europe and Canada, rBGH is banned due to concerns that these hormones are linked to an increased risk of estrogen-related cancers in humans—like breast cancer.

The most well-known dairy sensitivity is called a lactose intolerance. The lining of the microvilli (the shags) produces the digestive enzyme lactase. When your intestines have increased inflammation for any reason, such as eating gluten with a gluten sensitivity, the amount of lactase enzyme is reduced dramatically. Without this enzyme, we develop a lactose intolerance. About 50 percent of people with celiac disease also have a lactose intolerance, which may contribute to persistent symptoms even when they're following a gluten-free diet.[41] If they continue eating dairy products while following a gluten-free diet, they will continue to make antibodies to gluten. This is called *cross-reactivity*. Yet if they can maintain a gluten-free diet for 1 year, inflammation subsides and lactase production naturally increases. When this happens, lactose can be broken down and the intolerance disappears.

Eighty percent of the protein in cow's milk and 20 to 45 percent of the protein in human milk come from *casein*. Casein is a difficult protein to digest. That's why bodybuilders drink casein protein shakes at night before going to sleep. It takes hours for casein to break down in your intestines, which allows the gut to deliver small amounts of muscle-building amino acids to your muscles all night long. The immune system reacts to dairy in different ways, depending on which component of dairy your body sees as an irritant. For example, one of the components of poorly digested dairy are molecules called *casomorphins*. These peptides bind to opiate receptors in the brain and are associated with sudden infant death syndrome (SIDS), the histamine release of food allergies, stimulation of high-fat food intake, and cognitive dysfunction from ADHD to autism.[42] When your immune system decides that casomorphins are a problem, you will make antibodies called casomorphin antibodies. Casein is also added to some nondairy alternatives like rice milk as a preservative. Exposure to high levels of casein can lead to an immune response of inflammation similar to the immune system reactions to gluten.

Dairy can contribute to many autoimmune symptoms and conditions and might push you further on the autoimmune spectrum. Some consider it to be a silent autoimmune response because it is difficult to connect the dots between dairy consumption and symptoms for the average person. Yet dairy consumption is linked to autoimmune conditions like acne, Hashimoto's thyroiditis, lupus, and diabetes. For example, it's commonly known that for infants at high risk for type 1 diabetes (from a family history), parents are advised to avoid feeding their babies all cow's milk products for the first year of life—because if the baby does eat cow dairy that first year, there is a higher risk of the child developing type 1 diabetes.[43]

Along with gluten and sugar, I recommend that you remove dairy from your food choices for the 3-week program, because so many people are intolerant to it. However, if you can safely reintroduce dairy into your diet following the Transition Protocol, choose products that are clearly labeled organic and "No rBGH."

Lipopolysaccharides (LPS):
The Silent Trigger That Lives inside Us

Can you imagine that there is a condition in the United States that kills more people than cardiovascular disease every year, yet you've never heard of it? Unlike the environmental exposures we've been discussing that come from the foods we eat, there is a toxic exposure that's already in your body. Lipopolysaccharides (LPS) are components of bacteria, primarily found in the gut. LPS molecules can initially be found in the cell walls of certain types of infectious bacteria. When the infectious bacteria are destroyed by the protective, good bacteria that reside in the gut, the remnants of that bad bacteria are free floating in the intestines. When they remain in the gut, they are usually not a problem. If LPS penetrates the epithelial wall, they get into the bloodstream, and then you have a problem.

Endotoxins are poisons produced inside the body. LPS is one type of endotoxin, but because it is so prevalent, many authors and even some dictionaries say that they are one and the same. As you learn more about detoxification and creating a healthier environment inside your body, you'll hear the word *endotoxin*. Do not be confused by it; it almost always refers to high concentrations of LPS.

A high-fat diet, including but not limited to a high consumption of palm and corn oils, facilitates moving LPS into the bloodstream, literally on the backs of these dietary fat molecules. It's called *lipid raft transcytosis* (like a boat). Why would the body ever let this happen? Well, it turns out that small amounts of LPS in the bloodstream trigger the production of an anti-inflammatory hormone called adiponectin (the anti-obesity hormone). However, large amounts trigger much more inflammation than the body can handle, and then here comes the inflammatory cascade. One of the ways to prevent LPS accumulation is through the good foods you'll choose, including the healthy fats featured in our program, which will avoid this mechanism.

There are two primary compounds, among others, known to cause intestinal permeability (aka, the leaky gut, which we'll talk about next): gluten and LPS. When LPS enters the bloodstream, it travels everywhere. If it deposits in the brain, it triggers inflammation in the brain (sadly, that's what killed my mother: toxic metabolic encephalopathy). If it deposits in the joints, it triggers inflammation in the joints (arthritis and rheumatoid arthritis).[44] There is no organ or tissue that is immune to the effects of LPS, and it has been linked with many chronic symptoms. Where is your weak link? Remember, body language never lies. Can you hear your body telling you where its weak link is?

In small amounts, LPS may cause fever, altered resistance to bacterial infection, and leucopenia (a low white blood cell count), among other symptoms. In large quantities, the Centers for Disease Control and Prevention (CDC) tells us that it reduces bloodflow into any tissue, causing between 175,000 and 200,000 deaths annually. The CDC notes that perhaps a half-million people are affected annually by this mechanism, yet no one talks about it.[45] That's because there is no profit in addressing LPS: There's no drug to fix it.

LPS exemplifies the autoimmune spectrum. When LPS remains in your gut, it doesn't noticeably affect your health. But the moment it enters the bloodstream, it triggers the inflammatory process. As you can see from this chart, LPS can detrimentally affect many disease processes, in the same pattern. As LPS levels increase, inflammation increases and symptoms increase in severity. Left unchecked, it can be fatal. In Chapter 5, you'll learn how you can test for your current levels of LPS. Then you'll learn the lifestyle changes you can make to shut down this mechanism.

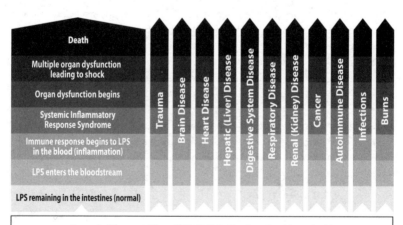

For each of these conditions, LPS in the intestines is no threat to our health. As the concentration of LPS increases in the bloodstream, the greater the degree of inflammation, tissue damage/dysfunction, and eventual death.

MEET NANCY

Nancy never left the house without a packet of tissues. She suffered from chronic allergies but could never figure out exactly what she was allergic to. She was also constantly battling her depression, and although she didn't think of herself as someone who had digestive problems, she always felt bloated. The comforting allure of a box of doughnuts, a pint of ice cream, a bowl of noodles, or, when things were really bad, a roll of raw cookie dough was often too hard to resist and seemed to calm down her anxiety. She dressed to hide her weight gain in public, hoping to pass invisibly through life. She didn't even consider dating. She had lost interest in men anyway, despite being only 28 years old.

To the average doctor, Nancy was a classic depressed patient who needed a prescription for antidepressants, perhaps some antianxiety medication, and a good weight-loss and exercise program. But here's what most doctors miss with people like Nancy: Her depression, anxiety, and weight gain were actually the result of immune responses that were causing chronic inflammation. Nancy, like so many women, had a constellation of symptoms that all pointed to one culprit: a systemic inflammatory cascade.

When Nancy came to my office, I ran an antibody test to determine the cause of her problems. I discovered that the culprits for her immune reaction were a sensitivity to gluten and dairy and elevated levels of LPS in her blood. These molecules were activating her immune system. But how did these molecules enter her bloodstream? The answer was the third factor: intestinal permeability.

With the proper testing and treatment, a gluten- and dairy-free diet, and the nutrition to heal her intestinal permeability, Nancy's antibody load to LPS reduced within 6 months. She stopped throwing gasoline on the fire (by removing gluten and dairy), and her symptoms began lifting within the first 2 weeks as her inflammation subsided. Within 6 months, she was down two dress sizes and came back to see me, vibrant with life.

FACTOR 3: INTESTINAL PERMEABILITY (AKA LEAKY GUT SYNDROME)

*The state of health or the state of disease is
the combination between what we are—meaning what
genetically makes us the way that we're engineered—and
the environment that's around us. And the gut is the point
of entry in which these two elements meet.*

—ALESSIO FASANO, MD

The digestive system has two closely related purposes. First, healthy digestion processes food so that beneficial, life-sustaining nutrients can enter the bloodstream and circulate through the body. At the same time, the digestive system filters out toxins or irritants and prevents them from being absorbed into the blood. A leaky gut, however, allows certain incompletely digested material and toxins like LPS to enter the bloodstream. Exactly which materials "sneak through" depends on how leaky someone's leaky gut happens to be.

To understand leaky gut, you must understand the anatomy of the small intestine, which is where the real work of digestion occurs. In the small intestine, food is broken down into molecules that will either continue through the digestive tract to be eliminated from the body or else pass through the lining of the small intestine into the bloodstream. The epithelial lining of the intestines is only one cell thick. It functions like cheesecloth: Only small molecules are supposed to get through into the bloodstream. One of the reasons that the small intestine is 20-plus feet long is that some foods are more difficult to digest and be broken down into particles small enough to fit through the cheesecloth. When the cheesecloth gets torn, however, due to inflammation, then larger molecules, called *macromolecules*, can get through the cheesecloth and into the bloodstream before they have been completely broken down into the raw materials to rebuild our bodies.

When these macromolecules enter the bloodstream, the immune system says, *Whoa, what's this? I don't recognize this big thing as a nutrient I can use to make new bone cells or muscle cells. I better fight this.* Now your body makes antibodies to these macromolecules. If it's tomatoes, you now have elevated antibodies to tomatoes. If it's gluten, you make antibodies to A-A-B-C-D, and now we're back to the concept of molecular mimicry. Your bloodstream has become a river of toxicity. Your immune system, again, in an effort to protect you, creates collateral damage wherever your weak link is. These are the people who do a food allergy test and come back with positive results to 15 foods, and they say, "OMG, that's everything I eat." Of course it is; your immune system is trying to protect you from the toxic macromolecules that entered the bloodstream too early—before they were fully digested.

Now with all three factors—genetic susceptibility, exposure, and leaky gut—you are faced with a flood of inflammation initiating the autoimmune spectrum. In all cases of autoimmune disease, increased permeability appears to precede.

Dr. Alessio Fasano, the chair of pediatric gastroenterology at Massachusetts General Hospital, who trains every pediatric gastroenterologist who graduates from Harvard Medical School, shared this analogy with me that perfectly describes this mechanism. Imagine the Great Wall of China is made of a single layer of cells. The Great Wall was built to keep the enemy outside, but every few hundred yards there are checkpoints where people can come and go, under tightly controlled surveillance. These checkpoints in the intestine are called tight junctions. When the checkpoints are well maintained, you won't have an enemy invasion. But once something goes wrong, and there is a breach of this checkpoint, an uncontrolled passage of instigators can come through and create damage.

When you are constantly eating foods that you can't digest properly, like gluten, you increase the inflammatory bonfire in your gut. This will reduce the beneficial bacteria in your gut and encourage the growth of bad bacteria and undesirable yeast. The environment of imbalanced flora in the gut is called *dysbiosis*. These bacterial changes cause food to ferment in the intestines instead of being digested, creating gas and bloating. Worse, the new bacteria and yeast are recognized by the immune system as another offending invader, creating a new inflammatory response in the digestive tract, and the tissue damage causes more tears in the cheesecloth, leading to more intestinal permeability, more immune response in the bloodstream, more inflammation throughout the body, and more symptom development at your weak link.

As long as the leaky gut persists, you will experience inflammation and symptoms. Low-grade fever, general fatigue, and inconsistent gut pain are common complaints of leaky gut syndrome. Seemingly out of nowhere, you are now more susceptible to seasonal allergies, rashes, or even autoimmune diseases like rheumatoid arthritis, systemic lupus, or Hashimoto's thyroiditis. Any of these, and many others, might be your weak link.

Of the many factors that may contribute to intestinal permeability, the ones that have been identified to consistently fuel this fire are stress, gluten, and excessive lipopolysaccharides (LPS). In one 2015 study published in the journal *Nutrients*, researchers found that all humans develop intestinal permeability whenever they're exposed to gluten, regardless of whether or not they have celiac disease or a gluten sensitivity.[46] Gluten will trigger a temporary leaky gut within 5 hours of eating. Usually, the gut will heal by itself, but for people with celiac disease or gluten sensitivity, within 36 hours the damage will not clear up by itself. The fastest-growing cells of the body are these same epithelial cells of the intestine (your cheesecloth). It's constantly repairing itself to the point where your body creates a completely new lining every 3 to 7 days. So when you have toast for breakfast, you tear the cheesecloth, but it heals. You have a sandwich for lunch, you tear the cheesecloth, but it heals. You have pasta for dinner, tear the cheesecloth, but it heals. Croutons on your salad, tear the cheesecloth, but it heals. Day in and day out. In the United States, the average consumption of wheat is 132.5 pounds per person per year. Now, I don't eat any. That means you're eating 265 pounds, and every bite tears your cheesecloth, but it heals. Until one day you can be 2 years old, 22 years old, or 62 years old, and your cheesecloth won't heal anymore.

What happened? Why did your body let you down? Researchers refer to this moment as *loss of oral tolerance*. Your body can no longer accommodate the degree of toxins you are exposed to—whether it's food, toxic chemicals, heavy metals, or stress. Now you have *pathogenic intestinal permeability*, the leaky gut, and now the autoimmune spectrum will begin to affect wherever your weak link is.

The good news is that intestinal permeability is completely reversible.

(continued on page 64)

SAMANTHA'S STORY, PART 2

I introduced you to my patient Samantha in the last chapter. I first met her after she was diagnosed with antiphospholipid syndrome and lupus, which came 3 years later. When I started working with her, she was 31 years old. One of the first things I did was take down her family history. I was specifically looking to find out if she had a genetic component to her autoimmunity. Samantha told me that neither blood clots nor lupus ran in her family, though her parents did have other symptoms and conditions that fell on the autoimmune spectrum. In fact, both her parents had evidence of gluten-related disorders that were manifesting with different symptoms than the ones she experiences.

I wasn't surprised, as I know that everyone has a different weak link, a genetic expression that may be different than other members of the same family. That's the story of epigenetics, which is how the environment triggers the expression of DNA. While Samantha and each of her parents shared similar DNA, her parents weren't affected by the environment in the same way she was, because their genes were either turned off when hers became turned on, or hers became turned on as theirs stayed shut off, which allowed for the expression of the illness presenting in different ways. Remember the example I gave earlier about identical twins? This is the same mechanism.

I asked Samantha about her own food sensitivities. We discovered that she had multiple food sensitivities, with gluten being especially debilitating. Samantha told me that before she went off of gluten, she had severe constipation and bloating (remember, she had been told as a child that bowel movements once a week were "normal"). She grew up eating gluten every day in just about every meal. But once we got her off gluten, her weight dropped so much that what she thought of as her "athletic booty" turned out to really be a "gluten booty." She also noticed that she had more energy and more mental clarity when she was gluten-free, and when she accidentally exposed herself to gluten from cross-contamination, the symptoms mostly affected her thinking. Samantha told me that she now gets brain fog or feels like she is drunk when she is exposed to gluten due to cross-contamination.

I found out that she had already been avoiding cow's milk products, and she thought she was doing the right thing when she drank goat's milk or sheep's milk. With proper diagnostic testing, I was able to determine that she had a systemic inflammatory response to casein, which is present in all animal milk. When she stopped eating these non-cow dairy products, she did much better.

I recommended that Samantha avoid sugar, but she told me that she had already eliminated it from her diet back in 2012. She told me every time she ate anything with sugar, including fruit, either a bladder infection or a yeast infection would flare 2 or 3 days later. I told her that this was common for people who had chronic yeast infections, where one fruit serving could be the straw that broke the camel's back, producing symptoms. I recommended that she continue being vigilant about her food choices.

Last, I evaluated her for intestinal permeability. She told me about the stomach cramps she always had as a child, even though it was never diagnosed as leaky gut syndrome. I assured Samantha that when she got herself off of all animal milk, she'd find that her stomach pains would diminish. The fact is, goat's milk protein is six times the size of human breast milk protein and very difficult to digest. Although it is not as difficult as cow's milk to digest, it can still be very difficult, especially for sensitive individuals.

I also assured Samantha that her overall health was going to improve because she had finally found a doctor who understood the autoimmune spectrum. The advice she had received in the past, while well intentioned, simply wasn't well informed. Remember, it takes 17 years for the latest research to trickle down to clinical practice. New research about the autoimmune spectrum is coming out every day, but most doctors simply don't have the time to read it. My job is to bring this research to them, and ultimately to you. So like Samantha, you're also in good hands. Vibrant health is your birthright.

You do not have to suffer with the symptoms of a leaky gut or the systemic complications it can cause. By following my program, you are going to remove the most common environmental exposures, which will reduce inflammation in your gut and allow your epithelial lining to recover. Again, you can arrest the development of autoimmune disease by healing a leaky gut.

NEXT STEPS

Intestinal permeability is one of two factors that help us see why we need to focus on our gut health in order to avoid or reverse autoimmunity. The second factor, which is arguably of equal importance, is the state of our microbiome: the mix of both good and bad bacteria that live in our gut. In the next chapter, we'll explore this new frontier and see what the latest research is showing pertaining to the connection between your microbiome and how you look, feel, and think.

> To listen to my podcast on how gluten is connected to autoimmunity, or watch my webinar slides, go to AutoimmunityPodcast.com.

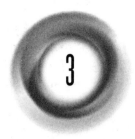

3

THE ABSOLUTE NECESSITY
OF A HEALTHY MICROBIOME

Imagine for a moment that you are a well-respected family physician. You've been practicing medicine long enough to have seen many of the youngsters you've stewarded through life grow up to be adults, and you have watched their parents age. You think you know all the ins and outs of the human body because you've treated every illness. Yet one day you attend a seminar for postgraduate education credits, and all of a sudden you're presented with startling new information: Researchers have just discovered a new organ in the human body, and it controls every aspect of your health.

This exact revelation is happening in medical offices across the country as scientists come to know more about the microbiome. The microbiome is the community of bacteria, yeasts, and viruses that live in the gut. In the last 10 years, it has begun to be recognized as an essential factor in overall health. Thanks to advances in science and technology, researchers have found that the microbiome is critical for more than digesting food: It is the control center for the entire body. As unbelievable as this statement sounds, that's the fact, Jack!

The microbiome is linked to manufacturing vitamins, regulating metabolism and blood sugar, and influencing both genetic expression and brain chemistry. For every message from the brain to the gut there are nine messages from the gut to the brain. These messages control the brain's response to stress, brain hormone production, the activation of the brain's own immune system, the growth of new brain cells (neurogenesis) and the adaptability of these new cells to learn (neuroplasticity), plus other functions.

The microbiome is the hottest topic in medical research today. In 2007, 396 new research papers were published on the subject. In 2015, that number was 5,512. That's 5,512 teams of researchers who spent months and months studying this topic, writing papers, submitting them for publication, and then being published. If you Google "microbiome" today, you'll see a listing of more than 19,000 recent studies, and each year brings new discoveries. For instance, we now know that we each are hosting a completely unique microbiome that comprises trillions of bacteria of several hundred species. The vast majority of microbes harbored in our intestinal tracts are thought to have beneficial effects, and while there are many different types of bacteria, they primarily fall into two big groups. The Bacteroidetes are supposed to be the dominant group that we host. The second group is the Firmicutes, and we're not as happy to have these as dominant houseguests. Individually, these Firmicutes bacteria aren't dangerous, but in high concentrations, they overwhelm the Bacteroidetes and take over, and the imbalance they create causes health problems—such as being a primary contributor to resistant obesity.

Your microbiome can weigh up to 5 pounds—nearly twice as much as the brain—and each bacterium it hosts is a living organism made up of cells and genes. Get this: There are between 100 to 150 times more genes found in your microbiome than the 23,000 genes found in your human DNA. Because of this, many experts have come to think of the microbiome as less like an additional organ in the body and more like a whole other organism with a life of its own. It's a conversation that I often have with my colleagues after we've been teaching about autoimmunity. We start wondering, "Are we humans hosting a whole lot of bacteria, or are we bacteria having a human experience?" We appreciate that we are living with a parallel civilization inside of us, each assisting the other.

There are also 10 times more cells of bacteria in our gut than all the cells in the rest of the body put together. We know this because of the shape of our intestines. Remember, the intestines are a tube 20 to 25 feet long lined with microvilli, the shag carpeting that aids in digestion. If you could flatten out the microvilli, the surface of our intestines would be the size of a tennis court. We need that much surface in the gut because there's so much activity going on. And covering every inch of that surface are bacteria, packed in between each of the shags.

If you were born via natural childbirth, you inherited your microbiome from your mother. In the last month of pregnancy, the mother's body starts colonizing the vaginal tract with high concentrations of *Prevotella* bacteria, which covers the baby during childbirth. These bacteria carry a message down to the baby's gut, preparing it to create the digestive enzymes that break down breast milk and use it efficiently.

If you were born via a cesarean section, all bets are off. Instead of Mom's good *Prevotella* bacteria, you were instantly exposed to a plethora of foreign bacteria resting on Mom's skin and in the air of the delivery room, and you consequently have a higher risk of disease over the course of your life, and possibly a lower IQ.[1] In the most recent and largest study to date reviewing the birth information of 750,569 children born by C-section, children delivered by both acute (meaning "necessary for the baby and/or mother's health") and elective C-section had an increased risk of asthma, laryngitis, and gastroenteritis (inflammation of the intestines). Children delivered by acute C-section had an increased risk of ulcerative colitis and celiac disease, whereas children delivered by elective C-section had an increased risk of lower respiratory tract infection and juvenile idiopathic arthritis. The effect of elective cesareans was higher than the effect of acute cesareans on the risk of asthma.[2] I have met a number of ob-gyns who tell me that when they have to do a C-section, they will swab the mother's vaginal canal with something similar to a Q-tip and then rub the swab inside the newborn baby's mouth. They're trying to get some of the protective, instructional microbiota (like *Prevotella*) into the baby at birth any way they can. Although there have been no long-term studies on this technique that I am aware of, it's rational to assume it does reduce the cesarean babies' future risk of numerous diseases, including autoimmune diseases. Of course, if a C-section is medically necessary, it is much more important to protect the baby's and the mother's lives than to worry about potential future health risks.

The microbiome is a primary component of the immune system in the gut. Seventy percent of our entire immune system resides in the gut, and the microbiome comprises the majority of that immune system. It's the modulator, or controller, of how the immune system in the gut operates. Just like a national guard is part of a police force yet works in its own unique way, the microbiome is a part of the immune system yet works in its own unique way.

Like the immune system, the microbiome is a collection of cells that function in unison with the gut immune cells that are designed to promote health, but when it becomes unbalanced, this can initiate disease.[3] We know that each of us has a unique microbiome that is influenced by genetics, our environment, and our dietary selections. There is a close relationship and an exchange of information between the gut bacteria and your immune cells sitting on that same gut wall. It is the initial part of your arsenal to control offending invaders.

Your antecedents—how you've lived your life so far—have a profound effect on the composition and diversity of your microbiome, much like it affects the immune system.[4] While others may tell you that aging is correlated with poor function and disease, this doesn't have to be the case. Addressing the microbiome is one important way for you to see reversals in many of the diseases related to deterioration, including atherosclerosis, colorectal cancers, organ atrophies, and serious infections.

WHEN BACTERIAL IMBALANCE OCCURS

Hippocrates made the statement thousands of years ago, "All diseases begin in the gut." We are just now able to confirm how right he was. The composition of the microbiome can shape a healthy immune response or predispose you to disease.[5] When your microbiome is poorly fed and cared for, harmful bacteria and fungi take over, making you more susceptible to chronic illnesses. When blood tests identify that you are on the autoimmune spectrum, it indicates a catastrophic failure of the microbiome allowing too many pathogenic bacteria (bad guys), which activate genes for inflammation and intestinal permeability.

Alessio Fasano, MD, believes, as I do, that a primary source of offending invaders that set off the autoimmune response is the imbalance of bacteria that live within us, increasing our risk for heart disease, cancer, stroke, Alzheimer's, diabetes, and other life-threatening autoimmune diseases. Hosting an unbalanced microbiome can also lead to depression, anxiety, memory loss, brain fog, and mood swings.

As we learned in the last chapter, genes don't predict disease. Instead, they identify the weak links in your chain where disease may develop (depending on how hard you pull on the chain). The bacterial genes of the microbiome influence our own genetic expression through epigenetics, which we discussed in the last chapter. For example, the bacteria in the microbiome help digest amino acids from foods and convert them into different brain hormones, called *neurotransmitters*. These neurotransmitters control everything from brain speed to mood to metabolism, which is how we can link the health of the microbiome to obesity: The availability of specific types of bacteria is one of the primary criteria to examine when people are unable to lose weight, even on calorie-restricted diets. If you've sincerely tried to count calories or diligently followed specific weight-loss programs and didn't get the results you wanted, it's very likely that the bad bacteria in your microbiome are acting as an emergency brake, holding your body back from losing weight.

An imbalanced microbiome pulls on our chain, so wherever your weak link is, that's where the link will break and leave you vulnerable to developing health problems. That's what's meant by a genetic vulnerability—not that you are destined to get such-and-such disease, but rather that if increased inflammation pulls at the chain too hard, then your genetic weak link will manifest. What's more, an imbalanced microbiome creates an inflammatory environment that will eventually be the last straw, creating intestinal permeability (the leaky gut), which allows food macromolecules (such as gluten) to sneak through the leaky gut into the bloodstream, which triggers an immune response to that food molecule. An abnormal microbiome will create inflammation and can cause intestinal permeability all by itself, even with a squeaky-clean diet. This is a major reason why some people who avoid the foods they are sensitive to may not feel better right away—they still have an ongoing inflammatory cascade in the intestines created by the imbalanced microbiome. The imbalanced microbiome is the environmental trigger pulling on your chain. However, your microbiome can begin to change in as few as 3 days when you change what you eat.

We learned in Chapter 2 that epigenetics controls how our genes express themselves. The major driver of epigenetic expression is the microbiome. It is the largest environment we deal with every day. It's interesting to me that humans are the dominant species on the planet, yet our genetic structure is so simple. For example, humans are made of about 23,000 genes. Compare us to a worm, which has 90,000 genes. So they're much more complicated than we are. Yet I believe that we don't have to argue too much that worms and human beings have different levels of sophistication in terms of what they're capable of doing.

So where does our sophistication come from? It comes from the fact that we really are made of two genomes. The human genome is fixed and rudimentary. You cannot change it. Then we have the microbiome, which contains 100 to 150 times more genes than the human genome. Genes control function. That means that the microbiome has 100 to 150 times more influence on our daily function than the human genome.

MEET THE PIMA INDIANS

The Pima Indians, Native Americans who have historically lived in the American Southwest near Mexico, pose an interesting question about microbiome and its impact on health. These indigenous people have lived in this arid part of the country for hundreds and hundreds of years. Driving through the area today, you can still see that there is nothing growing in the desert to eat, yet these people survived. One explanation for their survival is known as the *thrifty gene theory*: The Pima evolved to be very efficient with their food intake and were able to optimize their calories. The Pima used every calorie of food they took in or stored it for later use. When there isn't much to eat, you either adapt and get the most bang for your buck out of your efforts to harvest food, or you're malnourished and weakened, and you have a tougher time surviving. The ones who survived had offspring who had their parents' strong genes. Those who weren't very good at utilizing calories couldn't acclimate to their harsh environment.

The major difference between the successful Pima and those who didn't survive was their microbiome. Their survival was dependent on developing a microbiome high in Firmicutes, the group of bacteria that hoard calories. Over time, these Firmicutes influenced the Pima DNA, so that their offspring also carried high levels of Firmicutes. In this example, the term "thrifty gene" doesn't apply to the Pima people's DNA but to the DNA of the bacteria.

Now fast-forward to today, where the Pima are no longer eating their ancestral diet and instead eat the standard American diet: They live on convenience food and junk food, not many vegetables, way too much sugar and bad fat, etc. The result is that the Pima are still hoarding their calories, and by the age of 35, 50 percent of Pima adults have diabetes, and 95 percent of those with diabetes are overweight and are at a higher risk of cardiovascular disease, high blood pressure, and dementia. Even though food is no longer scarce, their thrifty genes in their microbiome still send the message to hoard calories more efficiently that the rest of us can. This is why their rate of diabetes is far higher than the average in the United States. This time, their "thrifty gene" and microbiome are working against them.

THE ORIGINS OF DYSBIOSIS

When the intestines contain the right balance of good and bad bacteria, they are described as being in a state of *symbiosis*. An imbalance in the microbiome is referred to as *dysbiosis* and is a primary source of inflammation in the gut and throughout your body. Dysbiosis can result from a deficiency of good bacteria or an overgrowth of harmful organisms, including unfriendly bacteria, yeast (candida), and protozoa. The composition of the microbiome is highly influenced by our environment. First and foremost, it is affected by dietary choices, because these bacteria eat our leftovers.

Most of us have abnormal microbiomes from adhering to the standard American diet of low-nutrient foods and living a sedentary lifestyle. The foods you eat profoundly influence the types of intestinal flora you carry and their behavior. This in turn affects how you burn and store calories and produce energy, and it determines the number and amount of neurotransmitters (brain hormones) you make, which in turn controls your moods and behaviors as well as your risk for disease. For example, foods containing gluten, casein (a protein found in dairy), and corn are thought to have endotoxin-like effects that can contribute to dysbiosis. What's more, about 75 percent of the food in the average Western diet is of limited or no benefit to the microbiome, especially for the bacteria found in the lower gut. Most of it, composed specifically of refined carbohydrates, is already absorbed in the upper GI tract, and what eventually reaches the large intestine is of limited value, as it contains only small amounts of the minerals, vitamins, and other nutrients necessary for maintenance of the microbiota.[6]

Every cell in your body reproduces itself. As we've already learned, we have an entire new body every 7 years. Some cells reproduce rapidly, some are quite slow. The fastest-growing cells in your body are found in the lining of your intestines. You have a completely new lining every 3 to 7 days. It's like a snake shedding its skin—new cells replace the old ones quickly. The fuel for those cells to reproduce is called *butyrate* or *butyric acid*.

Butyrate is a by-product of digestion involving good bacteria feeding on vegetable fiber. If you're not eating enough vegetables or if you don't have the right microbiome, you won't make enough butyrate. This is one of the more important reasons to eat a variety of vegetables—to supply the starches needed for our "good bacteria" to feed off of and make butyrate.

If you do not have enough butyric acid, your cells are still going to reproduce, but you are building your house out of straw instead of brick. You're still going to make new cells every day, but if you don't have enough of the right raw material, your cells will be weak. However, the right amounts of butyrate can (1) build strong, healthy colon cells that have a much better chance of functioning normally, (2) allow both the intestinal wall cells as well as intestinal immune cells to calm down and rest in a state of "ready to protect when needed," and (3) reduce the inflammation that is a primary trigger in developing obesity.[7] Many studies site a correlation with building your house out of straw instead of brick to a vulnerability in developing colon cancer. Having the right amount of butyrate is protective against the development of this type of cancer.

Remember the triad of development for autoimmune disease, which includes intestinal permeability? Here's exactly where food selection becomes important. The foods you eat play a major role in determining if you have enough butyrate. If you have enough butyrate, you help heal intestinal permeability, the gateway in the development of autoimmune disease.

Autoimmune disease is particularly prevalent in the Western world because our diet has so significantly damaged our microbiomes. In a 2010 Italian study, researchers compared stool samples of African tribal children to children living in Europe, and they found dramatic differences. The children in the African tribes who still eat the way their ancestors ate don't end up with many of our most common autoimmune

African Village Children

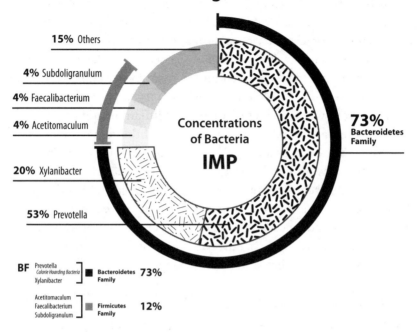

15% Others

4% Subdoligranulum

4% Faecalibacterium

4% Acetitomaculum

20% Xylanibacter

53% Prevotella

Concentrations
of Bacteria
IMP

73%
Bacteroidetes
Family

| BF | Prevotella *Calorie Hoarding Bacteria* Xylanibacter |] | ■ **Bacteroidetes Family** | **73%** |
| | Acetitomaculum Faecalibacterium Subdoligranulum |] | ▨ **Firmicutes Family** | **12%** |

European Union Children

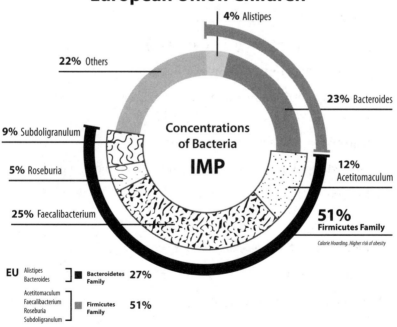

4% Alistipes

22% Others

23% Bacteroides

9% Subdoligranulum

5% Roseburia

25% Faecalibacterium

Concentrations
of Bacteria
IMP

12%
Acetitomaculum

51%
Firmicutes Family

Calorie Hoarding. Higher risk of obesity

| EU | Alistipes Bacteroides |] | ■ **Bacteroidetes Family** | **27%** |
| | Acetitomaculum Faecalibacterium Roseburia Subdoligranulum |] | ▨ **Firmicutes Family** | **51%** |

conditions (like allergies, asthma, eczema, acne, rheumatoid arthritis, psoriasis, or multiple sclerosis). The difference is the microbiome. The African children have a much higher rate of good bacteria and a limited amount of bad bacteria, as well as a unique abundance of good bacteria that were completely lacking in the European children. The researchers hypothesized that the African children's microbiome allowed them to maximize energy intake from fibrous plant foods (producing higher butyrate levels) while protecting them from inflammation.[8]

In the diagram on page 73, the European children have a four-fold increase in the calorie-hoarding Firmicutes family of bacteria. The African children have higher concentrations of the Bacteroidetes family, which is a critical component of a healthy microbiome with low vulnerability to developing autoimmune disease. So while we in the Western world may have advanced in our knowledge of the comforts and safety of life, we are just learning that the balance of the microbiome is the key to a disease resistant, slim, and healthy body.

SYMPTOMS OF DYSBIOSIS

When the digestive system is out of balance, the following symptoms may occur:

- A sense of fullness after eating
- Amenorrhea (absence of menstruation)
- Bloating, belching, burning, flatulence after meals
- Chronic intestinal infections, parasites, yeast, unfriendly bacteria
- Chronic vaginitis (vaginal irritation)
- Dilated capillaries in the cheeks and nose in the nonalcoholic
- Fatigue
- Greasy stools
- Indigestion, diarrhea, constipation
- Iron deficiency
- Nausea or diarrhea after taking supplements

- Postadolescent acne or skin irritations (including rosacea)

- Rectal itching

- Skin that bruises easily

- Systemic reactions after eating

- Undigested food in the stool

- Weak or cracked fingernails

Dysbiosis and Antibiotics

Dysbiosis can also be caused by medications, primarily the use and abuse of antibiotics. Interestingly, the epidemic of autoimmune disease coincides with the introduction of antibiotics. Taking an antibiotic is like dropping a bomb on your microbiome: The drug damages or destroys everything in its path, including both good and bad bacteria. Over time, the bad bacteria become resistant to the antibiotics, prosper, and create an imbalance in our intestines, triggering inflammation that goes systemic. In a meta-analysis of 4,373 papers, researchers concluded that individuals prescribed an antibiotic for a respiratory or urinary infection develop bacterial resistance to that antibiotic. The effect is greatest in the month immediately after treatment but may persist for up to 12 months.[9] So if you're experiencing recurring ear, sinus, or lung infections, it may be caused by the fact that your body is no longer responding to the medication your doctor is prescribing.

Antibiotics definitely have their place in medicine. They effectively treat bacterial infections. But when they are overused, or if your immune system is busy fighting off other offending invaders, they can cause more problems because they kill all bacteria, good and bad.

Unfortunately, the last 3 decades have seen the overuse of antibiotics in both the medical community as well as conventional farming. This has resulted in a systematic depletion of the good bacteria in our intestines. Seventy percent of our immune system is found in the intestines, and our primary protection from colds, flus, viruses, cancer cells, and more is supposed to come from the beneficial bacteria naturally occurring in our gut. When the good bacteria are further reduced from a dose of antibiotics, inflammation increases, intestinal permeability increases, and we are at a higher risk of infection and disease.

Often, antibiotics are prescribed to treat illness they are not created to address. Antibiotics can't treat a cold or a yeast infection. In fact, the reason why so many children do not resolve their ear infections with antibiotics is because 14 to 28 percent of ear infections are caused by fungus or yeast, not bacteria.[10]

All of us are exposed to antibiotics, whether by prescription or not. Farmers spray their vegetables with antibiotics, and animals like cows and chickens are given antibiotics to make them stronger. Antibiotic residue is in meat and poultry products, vegetables, and our water supply. It is so very challenging to understand how governmental agencies that are supposed to be protecting us allow the indiscriminate use of these powerful drugs in so many situations where they are not necessary. There is no reason on earth why we should be spraying our vegetable crops with antibiotics and thus dripping gasoline on the inflammation fire every time we eat them. This is another reason why supposedly healthy foods have become unhealthy for us. Any part of our food chain that is treated with antibiotics results in an inflammatory food.

Another problem with antibiotics is that they stimulate the production of biofilms, a type of polymer (hard plastic) that bacteria produce to protect themselves. It's like a force field created to protect bacteria. Biofilms prevent antibiotics from reaching bacteria. According to a CDC 2013 report, antibiotic-resistant bacteria cause more than 23,000 deaths per year in the United States alone. This is one of the ways that superbugs, or bacteria that are resistant to antibiotics, are created (the second way being a lack of competition for resources in the gut). The National Institutes of Health says that it can now take up to 100 times the standard dose of antibiotic to kill a bacterium if it has a strong biofilm. This is why you may be taking more antibiotics than before to fight off an infection. The longer we have low levels of bacteria in our bodies that shouldn't be there, the more likely the biofilms will develop.

Dysbiosis and Stress

Last, dysbiosis can be caused by stress, ranging from environmental exposures such as pollution, chemicals, radiation, and low-quality,

Meet Paul

After dental surgery, my friend Paul was given a prescription for antibiotics to ward off potential infections. Soon afterward, Paul noticed some unpleasant changes in his health. He started feeling bloated most of the time, and he felt like a cold was coming on every 4 to 6 weeks. The fatigue that followed was taking longer and longer to lift.

Paul's deteriorating health took away his motivation to exercise, and he gained a little more than 10 pounds. When the joints in his body began to feel achy all the time, he assumed it was from the lack of activity. What he mostly wanted to do every day was to stay home and watch TV. When he couldn't get off the couch for 2 days in a row, his wife sent him into my office.

Paul told me what was going on, and I realized that his achiness was stemming from inflammation in his joints caused by LPS infiltration from intestinal permeability that was caused by the antibiotics. Paul didn't realize that the antibiotics he had taken had triggered an internal crisis in his body (dysbiosis), and his microbiome was sending a crisis message. It signaled the immune system to create inflammation, causing intestinal permeability, allowing LPS to get into his bloodstream, which deposited in his weak link—his joints.

Upon testing, we confirmed that Paul's LPS levels were quite elevated. Even though Paul didn't think he was sensitive to dairy or gluten, I asked him to take a 3-week break from both, just to see. To his surprise, even before the 3 weeks were over, his joint pain decreased and he went back to exercising while he followed my gluten-free, dairy-free, sugar-free diet. Within 6 weeks, he had lost the added weight. He told me, "Dr. O'Bryan, I finally feel like myself again. I understand what you were saying when you told me to listen to my body."

nutrient-poor foods to the stresses of our everyday lives, including dealing with not feeling well. Stress has become such an ingrained part of our day that it's no wonder our microbiomes are a mess.

Our understanding of stress and how it affects the body was first noted by Hans Selye, MD, PhD, a Hungarian physician who also earned a doctorate in organic chemistry. In the 1950s and 1960s, Dr. Selye first explored the critical concept of the adrenal glands as our first line of defense against stress. Whether we face chemical, emotional, or physical stress, our adrenal glands allow us to respond in a healthy way. They are in charge of determining when to activate the famous "fight, flight, or fright" response.

Dr. Selye and other scientists at the time already knew that there are two different nervous systems in our body: the parasympathetic nervous system and the sympathetic nervous system. When you are in a stress mode, the fight, flight, or fright response kicks in, and your sympathetic nervous system is activated. Dr. Selye pointed out that our bodies are designed just like those of our ancestors, going back tens of thousands of years ago when we lived on the savannas of Africa, which means that we respond to the stresses of life just like our ancestors did. Here's an example: One of the physiological manifestations of fight, flight, or fright is a reduction of bloodflow to the skin. When our ancestors were in a stressful situation (hunting, fighting an animal) and the sympathetic nervous system was the dominant functioning system at that moment, there would be a reduction in bloodflow to the skin. Why? So that we wouldn't bleed excessively when we were fighting for our lives. Fast-forward to our everyday, stressful lives. When we are in a sympathetic dominant state, which we are most of the time, we have a reduction in bloodflow to our skin. How might that manifest? Acne, psoriasis, or vitiligo (loss of pigment causing white patches in the skin). We could go through every system in the body and demonstrate similar lifesaving, protective responses that occur in a sympathetic dominant state. But we're not supposed to live like this 24/7.

How often were our ancestors exposed to extreme stress, requiring a fight, flight, or fright response? Not very often. We can imagine that occasionally their lives would be in danger or that they would need to be hyperalert. Yet they lived in tropical climates where nothing but organic food grew year-round. That's why we have a stress response to chemically laden and often genetically modified foods. Our forebears didn't need a coat to keep them warm in the winter. That's why when we feel cold, it puts stress on our system, activating an adrenal response.

We know that we're supposed to live a relatively mellow life and rarely activate our adrenal glands because they are in fact very small. In a healthy pair of adrenals, each gland is the size of a walnut. If we were supposed to be stressed all the time, wouldn't the organ be larger, like the heart?

Yet in the crazy lifestyle that we live today, we're under tremendous stress, operating almost constantly in a sympathetic dominant state, taxing our bodies, and creating a continual stress response. On autopsies of people who die of disease, it's been found that the adrenal glands were completely overused and had shrunk to the size of a peanut. Yet on autopsies of same-age people who died of trauma (like a car accident) but no disease, the adrenal glands were the size of a walnut. How in the world could peanut-size, shrunken glands support our crazy life? They can't. That's why we don't respond to stress well: We've worn out the stress response system, and the toll shows wherever we have a weak link in our chain.

As a medical student, Dr. Selye observed that patients suffering from different diseases often exhibited identical signs and symptoms. In his words, they were "stressed." The signs of severe adrenal stress include dizziness upon standing too quickly; having to wear sunglasses even on cloudy days; increased pulse rates; shorter, quicker breathing; and recurrent muscle tension.

He later discovered the general adaptation syndrome, a response of the body to demands placed upon it. Dr. Selye was the first to point out that stress induces hormonal autonomic responses. Over time, these hormonal changes, if excessive, can lead to physical manifestations. He was the first to identify that excess stress wears out the body and causes disease. His definition of stress was anything that activates a sympathetic nervous system response, whether it's chemical, physical, or emotional.

In a 1955 article in the medical journal *Science*, Dr. Selye showed how arthritis, stroke, and heart disease are all affected by stress-induced overworked adrenal glands. His research was conducted on mice, and he was able to demonstrate how changing their environment by adding recurring stress could alter them physically. One mouse was allowed to lead a normal mouse life in the laboratory. The other was worked hard by constantly being placed on a hamster wheel or by being thrown into water above its head, swimming to exhaustion. The result was that the adult relaxed mouse was twice the size of the stressed mouse. It had a beautiful coat, whereas the stressed mouse was half the size and looked wiry. It developed disease and died earlier.

Dr. Selye identified the stages of adrenal function. Normal adrenal response is referred to as *sympathetic dominance*. When the fight, flight, and fright response occurs day in and day out, our adrenals go into a state of adrenal fatigue, and their response is less thorough. When the fight, flight, or fright response continues, we go from adrenal fatigue to adrenal exhaustion, and it becomes difficult to elicit an adequate response. When the fight, flight, or fright response continues further, we go into a state of adrenal depletion and we are unable to respond. Now the stress we are being exposed to cannot be addressed or diffused by our stress hormones, and it hits our body full force. This means that when you have a stressful life and you've worn out your adrenal glands, another organ has to deal with each particular stress. For some people, the thyroid takes over, but then you start taxing your thyroid, especially if it is the weak link in your health chain. If you can no longer make adequate amounts of the adrenal hormones that deal with sugar intake, known as *glucocorticoids*, the blood sugar regulating system that has to pick up the slack is the pancreas, which responds to the stress by making more insulin. Over time, you develop insulin resistance. Then here comes diabetes, and you are on the autoimmune spectrum.

We are supposed to live in a state of parasympathetic dominance. Because of our lifestyle today, we are living in sympathetic dominance all the time. We're constantly on alert in everyday life, so much so that most people, especially those who have been diagnosed with autoimmune disease, have gone from adrenal fatigue to adrenal exhaustion to adrenal depletion. The result is that stress hits you much harder and more often. If you're feeling burned out, it's because you are. And so is your body's ability to be resilient. Without the mechanism to return to a parasympathetic dominant state, you become extremely vulnerable to developing any disease, depending on your weak link.

What organ controls the entire relationship of how our bodies respond to the stress of life? You might think from this discussion that it was the adrenal glands. Doctors used to believe that until just 5 years ago. Now we know that the microbiome is the central computer directing the microbiota-gut-brain (MGB) axis.[11] The microbiota sends chemical messengers to the brain along the spinal cord and through the bloodstream. These messages instruct the hypothalamus how to respond to perceived stress. The hypothalamus tells the pituitary glands which stressors are the priorities, which then sends messages telling the organs what hormones to produce.

Here's an example. It's April 14. You haven't done your taxes, and you have a sinking feeling in your stomach. You wake up in a sweat. You might notice that your pulse is up as you try to figure out a strategy to get the work done. Inside your body, a healthy microbiota begins taking charge. It sends a message to the hypothalamus, which sends a message to the pituitary glands, who send a message to the adrenals to produce more glucocorticoids. You need these because an increase in glucocorticoids increases your alertness so you have more brainpower to stay up late and finish filing your taxes. When you are in the midst of doing your taxes, you'll notice that sinking feeling is gone. Your microbiota is no longer sending a stress message because you are deep in the stress response and acting appropriately.

However, if your microbiota is out of balance, the anxiety you woke up with wouldn't go away and might even increase while you filled out the paperwork. You don't have the support in your gut needed to keep your brain calm. In fact, the severity of the stress response is 2.8-fold higher, producing stress hormones when you don't have the right microbiota.[12]

You can decrease intestinal permeability by lowering your stress levels. As we learned in Chapter 2, activation of the nervous system increases intestinal permeability.

Stress hormones weaken and damage the gut lining, leading to leaky gut. When you have intestinal permeability, the lipopolysaccharides from the gut breach the cell wall and get into general circulation, stimulating more immune cells, which in turn send a message back up to the brain, which creates more stress, activating the immune response and producing more inflammation. Intestinal permeability maintains the cycle, but the excessive stress in our lives will trigger intestinal permeability all by itself. Our bodies were designed to run as smoothly as a Rolls-Royce, but our lifestyle has them running like Ramblers.

Every doctor tells patients to reduce the stress in their lives. Realistically, we can't drop the stress in our lives overnight. We have kids, jobs, and a lifestyle that we're locked into. We can reduce the stress in our lives over time, if we have a plan to do it. However, how the body physically handles stress while we're in transition to a lower-stress life is where we can make an impact now. We can shore up the microbiome so that when stressful situations happen, we have more resilience to handle it better. If you can get your body healthier, your body will allow you to manage your stress more effectively.

For example, I've never been a great sleeper. On a typical night, I used to sleep about 5 hours. One of my primary concerns from a health perspective has been my sleep, because I know how critically important shut-eye is to cellular regeneration: You heal when you sleep, so if you don't sleep, you don't heal well. But once I balanced my microbiome, my sleep improved. I can now sleep 6 or 7 hours solidly, without making any other changes to my lifestyle. And because I'm better rested, my body heals quicker, and I can handle the daily stress of life much better.

THE MICROBIOME'S ROLE IN HARNESSING LPS

As we saw in Chapter 2, the microbiome protects us from lipopolysaccharides (LPS), which are detrimental to the health of the immune system. LPS are one of the most-studied and most-destructive aspects of an unhealthy microbiome. One of the main jobs of the microbiome is to keep LPS in check. Here's the problem with LPS and why they cause so much damage: When we lose the protective dominance of good bacteria in the microbiome (which almost all of us have lost), the amount of LPS produced is overwhelming to the body, and—as we learned in the last chapter—causes inflammation.

One of the essential features of a healthy microbiome is its production of *bacteriocidins*, enzymes that destroy unfriendly bacteria. With the development of an unhealthy microbiome due to unhealthy food choices or antibiotics, our protective capacity diminishes and LPS flourish. Now you have a mess in the gut, and the LPS penetrate the walls of the intestines, triggering the systemic inflammatory cascade. How can we prevent this? By reestablishing a healthy microbiome.

SUPPORTING A HEALTHY MICROBIOME

I was recently asked the following question during an interview: "What's the one thing you would do, more than anything else, if you were going to focus on being healthy?"

My recommendation is to focus on creating a healthier microbiome. All the little steps that are easy to implement will add up to having a robustly healthy microbiome. Nothing is more important to the function of your body. Nothing has more control. Nothing impacts more of your tissues and organs than the microbiota. It's the big kahuna.

Luckily, the microbiome can easily be rebalanced. In just a day or two of changing your diet, you can begin to change and reduce dysbiosis. First, avoid the foods you may be sensitive to. When you have food sensitivities, the immune system responds with an inflammatory cascade in the gut. Every forkful can have a detrimental effect on your microbiome, even if you don't feel bad as you eat it. The inflammatory cascade kills off the good bacteria, and pathogenic bacteria begin to prosper, creating an imbalanced environment in the gut. For example, in one study of celiac children, 39 percent had abnormal bacterial growth in their intestines, and many of these bacteria were never before identified in humans. When the offending gluten was removed for 2 years, the unknown bacteria disappeared for 81 percent of the children.[13] This shows that when you remove the foods you are reacting to—beginning with gluten, dairy, and sugar—you can positively affect your microbiome.

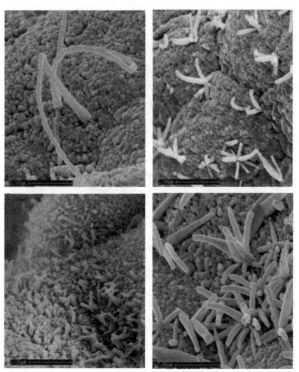

The rod-shaped bacteria in these photographs were previously unknown but often occur in more than one-third of children with celiac disease. Reprinted with permission from Macmillan Publishers Ltd: The American Journal of Gastroentology, 2004.

Fix #1: Foods That Support a Healthy Microbiome

My Transition Protocol includes better food selection, probiotics, and prebiotics to help restore a healthy microbiome. The foods that support the microbiome are grouped into four categories.

1. **Choose foods high in polyphenols—colorful, high-fiber fruits and vegetables.** Polyphenols are micronutrients found in the bright colors in fruits and vegetables and have an incredibly beneficial effect on the microbiome.[14] You may have heard of resveratrol, found in red wine, and the benefits of dark chocolate or green tea. It's the polyphenols that provide much of these foods' health benefits. Polyphenols occur within a diverse class of plants and are associated with strong-colored fruits (like berries) and vegetables (like red tomatoes). Fruits and vegetables that are high in polyphenols have the same dark color throughout. While eggplants have a nice, dark skin, the flesh is white, so it isn't a high polyphenol choice. A better choice would be dark, leafy greens like spinach or kale.

   The most exciting information about polyphenols is that studies have shown the interaction between polyphenols and the microbiome is bidirectional: Gut microbes affect the absorption of polyphenols, which then affects the growth of bacteria, which then affects a 75 percent reduction in cardiovascular disease.[15] In 2003, the *British Medical Journal* published a paper titled "A Strategy to Reduce Cardiovascular Disease by More Than 80%." The authors of the paper did a meta-analysis in which they pooled together benefits of separate drugs. Using this logic, they concluded that a "polypill" made up of a statin to reduce cholesterol, three blood pressure medications, a baby aspirin, and folic acid would reduce the risk of cardiovascular disease by more than 80 percent. This was published on the front page of most newspapers in the country. Interestingly enough, the authors had filed a patent for this polypill. Eight months later, a second paper appeared in the *British Medical Journal* titled "The Polymeal: A More Natural, Safer, and Probably Tastier (Than the Polypill) Strategy to Reduce Cardiovascular Disease by More Than 75%." Using the same logistical analysis, the researchers demonstrated that eating cold-water fish four times per week, as well as eating foods high in polyphenols like dark chocolate, garlic, almonds, a pound of vegetables, and red wine every day, reduces the risk of cardiovascular disease by 75 percent. The estimated life expectancy free of cardiovascular disease increased by 9 years for men and 8.9 years for women.[16]

In Chapter 7, you'll receive complete instructions on how to add polyphenols into your diet every day, including salads filled with greens and crunchy, colorful cruciferous vegetables. It is the insoluble fiber in these vegetables that the bacteria thrive on that promote being lean and healthy. Other foods high in polyphenols can be eaten every day, but in moderation, including fresh garlic, fresh raw almonds, and 70 percent cacao or higher dark chocolate. Cocoa has been shown to influence the microbiome toward a more health-promoting profile by increasing the relative abundance of good bacteria.[17] What's more, chocolate is thought to modify intestinal immune status, lowering the expression of IgA antibodies.[18]

GO AHEAD, EAT CHOCOLATE EVERY DAY

Eat a little dark chocolate every day to increase your intake of polyphenols and prebiotics. Take a square of the very best dark chocolate (at least 70 percent cacao) that you can get and put it on or under your tongue. Don't let it touch your teeth. Let it sit there without chewing, so that it slowly dissolves in your mouth. In this way, you saturate your taste buds to send the message "chocolate is here" to your brain via the oral thalamic tract that leads from the mouth right up to the brain. Chocolate stimulates the production of endorphins and enkephalins, which are 200 times more powerful than morphine in how they stimulate the feel-good sensors in your brain.

If you eat that one square of chocolate every day and let it melt in your mouth for about 2 minutes, you'll most likely feel very satisfied. If you want more, go ahead and have another piece. I've never ever, ever had a patient want more than two squares if they follow this method. This way, you can have dark chocolate every day and not gain weight or throw your blood sugar out of balance.

2. **Choose the right carbohydrates—avoid processed carbohydrates that feed bad bacteria:** chips, French fries, breads, white rice, cookies, crackers, desserts, and sugars. These foods put your body in a chronically hungry, metabolically damaged, fat-storing mode. Eating them can increase your risk of intestinal permeability and may alter the makeup of your microbiome, upsetting the balance between "friendly" and "unfriendly" bacteria.

However, eating good carbohydrates can actually reduce obesity by increasing beneficial bacteria. In 2006, microbiologist Liping Zhao, PhD, conducted an experiment on himself to replicate findings that showed a link between obesity and the microbiome in mice. At the time, Dr. Zhao was overweight and in poor health. He adopted a diet that included whole grains (brown rice) along with two traditional Chinese medicine foods: Chinese yams and bitter melon, both of which contain a particular type of indigestible carbohydrate (a prebiotic that encourages the development of one form of good bacteria, *Faecalibacterium prausnitzii*). He monitored his weight loss as well as his microbiome. Two years later, he had lost a total of 44 pounds by restoring his good bacteria.[19] In a 2016 study from the Department of Twin Research and Genetic Epidemiology at King's College London, it was found that the bacteria produced by eating these same foods (*Faecalibacterium*) is significantly associated with reduced frailty.[20] This is important, because frailty is a useful indicator of overall health deficit, describing a physiological loss of reserve capacity and reduced resistance to stress.

Carbohydrates containing artificial sweeteners promote unhealthy gut bacteria that cause obesity. In one study, the sugar substitute saccharin was shown to alter the function of 115 different pathways in the gut because of the microbiome controlling glucose tolerance, leading to obesity. The bacteria that aid in the digestion of saccharin turn the switch on to store energy as body fat and alter the gut microbiome.[21]

3. **Eat grass-fed red meat and healthy fats.** When you eat healthy fats, including the fats found in avocados, olive oil, coconut oil, nuts, fish, free-range poultry, and grass-fed beef, there is no evidence of lipid raft transcytosis (discussed in Chapter 2), which is responsible for moving LPS into the bloodstream. In Chapter 7, you'll learn more about choosing the best fats for this program.

4. **Eat one forkful of fermented foods every day.** A hundred years ago, people thought yogurt was healthy for you but were not exactly sure why. We now know that it is because of the fermentation of the bacteria in milk: Every time you eat yogurt, you get a dose of good bacteria. However, because so many people have a dairy sensitivity, and because the quality of most pasteurized yogurts found at the grocer is so poor and low in beneficial bacteria by the time it reaches your table, we are going to focus on eating fermented vegetables and drinks like kefir (a cultured/fermented milk), KeVita (a cultured/fermented coconut water), and kombucha (a fermented tea) to encourage the growth of good bacteria in your gut.

Fermented foods are those that grow bacteria in them or on them. They are some of the best detoxifying agents available. The beneficial bacteria in these foods are capable of drawing out a wide range of toxins and heavy metals. The ancient method of fermenting unlocks nutrients from food, breaks down some of the starches, and adds beneficial bacteria and enzymes to every bite. Fermented foods are a better choice than over-the-counter probiotic supplements. Not only do fermented foods provide a wider variety of beneficial bacteria, they also give you far more of them. For example, most probiotic supplements contain fewer than 10 billion colony-forming units (CFUs). But fermented vegetables can contain 10 trillion CFUs of bacteria. Literally, one serving of fermented foods is equal to an entire bottle of a high-potency probiotic. Every day, you need to eat just a little bit, such as one forkful of fermented foods like sauerkraut and kimchi, both made from cabbage. You can purchase fermented vegetables or follow the recipes in Chapter 10 to make your own. If you find that you have a little gas or bloating after eating fermented vegetables, it is a biomarker of dysbiosis (abnormal gut bacteria in high concentration). It doesn't mean the fermented foods are bad for you; it means your threshold for digesting them is very low. So reduce your dosage: Try a tablespoon of sauerkraut juice on your salad with your normal salad dressing so that the taste isn't so strong. Next week, try 2 tablespoons per day. This is an example of transitioning—you are taking an accurate evaluation of where your body is currently functioning and moving it in the direction of better functioning.

Fix #2: Probiotics

Probiotics is the term for the good bacteria in your gut. For a healthy microbiome, probiotics need to be the majority of all your gut bacteria. There are thousands of different types of probiotics, and each is defined by its genus (for example, *Lactobacillus*), by its species (such as *rhamnosus*), and by its strain designation (often a combination of letters or numbers). The concept of a bacterial "strain" is similar to the breed of a dog—all dogs are the same genus and species, but different breeds of dogs have different attributes, and different breeds are good for different tasks. You don't bring a Chihuahua to your door if you need a Rottweiler.

The use of probiotic supplements is still in its infancy. We really don't know exactly how to use them to create a healthier microbiome. We do know that they work to balance immune function and decrease inflammation by helping you maintain a healthy environment in the gut. They are available as nutritional supplements that increase beneficial bacteria in the gut and crowd out bad bacteria. They can also heal intestinal permeability. Different strains of even the same species of probiotics can vary in their specific bacteria.

Probiotics are most effective when they are combined with a high-fiber diet that features lots of vegetables every day (remember the Polymeal). Vegetable fiber is critical for creating butyrate, which, as we discussed earlier, is the fuel for the fastest-growing cells in the body: the inside lining of the intestines. This is a critical concept and the reason why I don't encourage fiber supplements, because I have never found a study where fiber supplements increase butyrate levels. The right fiber acts as a fertilizer that helps the probiotic grow and proliferate good bacteria in your microbiome. And because probiotics interact with the digestive system, each strain performs differently depending on your gut's unique environment. This means that one type of probiotic doesn't work the same for everybody. To find the supplement that will work best for you, choose a broad-spectrum, high-potency probiotic. "Broad spectrum" means that it contains more than one strain of probiotics. You might try different formulations to find the one that works best for you. Your test results that we'll investigate in Chapter 5 will guide your selection based on your own deficits.

When purchasing probiotics, follow the guidance of the International Scientific Association for Probiotics and Prebiotics. They recommend

SAMANTHA'S STORY, PART 3

My patient Samantha's microbiome was directly affected by the antibiotics and other drugs she was given to treat her acne as a teenager. Later, during her lupus treatments, the steroids and chemotherapy medications pushed her microbiome over the edge. By the time I met her, her stress levels were high, which contributed to the problem as well. Aside from the damage caused by her food sensitivities, she suffered from constant bloating, which was a direct result of the gut imbalance. Even though she wasn't really overweight, she told me that she always felt heavy, almost dense, but just assumed that feeling was normal.

I started Samantha on a simple plan of incorporating fermented foods into her diet. I explained that she doesn't need a whole lot of them, just a little bit every day. Everyone finds the right balance. With fermented foods, too much is too much, and too little is not helpful at all. I usually start adults at 1 tablespoon per day and have them rotate the fermented food choices: one day sauerkraut, one day kimchi, one day miso soup, etc.

Samantha was able to calibrate what she needed and responded to the fermented foods very positively. When I asked her how she felt, she told me, "I'm eating a half cup of sauerkraut every day with my lunch. It's been very helpful and nourishing, and it's caused a detox on some level. And it's allowed me to slowly add back foods into my diet that I used to avoid. Now that my gut is more balanced, I can eat certain fruits again without pain or gas. And I don't have bloating anymore. My friends have noticed that I've lost some of my curves, but I realize that was just bloat. I even feel lighter."

I also recommended that Samantha take prebiotics, which would work in concert with the fermented foods. Prebiotics and probiotics help to create an alkaline environment in the gut that reduces inflammation.

that you look for supplements that list the following information on their packaging:

- Strain
- CFUs (colony forming units). How many live microorganisms are in each serving? When does the product expire? Packaging should ensure an effective level of live bacteria through the "best by" or expiration date.
- Suggested serving size
- Health benefits
- Proper storage conditions
- Corporate contact information

Fix #3: Prebiotics

Even the best of dietary intentions can cause problems. A gluten-free diet may actually contribute to dysbiosis. When you follow a gluten-free diet, you remove many of the carbohydrates necessary to feed good bacteria. Gluten-free foods are not known to contain healthy prebiotics. You are in effect starving your own bacteria unless you replace the gluten with prebiotics.

Prebiotics are food components that cannot be digested by the body but are consumed by the beneficial bacteria to help them function. Chocolate or cocoa is considered a prebiotic that is also rich in polyphenols.[22]

NEXT STEPS

Now that you understand the different factors that push on your immune system, it's time to see what health issues you may be dealing with, even if they are on the very beginning of the autoimmune spectrum. The next chapter features two quizzes—but don't worry, they're fun. Our first goal is to identify what is currently occurring in your body, and the earlier we can do this, the better. Then you can learn to arrest the development of damage *before* you have a diagnosable disease. The tests in Chapter 4 are critical for understanding how you will manifest optimum healing.

DETERMINING YOUR PLACE
ON THE AUTOIMMUNE SPECTRUM

The first step to determining if you are already on the autoimmune spectrum—and if you are creating a leaky gut—is to assess your current health. The type of checkup I subscribe to is one based on functional medicine. This is important to know because not all health assessments are equal.

I believe the functional medicine approach to health care is the most comprehensive way of addressing health complaints. Functional medicine investigates the underlying causes of disease by using a systems-oriented approach. This means we evaluate every system of your body to see if it's contributing to your health problem. To do this, we work together, creating a holistic partnership between the patient and the practitioner. In this way, we can treat both the symptoms and the causes of disease. For example, my role on the faculty of the Institute of Functional Medicine is to teach about intestinal permeability (the leaky gut)—where it comes from, what triggers it, and how to address it.

Functional medicine practitioners range from acupuncturists to cardiologists, chiropractors to psychologists, nutritionists to endocrinologists. No matter what your health-care providers' initial area of expertise is, they can become trained in functional medicine. This training teaches them to listen to their patient's health and family histories and look for the interplay among genetic, environmental, and lifestyle factors that could initiate health complaints and the development of complex chronic disease. By shifting the traditional disease-centered focus (treating the symptoms of the disease) to a more whole patient-centered approach, functional medicine addresses the whole person, not just an isolated set of symptoms.

I compare the difference between functional medicine and traditional medicine to taking a flight on an airplane. When you are initially seated on the plane, you may look out the window. All you can see is the plane at the gate next to you, and maybe the baggage handlers throwing the bags on the conveyor belt. You have a limited view; you can't see beyond what is right in front of you. Your limited view represents traditional medicine—the experts and specialists who are board certified in their area of expertise, such as cardiology, pediatrics, internal medicine, psychiatry, etc. These doctors view their world, and their field, by what's in front of them.

But as the plane pushes back from the gate and you're looking out the window, now you can see the runway. Perhaps it's the fall and the leaves on the trees just past the runway are turning colors. As the plane takes off, you notice that there is an entire forest beyond the airport that you couldn't see before. Oh look, there's a lake, and a skyline in the distance. As the plane climbs into the sky, your view keeps expanding and you see a bigger picture. Finally, you're at cruising altitude and you have what I call the 30,000-foot view. Now you can observe the lay of the land. You have a big picture of what's there in front of you. That's functional medicine: addressing the whole person by seeing the 30,000-foot view of the patient's body's current function, or lack of, and where the problems might have originated.

Functional medicine allows us to view autoimmunity in a more comprehensive way than traditional medicine does. The same symptoms might derive from many different sources. For instance, intestinal permeability may be initiated by chronic constipation, but why? In some people, constipation may be caused by a simple and obvious source, such as food sensitivity. For others, there might be physical or emotional abuse in their past, producing a constant flood of stress hormones that's causing the gut to be so tight and tense that they are chronically constipated. Yet for others, a childhood history of antibiotic use for recurrent ear infections may have created a poor microbiome that is butyrate deficient, producing a lack of movement in the colon. If we were to treat the constipation with laxatives, which helps in the short term, the underlying mechanism causing the constipation would continue and likely produce worse symptoms in the gut over time.

On the other end of the autoimmune spectrum are diseases, which can also be viewed from a functional medicine approach. If you have been diagnosed with an autoimmune thyroid disease, such as Hashimoto's thyroiditis, a traditional medicine approach may well include a prescription for thyroid hormones to help reduce the symptoms of a poorly functioning thyroid. There is no question that extra hormones are likely of value to help with your symptoms, but they usually do not address what is causing the thyroid dysfunction in the first place.

The functional medicine platform includes addressing your health from a lifestyle perspective, including what happened to you up to this point that may have set you up for a thyroid problem and may be a continual fuel keeping the thyroid not working up to par. By investigating the reasons behind your thyroid issues, we might unearth several different causes of the dysfunction, each of which can be addressed.

- A sensitivity to gluten. It has been found that 43 percent of people diagnosed with Hashimoto's thyroid autoimmune disease also have a gluten sensitivity.[1] Eating foods with gluten may be the gasoline on the fire that fuels this autoimmune disease. Once you remove gluten from your diet, your thyroid function may return, without the need for additional hormone therapy.

- A sensitivity to chlorine (even trace amounts found in drinking water) not only impacts thyroid function dramatically after years of chlorine accumulation[2] but also affects the developing brain in utero, during infancy, and in the toddler years.[3] If you discover this sensitivity, a few small lifestyle adjustments may help your thyroid work much better, including something as simple as installing one chlorine filter for your drinking water and another for the showerhead. During a hot shower, we inhale the steam, and the chlorine goes right through our lungs into our bloodstream.

- Exposure to small amounts of iodine 131 from nuclear fallout radiation. There have been 1,054 nuclear tests conducted in the United States (including 216 atmospheric, underwater, and space

REALITY CHECK!

When I ask any of my patients how they feel, the majority say, "I'm fine." Then I ask, "How's your energy?" and they still say, "Fine." Then I ask my favorite question:

"On a scale of 1 to 10, 10 is the amount of energy you think you should have, and 5 is half as much. Do you know your number? But wait, take your willpower out of the equation. What's your number now?"

The look on their faces when they remove their willpower from the equation is startling. The smiles disappear, because the reality check is that they are usually a 5 or less. And that's not great. Having half the energy you think you should have to live your lifestyle is a reality check. It sets you up for the autoimmune spectrum.

So when you're filling out this chapter's quizzes, don't settle for "fine."

tests), which have inadvertently put many US citizens born after 1946 at high risk of developing Hashimoto's thyroiditis and eventual thyroid cancer.[4] Other radiation exposures have occurred at Chernobyl, in the former Soviet Union, and more recently in Fukushima, Japan. Iodine 131 (nuclear fallout) in small amounts carried on atmospheric currents is one of the environmental triggers—in the triad of genetics, exposures, and leaky gut—that can instigate the development of autoimmune thyroid disease. If this was the cause of your problem, you would benefit from a detoxification program to reduce the elevated iodine levels in your body.

Knowing the causes of various diseases can be overwhelming at times. That's why it's so important to have a big-picture overview as a patient and to work with a functional medicine practitioner as part of your health-care team, who can help you dial in the specific areas to investigate. You have to first determine where your problems are coming from in order to resolve them completely, instead of just alleviating symptoms temporarily.

ARE YOU READY FOR CHANGE?

I know that change is not easy, but it also is not impossible. The lifestyle changes in the Transition Protocol take commitment and patience. We all want to be healthier, and we know that we have to do something in order to make these changes. You probably bought this book (thank you!) because something in your life is not working. Just remember that change is an ongoing process.

More than 20 years ago, alcoholism researchers Carlo C. DiClemente, PhD, and James O. Prochaska, PhD, introduced a model to help professionals understand their clients with addiction problems and motivate them to change. Their model is based not on abstract theories but on personal observations of how people went about modifying lifestyle behaviors, specifically for smoking, overeating, and drinking. Functional medicine practitioners use this model, as it is quite relevant to making lifestyle changes that can enhance health.

In their book *Changing for Good,* Drs. DiClemente and Prochaska and John C. Norcross, PhD, described what they learned when they studied more than 1,000 people who were able to positively and permanently alter their lives without psychotherapy. They found that change does not depend on luck or willpower. Instead, it is a process that can be successfully managed by anyone who understands how it works. Once you determine which stage of change you're in, you can create a climate where positive change can occur, maintain motivation, turn setbacks into progress, and make your new beneficial habits a permanent part of your life.

The five stages of change are:

- **Precontemplation:** Individuals in this stage are not even thinking about changing their behaviors. They haven't seen that their lifestyle is a problem affecting their health.
- **Contemplation:** Individuals in this stage are willing to consider the possibility that they have a health problem, and the possibility offers hope for change. However, in this stage, people are often highly ambivalent. They are on the fence. What lets me know if someone in this stage will ultimately be successful is if he or she shows skepticism ("I don't believe this, but I'm willing to look at more information") rather than cynicism ("I don't

believe; it's untrue"). Contemplation is moving in the right direction toward change, but it is not a commitment.

- **Determination:** Individuals in this stage will make a serious attempt to improve their lifestyle behaviors in the near future. They are ready and committed to action because they have garnered enough information (from reading this book and taking the quizzes in this chapter) and are now convinced that behavioral change may improve their health.

- **Action:** Individuals in this stage put their plan into action, making changes to their diet through the Transition Protocol. In a few weeks, they start to see results, and nothing succeeds like success. A person who has implemented our plan begins to see it work and experiences a positive change in health.

- **Maintenance:** I tell my patients all the time that humans are the only species on the planet that finds something that works and then stops doing it. Change requires building a new pattern of behavior over time and sticking to it. It's common that when you're feeling great, you will be tempted to have a piece of birthday cake or a blueberry muffin, even though it's not gluten-free. However, after you eat it, I will bet that you won't feel so great anymore, and the value of maintenance will become obvious. It's human nature to blow it and go back to bad habits or old treats. Then we feel lousy, get back on track, and feel better. As you fall down and pick yourself back up again and again, the temptation of the birthday cake ("I'll just have a bite") will dissipate. After 6 months of maintaining your new lifestyle choices, the researchers found that old lifestyle habits no longer pose a significant danger or threat.

THE READY-TO-CHANGE QUIZ

Taking the Ready-to-Change Quiz (opposite) will help determine if you are truly to ready to start this program. I've found that the most successful people come to this point in the book at the determination stage: They're ready and excited, but they need guidance. This quiz will allow you to gauge your desire, receptivity, and commitment to improve your health.

We all would like to assume that we'll do whatever it takes to be healthy, but in reality, that's usually not the case. You may have the desire to be healthier but are stuck in the contemplation stage. To be successful in this program, your desires need to align with your determination. If you can answer these questions positively, you know that you are ready to make a change. If your answers reveal an unwillingness, you need to explore what beliefs are holding you back.

For many of my patients, what pushes them off the fence and into the program is seeing that they are currently on the autoimmune spectrum. It was an "OMG" moment for me when I discovered I had three different elevated antibodies in my brain that had the potential of causing multiple sclerosis, brain shrinking (atrophy), and a loss of balance as I aged (cerebellar degeneration).

Please answer all questions by circling the response that comes closest to how you feel right now. Then you can see what your most common reaction is to these best practices for enhancing health.

READY-TO-CHANGE QUIZ

To improve your health, how willing are you to do the following?

Significantly modify your diet

___ Extremely willing
___ Somewhat willing
___ Neutral
___ Somewhat unwilling
___ Not at all willing

Take nutritional supplements each day

___ Extremely willing
___ Somewhat willing
___ Neutral
___ Somewhat unwilling
___ Not at all willing

Keep a record of everything you eat each day

___ Extremely willing
___ Somewhat willing
___ Neutral
___ Somewhat unwilling
___ Not at all willing

Modify your lifestyle—things such as work demands

___ Extremely willing
___ Somewhat willing
___ Neutral
___ Somewhat unwilling
___ Not at all willing

Improve sleep habits

___ Extremely willing
___ Somewhat willing
___ Neutral
___ Somewhat unwilling
___ Not at all willing

Practice a relaxation technique

___ Extremely willing
___ Somewhat willing
___ Neutral
___ Somewhat unwilling
___ Not at all willing

Engage in regular exercise

___ Extremely willing
___ Somewhat willing
___ Neutral
___ Somewhat unwilling
___ Not at all willing

How confident are you about your ability to organize and follow through on the recommended health-related activities?

___ Extremely willing
___ Somewhat willing
___ Neutral
___ Somewhat unwilling
___ Not at all willing

How supportive are the key people in your life to your making these changes?

___ Extremely willing
___ Somewhat willing
___ Neutral
___ Somewhat unwilling
___ Not at all willing

ARE YOU ON THE AUTOIMMUNE SPECTRUM?

Autoimmunity affects people differently, depending on where the weak link in your chain is. There are more than 300 disorders associated with autoimmunity (see Chapter 1), and yet if you are on the earlier end of the autoimmune spectrum, you may not have any symptoms yet. The quiz on page 100 highlights the most common symptoms of inflammation, which triggers the autoimmune cascade. In this quiz, you will decipher how you feel. It's the subtle changes in your health that you need to account for, because they are the warning flags of greater health problems. Remember, you may be full force on the autoimmune spectrum, even if your symptoms are minor. People do not "feel" Alzheimer's in the earlier 20-plus years of its development.

My friend Alex sent me this e-mail recently that perfectly sums up the precontemplation stage and the importance of recognizing the subtle indicators of internal imbalances.

> *Tom, for the last 3 weeks, I began to notice something slowing me down. Then it shifted to having chest pains. In my yearly physical, we speculated on whether my health problems were gastrointestinal or a heart problem. So my doctor checked my cholesterol and triglycerides, and they were normal. [FYI, 50 percent of people who have a fatal heart attack do not have high cholesterol—why are traditional doctors only using cholesterol as the biomarker of high risk for heart disease?]*

Two weeks ago, when I was in Las Vegas with my kids, I noticed that I labored from the hotel to the car. Gradually, the pain started setting in when I was carrying gear, and I had to sit down for a few minutes before moving on. During the weekend, I made sure that I moved in shorter movements and sat down as much as possible. On leaving the weekend, I experienced strong chest pain in carrying out my gear. I had to sit for a spell.

I played golf last Monday, all the while feeling a chest pain, but I labored through it and actually played well. It must be some gut problem, I rationalized. But then this Sunday night I felt a little off. By 3:30 a.m. on Tuesday, I woke with severe chest pain. I called my internist, who told me to get to the hospital as quickly as possible. I got in my car and drove furiously through red lights to the hospital in about 5 minutes, parked the car at the ER, and pressed for immediate attention.

They got me in to see the ER attending, who gave me a nitroglycerin tab that gradually took the pain away. Then it came back again and I thought, "What is going on?" The awareness came forth that I had been denying a heart problem. "I could not be having a heart problem. I am above it." Then they put me on a blood thinner, another drug, and got me into a hospital room. They scheduled me for an angiogram. Being aware that my heart was wanting to jump out of my body, I became quite impatient. Then I just started praying, surrendering to spirit, and saying my spirit's blessing over and over. When they rolled me into the operating room, I heard Andrea Bocelli playing in the background. WTF! Somehow I totally surrendered that if I died and that was meant to be, so be it.

After an hour and my being awake for the whole procedure, they told me that they had discovered a dominant artery that was 99.9 percent blocked. That might have explained why for the last 48 hours, just moving from room to room was difficult. They inserted a stent through an angioplasty procedure to open the artery. For the next hour or so afterward, I could feel my heart and wondered, "Did they do it right?"

A short time later, I started to feel the blood flowing again. After being discharged and home by 5:00 p.m., I am feeling healthier, and the blood is opening up the tight places in my body.

So it was a hair short of a heart attack. They called it a cardiac event. I will be on a series of drugs, some supposedly as long as I live. The likelihood is *that I will be healthier than recently as when I just became used to slowing down and attributed it to "old age."*

I now need to reassess my health life. Be grateful for what I have. But it's a wake-up call, as if I usually need them in my life. I keep thinking how often I thought you were an asshole, and all the time you were trying to save my life.

So what was the message I was trying to give Alex? I was trying to teach him about the subtle messages the body sends when you are on the autoimmune spectrum, but since he was in the cynic stage of pre-contemplation, he refused to listen to me or to his body. Had he taken these simple quizzes before, and then followed up with the right testing to confirm these findings, he would have discovered the inflammation pulling on the weak link of his chain, his heart blood vessels.

The following comprehensive and accessible quiz will show you where your weak link is and where you fall on the autoimmune spectrum. This quiz comes from the Institute for Functional Medicine. This is the same quiz I use with my patients. Answer these questions to the best of your ability. Think about how you have been feeling over the previous month. Rate each of the following symptoms based on how you feel most days, using the following scale:

> 0 Never or almost never have the symptom
> 1 Occasionally have it, effect is not severe
> 2 Occasionally have it, effect is severe
> 3 Frequently have it, effect is not severe
> 4 Frequently have it, effect is severe

MEDICAL SYMPTOMS QUIZ

HEAD

___ Headaches
___ Faintness
___ Dizziness
___ Insomnia

___ **Total**

EYES

___ Watery or itchy eyes
___ Swollen, reddened, or sticky eyelids
___ Bags or dark circles under eyes
___ Blurred or tunnel vision (does not include near- or farsightedness)

___ **Total**

EARS

___ Itchy ears
___ Earaches, ear infections
___ Drainage from ear
___ Ringing in ears, hearing loss

___ **Total**

NOSE

___ Stuffy nose
___ Sinus problems
___ Hay fever
___ Sneezing attacks
___ Excessive mucus formation

___ **Total**

MOUTH/THROAT

___ Chronic coughing
___ Gagging, frequent need to clear throat
___ Sore throat, hoarseness, loss of voice
___ Swollen or discolored tongue, gums, lips
___ Canker sores

___ **Total**

SKIN

___ Acne
___ Hives, dry skin
___ Hair loss
___ Flushing, hot flashes
___ Excessive sweating

___ **Total**

HEART

___ Irregular or skipped heartbeat
___ Rapid or pounding heartbeat
___ Chest pain

___ **Total**

LUNGS

___ Chest congestion
___ Asthma, bronchitis
___ Shortness of breath
___ Difficulty breathing

___ **Total**

DIGESTIVE TRACT

___ Nausea, vomiting
___ Diarrhea
___ Constipation
___ Bloated feeling
___ Belching, passing gas
___ Heartburn
___ Intestinal/stomach pain

___ **Total**

JOINTS/MUSCLES

___ Pain or aches in joints
___ Arthritis
___ Stiffness or limitation of movement
___ Pain or aches in muscles
___ Feeling of weakness or tiredness

___ **Total**

WEIGHT

___ Binge eating/drinking
___ Craving certain foods
___ Excessive weight
___ Compulsive eating
___ Water retention
___ Underweight

___ **Total**

ENERGY/ACTIVITY

___ Fatigue/sluggishness
___ Apathy/lethargy
___ Hyperactivity
___ Restlessness

___ **Total**

MIND

___ Poor memory
___ Confusion/poor comprehension
___ Poor concentration
___ Poor physical coordination
___ Difficulty in making decisions
___ Stuttering or stammering
___ Slurred speech
___ Learning disabilities

___ **Total**

EMOTIONS

___ Mood swings
___ Anxiety, fear, nervousness
___ Anger, irritability, aggressiveness
___ Depression

___ **Total**

OTHER

___ Frequent illness
___ Frequent or urgent urination
___ Genital itch or discharge

___ **Total**

___ **Grand Total**

REVIEW YOUR RESULTS

Add up your score in each category, and then add up those scores for a grand total. A grand total score of less than 10 is optimal. A score of more than 40 suggests the presence of significant inflammation pulling on your chain. The category with the highest score is likely the weak link in your chain.

CREATING YOUR TIMELINE

A functional medicine checkup includes every detail about your health, starting with your birth history; health in infancy, childhood, and young adulthood; vaccinations; fevers; antibiotic use; and more. It includes everything and anything that has happened that may have contributed to the "you" of today. When you're looking at how to stop the disease mechanism that is occurring in your body, it just makes sense that what has happened to you up to now may be critical information for crafting a unique and ideal game plan to reverse the autoimmune spectrum.

For every patient I treat, I create a timeline so we can easily visualize the development of the imbalance eventually causing the symptoms they now have. Many times an adult will come into my office with the symptoms of autoimmune disease, and we can trace the first symptoms back to when they were very young. Understanding your timeline allows you to grasp how far along you are on the autoimmune spectrum, because you will see how the earliest symptoms have progressed over time. It's usually a jaw-dropping experience when patients realize how it is all connected. Their current health symptoms began many years earlier.

In my office, the work begins as patients fill out a 26-page questionnaire after they take the Medical Symptoms Quiz, starting on page 100. The questions not only cover their own lifelong medical history but also their families', as genetics are critical to understand. Patients list their diet, relationships, and emotional state from a current and historical perspective. Then I take the data from the questionnaire and create a timeline: a linear document. When my patients see how their health events lay out on the timeline, they understand how their inflammatory symptoms have developed over time as well as how the symptoms are interconnected with one another. Showing them this document is one of the best ways to empower patients, as they recognize that healing is possible if they commit to making the lifestyle changes we'll discuss in the Transition Protocol.

My friends at LivingMatrix have created a mechanism for you. This free resource is revolutionary, as it has never been done before. You can create a completely comprehensive timeline and then find a functional medicine practitioner who understands how to work with you and your timeline. Visit LivingMatrix.com/TheAutoImmuneFix for more information to create a personalized timeline for each member of your family, and theDr.com to find a functional medicine practitioner.

You can also use the following chart to create your timeline. First, plug in the symptoms you have identified from the previous Medical Symptoms Quiz. See if you can determine when the symptoms started and how they have changed over time. Then dial down to the details of any chronic or recurring symptoms, or the minor pains that are more of an annoyance at this stage of your life. Your answers from the quiz above should point you toward areas of your health to explore. Really strive to determine when the first, most subtle changes to your health occurred.

Then think back to your youth and record on your timeline each major or minor physical or emotional health upset. Include what you did at the time to address each event. You can ask your parents or relatives if they have any information about your mother's pregnancy and delivery. The major events will quickly come to mind, like ear infections, repeated bouts of strep throat, or having your tonsils removed.

MY TIMELINE

Copy this chart into a journal if you need more space.

Age	Key Event	Treatment and Outcome

Then transfer this information onto a linear graph, using the following guide:

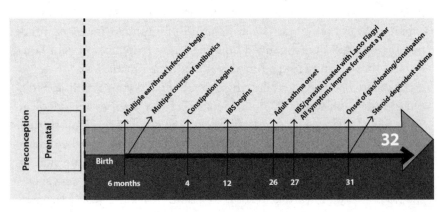

Reprinted with permission from Lisa Klancher K2Studios, LLC.

DIAGNOSING CELIAC DISEASE VS. NON-CELIAC GLUTEN (WHEAT) SENSITIVITY

My personal expertise comes through a thorough understanding of how gluten is a primary trigger of inflammation, which activates the genes for intestinal permeability, and the development of the autoimmune spectrum. As I showed in Chapter 3, important studies published in just the last 2 years clearly demonstrate that all people have a problem digesting the toxic gluten peptides from wheat, rye, and barley, whether or not they have symptoms when they eat it. We mistakenly believe that if we don't "feel" bad when we eat something, we do not have a problem with that food. We do not associate the headache we woke up with this morning—or our high blood pressure or our brain fog or lack of ability to think in school—with the food we ate yesterday. We just do not make that type of association. But it's important to realize that food sensitivity symptoms may not be obvious right after we eat the food. And those symptoms may not occur in our gut. They could show up anywhere in the body.

The typical diagnosis of celiac disease can take up to 11 years on average from the first presentation of symptoms—because the symptoms can be so mild or assigned to other causes. Worse, many people remain undiagnosed for their entire lives. Until the recent past, the only way to make a complete celiac diagnosis was to perform an endoscopy with a biopsy showing this autoimmune insult. Now we have much more sensitive blood tests than ever before, which we'll talk about in the next chapter.

The classifications of an endoscopy report are Marsh I, Marsh II, Marsh III (a, b, and c).

- Marsh I is labeled when you have increased inflammation. The shags of your microvilli are still there, but your intestines are full of inflammation, and there are lots of cytokines inside the shags.
- Marsh II is labeled when the shags are starting to wear down and the base membrane is swelling up.
- Marsh III is labeled when the shags have worn completely and you are left with flat Berber carpet instead of shag carpeting: total villous atrophy. Within Marsh III there are three stages: (A) partial villous atrophy, (B) subtotal villous atrophy, and (C) total villous atrophy.

Many other people can have a gluten-related disorder, with symptoms that present just like celiac disease, but an endoscopy does not show any damage. In 2009, a Swedish research team published the largest study ever on celiac disease and mortality in the *Journal of the American Medical Association*. The researchers looked at more than 350,000 biopsy reports and found 39,000 people with a diagnosis of celiac disease defined by total villous atrophy. They also found another 3,700 individuals who had an increase in their blood markers for celiac disease but no villous atrophy. The antibodies were elevated, but they did not have a positive biopsy. Then they found another cohort of 13,000 people who did not have positive bloodwork nor positive endoscopy but who had increased inflammation in the intestines.

All of these people were followed for 25-plus years. The researchers found that those who had been positively diagnosed with celiac disease—regardless of whether they were following a gluten-free diet—had a 39 percent increased likelihood of early death compared to someone who did not have celiac disease. Those who had positive bloodwork but negative endoscopy had a 35 percent increased chance of early death. So does it really matter if a celiac patient has total villous atrophy or just positive bloodwork with no villous atrophy? No, it doesn't matter if you are looking at the increased risk of early death. The percentages are almost the same. More important, those who had inflammation alone—meaning their bloodwork was negative, and their endoscopy was negative—had a 72 percent increased risk of early mortality.[5] Almost double. This is a critical concept that very few doctors know.

So many doctors have told their patients that if their endoscopy comes back normal (no villous atrophy), then it's fine to eat wheat. Yet the largest study ever done is saying that even if the endoscopy comes back normal and your shags are not worn down but you have positive bloodwork, you have a 35 percent increased risk of early mortality. This is why we must take positive bloodwork seriously, with or without villous atrophy.

But why double the risk of an early death without positive endoscopy or bloodwork? The reason is that very few doctors test for inflammation in the intestines—and thus the fire continues to roar, causing intestinal permeability that opens the floodgates for systemic inflammation. Wherever the weak link is in your chain, that's where the damage begins to accrue. If it's your brain, you can end up with dementia or Alzheimer's disease. If it's your heart, your future may include myocarditis or congestive heart failure or, like my friend Alex, arteriosclerosis. Your kidneys? Nephritis or recurrent bladder infections.

At what point should you consider taking action and trying a gluten-free diet? If we review the steps that lead to inflammation, it's clear to my mind that the answer is now.

THE AT-HOME TRIAL: COMMON SYMPTOMS OF A GLUTEN-RELATED DISORDER (WITH OR WITHOUT CELIAC DISEASE)

Talk with your doctor about comprehensive testing for celiac disease or a gluten-related disorder if you have, or had during your lifetime, any of the following symptoms (and add them to your timeline):

- Anemia (iron-deficiency) that does not respond to iron therapy
- Bone density issues ranging from osteopenia (mild) to osteoporosis (severe)
- Chronic anxiety or depression
- Chronic diarrhea or constipation
- Chronic fatigue
- Delayed puberty
- Failure to thrive or short stature
- Liver and biliary tract disorders (transaminitis, fatty liver, primary sclerosing cholangitis, etc.)
- Pain in the joints
- Pale, foul-smelling stool
- Pale sores inside the mouth
- Peripheral neuropathy
- Recurring abdominal bloating and pain

- Skin rash identified as dermatitis herpetiformis (DH)
- Tingling numbness in the legs
- Tooth discoloration or loss of enamel
- Unexplained infertility, recurrent miscarriage
- Unexplained weight loss
- Vomiting

If you have a disproportionally large forehead, it's another sign that you need to get tested for celiac disease. Studies show that 86 percent of celiac adults have an enlarged forehead.[6] An enlarged forehead is more of an indicator of celiac disease than any of the above common symptoms. Here's how researchers express the importance of it.

> The cranial facial morphology of patients with celiac disease reveals an altered pattern of cranial facial growth. This alteration is a clinical sign that should be included amongst the outside-of-the-intestinal manifestations of celiac disease. It has a frequency comparable to other signs and symptoms such as anemia, short stature, and is a better predictor of celiac than other signs such as recurrent aphthous stomatitis [cold sores in the corner of the mouth], recurrent miscarriages, and dental enamel hypoplasia.[7]

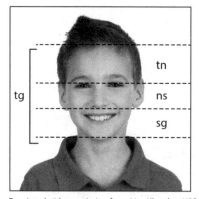 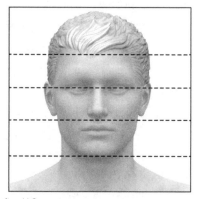

Reprinted with permission from Lisa Klancher K2Studios, LLC.

The ideal proportions of the human face are divided into three equal parts (see the illustration above, right). The forehead should make up the top one-third of the face. But in the photograph of the boy on the left, you can clearly see that his forehead, measured from the top of his eyes to his hairline, is larger than the other two sections of his face.

This is me (below). As you can see, I have a large forehead. A large forehead can be measured simply: All you need is a soft tape measure. Take a photograph of your own face, and then measure the distance between your chin and the base of your nose, your nose to the top of your eyes, and the top of your eyes to your hairline. You may find that, like I do, you have a large forehead.

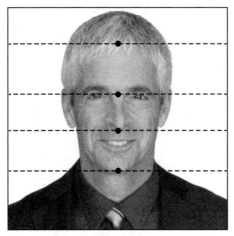

Reprinted with permission from Lisa Klancher K2Studios, LLC.

THE NEXT STEP

Once you see where you currently sit on the autoimmune spectrum, the blood tests listed in the next chapter will confirm your findings. Then start the Transition Protocol. After the first 3 weeks, you can retake the quiz. For the vast majority of my patients, they realize they're feeling so much better. If you are still not feeling as good as you should, continue to Transition Phase 2, and then take the quiz again when you are done. By this time, you should be seeing real improvements and be able to pinpoint which foods are making you feel forgetful, sick, fat, or tired.

One of my mottoes is "Base hits win the ball game." The prescription for addressing any symptom or condition on the autoimmune spectrum is not instant home runs or quick fixes. Instead, it's the daily wins of making the right food selections and caring for your body that will help you reverse autoimmunity. But you'll never know when to hit the ball if you don't look for the source of your health problems. That's the job of this book, to open up a new world of questions so you can answer the question "Where are my health problems coming from?" This paradigm is a whole new way of looking at health care beyond the "give me something for the symptoms."

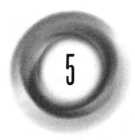

THE SCIENCE OF PREDICTIVE AUTOIMMUNITY

In the last chapter, you learned how to identify if you currently have symptoms on the autoimmune spectrum. But what if you could find out if your health was being affected before there was enough tissue damage to produce a single symptom? That's the science of predictive autoimmunity. In this chapter, you will learn how to test for all of the different factors that influence the immune system's production of antibodies to your own tissue: autoimmunity.

I'm a firm believer in identifying "what's brewing" in your body as early as possible. Knowledge is power, especially if you couple that knowledge with action. Science has moved forward to the point where we can identify an autoimmune spectrum long before it causes noticeable symptoms. When we can pinpoint which imbalances are occurring in our bodies, whether or not we currently experience symptoms, it gives us a window of opportunity to make informed decisions: "What do I do? Can I stop this from progressing? Can it be reversed?" This is why the world of predictive autoimmunity is of such value.

According to Professor Yehuda Shoenfeld, MD, one of the world's leading medical experts in autoimmunity, autoimmune diseases have incubation periods that range from as little as a few years to as long as 40 years. That's how long it may take before a person has enough tissue damage that would generate strong enough symptoms that warrant a trip to the doctor, and usually it takes multiple doctor visits before receiving an accurate diagnosis. For example, it takes an average of 11 years of suffering and visits to five different health-care practitioners before you get the right diagnosis of celiac disease.

Autoimmune diseases can be identified by testing properly for elevated levels of autoantibodies—the antibodies to your own tissue—that can tell doctors when a certain disease is "brewing," sometimes years before there is enough tissue damage to produce symptoms. I like to think of these autoantibody levels as messengers from the future. The groundbreaking 2003 research of Melissa Arbuckle, MD, PhD, which I introduced in Chapter 1, showed that autoantibodies are typically present many years before the diagnosis of autoimmune diseases like lupus. Furthermore, when these autoantibodies appear, they tend to follow a predictable course, with a progressive accumulation of specific autoantibodies before the onset of the disease, even while patients are still asymptomatic.[1] Her graphs that we reprinted in Chapter 1 tell the story: The antibodies for lupus were present years before the onset of disease.

Antibody levels of any type are also referred to as *biomarkers* because they measure body function. Doctors already use biomarkers to predict a host of illnesses. For instance, a biomarker of inflammation (hs-CRP) is a more accurate predictor of heart disease than having high cholesterol. These tests confirm why we know that you don't wake up with heart disease or Alzheimer's: The biomarkers are there years before the disease shows up.

Biomarker testing gives us a *positive predictive value* (PPV) when we are looking for the earliest stages of autoimmune disease. The biomarkers of predictive autoimmunity are the temperature gauges on the dashboard of your immune system. Some cars have only a hot light that turns on when the engine is overheating, but others have a gauge that inches up toward a red zone. When you see the needle climbing toward the red zone, it gives you notice to stop and get your engine checked. But if you have only a hot light on the dashboard, you do not get advance warning, and you don't know there's a problem until smoke is coming out of your engine. Those are your symptoms.

Predictive autoimmunity may seem to be almost magical, but it's not fortune-telling. It doesn't actually predict what the future will be. It identifies the direction your health is heading. What you will learn is that the lifestyle choices you make interact with your genetic vulnerabilities and determine whether or not your immune system is called into action. For example, one study showed that if you have elevated antibodies to your thyroid, especially postpartum, then you have a 92 percent PPV of getting Hashimoto's thyroid disease within 7 years. Now, you may not currently have symptoms of thyroid dysfunction, but if you test positively for elevated autoantibodies to your thyroid, those symptoms are coming.

If you have elevated antibodies to yeast in the intestines called *Saccharomyces cervisae*, you have close to a 100 percent PPV that you're getting Crohn's disease within 3 years. Having this information would give you a window of opportunity to do something about it.

In the following charts, the PPV category shows the percentage rate of likelihood as to whether you will develop a particular disease. The "years before clinical diagnosis" column shows how many years from the first identification of elevated antibodies that you could receive a diagnosis of that particular autoimmune disease.

SAMPLE SYSTEMIC AUTOIMMUNE DISEASES[2]

Disease	Antibodies	Positive Predictive Value (PPV)	Years before Clinical Diagnosis
Antiphospholipid syndrome	Antinucleosome antibodies Anticardiolipin antibodies Anti-β2 glycoprotein 1	100%	11
Rheumatoid arthritis	Rheumatoid factor Anticyclic citrullinated peptide	52–88% 97%	14
Scleroderma	Anticentromere antibodies Antitopoisomerase I antibodies	100%	11
Sjögren's syndrome	Anti-Ro and anti-La antibodies	73%	5

SAMPLE ORGAN-SPECIFIC AUTOIMMUNE DISEASES[3]

Disease	Antibodies	Positive Predictive Value (PPV)	Years before Clinical Diagnosis
Addison's disease	Adrenal cortex antibodies	70%	10
Celiac disease	Anti-tissue transglutaminase Anti-endomysial antibodies (HLA-DO2 or DO8 antigens)	50–60% (100%)	7
Crohn's colitis	Anti-*Saccharomyces cerevisiae* antibodies	100%	3
Hashimoto's thyroiditis	Antithyroid peroxidase antibodies (postpartum)	92%	7–10
Primary biliary cirrhosis	Anti-mitochondrial antibodies	95%	25
Type 1 diabetes	Pancreatic islet cell, insulin, 65 kD glutamic acid decarboxylase, tyrosine phosphatase-like protein	43%, 55%, 42%, and 29%	14

KEEPING TABS ON YOUR WEAK LINK

Predictive autoimmunity allows us to identify where the weak link in your chain is right now. As you've learned, these weak links have very little to do with how you feel. If the number one cause of getting sick and dying is the immune system attacking your own body, wouldn't you want to know what your immune system is currently attacking? If you want to stay healthy and prevent disease, you cannot rely exclusively on standard medical testing, which is designed only to identify disease—a point at which most doctors say it is often too late to reverse the disease. Traditional medicine cannot diagnose an autoimmune condition until it has destroyed most of the tissue or gland it is attacking (i.e., the thyroid gland, pancreas, joint tissue, myelin sheath). Meanwhile, you've progressed from being on the early end of the autoimmune spectrum to being at the end stage with an autoimmune disease. As Mark Houston, MD, says, "You can't really depend just on the risk factors anymore to define disease (smoking, being overweight . . .). You've got to measure the early indicators." He is referring to the biomarkers, or antibodies, listed in the charts above.

The blood tests described in this chapter are not included in the battery of testing most doctors will offer during an annual physical. However, I believe they are an essential addition to traditional medical testing, and I believe everyone should have a baseline set of biomarker tests, even if you are not currently experiencing symptoms. This is a revolutionary, groundbreaking testing protocol that can wipe away years or even decades of mystery, confusion, and loss of hope.

While no one has to pay for lab tests to follow my 3-week program, accurate, scientific blood testing is an excellent way to confirm the results from the quiz in Chapter 4 and to conclusively determine where you are on the autoimmune spectrum. You can also track your progress by continuing to monitor your autoantibodies. Many people believe that once they feel better, their health problems are gone. Nothing is further from the truth in the world of autoimmunity. Although eliminating the symptoms is a primary goal, even when there is symptom relief, we are still on the spectrum. The only way to know if you have silenced the autoimmune cascade is to retest. Otherwise, we may think that since our symptoms are controlled, we do not have to be as vigilant in following our doctor's recommendations. I have seen this happen many times over the years, where "surprise" flare-ups reappear seemingly out of nowhere. The problem was that the body hadn't fully healed, and when an irritant like gluten was reintroduced, the inflammatory cascade began again.

A classic example of this is celiac disease, where only 8 percent of people heal completely on a gluten-free diet, although many more will remark that they feel significantly better. According to a 2009 study published in the journal *Alimentary Pharmacology and Therapeutics*, 65 percent of celiac patients feel better but still have underlying, excessive inflammation in their intestines, causing intestinal permeability that opens a gateway to the development of other autoimmune diseases, even when they are following a gluten-free diet.[4] The remaining patients did not heal at all, even on a gluten-free diet (they may have had other compounding triggers that needed to be addressed). The advice for all celiac patients, then, is to get retested for the biomarkers of intestinal permeability. Without retesting, you will never know if you have completely healed. If your intestinal permeability has not completely healed, the damage will continue at that weak link (celiac disease) or at another weak link.

THE MULTIPLE AUTOIMMUNE REACTIVITY SCREEN

Aristo Vojdani, PhD, is a researcher who focuses on autoimmunity and has been my mentor in understanding how to use the immune system's biomarkers to see where the weak link in our chain may be, what link is currently being pulled way too hard (increased antibodies), and how to monitor the progress of treatment plans. He has devoted his life to measuring the action of our "armed forces."

In the past, blood tests that checked for elevated antibodies to your own tissue (an autoimmune mechanism) looked at one or two antibodies at a time. Such tests are prohibitively expensive. Dr. Vojdani's research has produced the first tests to check for a number of different tissues

Meet Mark

Mark was 44 years old when he first came to see me. His father died at 44 of a heart attack. His two older brothers also died in their early forties of massive heart attacks. When his last brother died, Mark was in his thirties, and his cardiologist, in an effort to keep him from his likely genetic fate, prescribed a statin drug even though Mark was by all appearances healthy.

Mark followed the doctor's orders and took the medication for more than 10 years. When he came to my office, he had a healthy 16 percent body fat and told me he exercised regularly. Mark said, "Dr. Tom, I feel perfect, and my doctors say I'm in great shape, but I heard about predictive autoimmunity. I want to do these tests."

I supported Mark's decision, and we ordered the blood tests. It turned out that even though he was taking a statin and keeping in shape, he still had elevated antibodies to his heart in three different categories. Elevated antibodies cause inflammation in the tissue. I told Mark that the test showed that his heart was slowly being killed off by his immune system. The statins were stopping the liver from making extra cholesterol, but they weren't stopping the tissue damage caused by his immune system attacking his heart. This likely was the mechanism by which his father and his two older brothers died in their forties of heart attacks: The unchecked inflammation pulled on the chain—in these cases, their hearts—until the link broke.

Doing these predictive antibody tests allowed us to investigate his immune response. The same blood panel showed that he had elevated antibodies for a sensitivity to many peptides of wheat, and he had intestinal permeability. Mark's genetics told the story of a history of heart disease, and the functional blood tests told us his "gateway" was open and the autoimmune process was in full force, affecting the weak link on his health chain, which was his heart. I immediately put Mark on my Transition Protocol, which included a gluten-free, dairy-free, sugar-free diet. I also advised him to take probiotics, prebiotics, and nutrients we'll talk about in Chapter 8 to heal his gut.

A year later, Mark came back to see me and we ran the blood tests again. This time, all of his heart antibodies were down into the normal range. This meant that his inflammation had subsided, and his body was healing. Mark said, "Doc, you saved my life."

(multiple weak links in the chain) at a fraction of the cost of traditional laboratory testing. His patented blood test panels do not address every autoimmune disease, only the 24 most common ones.

The following bloodwork must be ordered through a licensed health-care practitioner. Again, it will identify *if* you are on the spectrum for a particular autoimmune disease and if the process has begun where your immune system is destroying tissue, whether or not you have symptoms.

Your doctor may not be familiar with these tests. At my Web site, theDr.com/TheAutoimmunityFix, you can download information to take to your doctor when you want to discuss these tests.

Here is a list of the most common antibodies we currently check for in the most general screen. Once again, this is not a complete list—just the most common ones we see. If you are having symptoms in any of these areas, these antibodies may identify the trigger not only causing the symptoms but putting you on the spectrum for developing the disease. And if you've been diagnosed with a disease already, this test will give you a starting point from which you can recheck in 6 months or a year to see if the protocols you are following are working. You will be able to tell because the autoantibody levels should reduce.

Category I: Gastrointestinal System

Parietal Cell and ATPase Antibodies

The parietal cells in our stomach produce hydrochloric acid (HCl), which is essential in breaking down the foods we eat. As we age, it is common to lose the ability to make enough HCl. Elevated antibodies to parietal cells trigger inflammation, which reduces the function of the cells and lowers HCl production. This mechanism is the most common cause of vitamin B_{12} deficiency worldwide and is referred to as autoimmune gastritis or pernicious anemia.[5] Eleven percent of celiac disease patients have been shown to have elevated levels of parietal cell antibodies.[6] This is why some celiac patients have stomach issues, protein and vitamin deficiencies, and neurological problems, among other symptoms related to low stomach acid (hypochlorhydria).

Here is just one example of many that shows how HCl deficiencies affect the autoimmune spectrum (which can be caused by an elevated level of parietal cell antibodies). Multiple studies have reported a high incidence of stomach malfunction (specifically, low levels of hydrochloric acid and pepsin) in individuals with rheumatoid arthritis. These reports reveal that just replacing the "missing" hydrochloric acid and pepsin—without making any other changes—can significantly improve many cases of rheumatoid arthritis.[7]

DISEASES RELATED TO LOW STOMACH ACID (HYPOCHLORHYDRIA)

- Addison's disease
- Asthma
- Celiac disease
- Chronic autoimmune disorders
- Chronic hives
- Dermatitis herpetiformis (herpes)
- Diabetes
- Eczema
- Gallbladder disease
- Graves disease
- Hepatitis
- Hyper- and hypothyroidism
- Lupus erythematosus
- Myasthenia gravis
- Osteoporosis
- Pernicious anemia
- Psoriasis
- Rheumatoid arthritis
- Rosacea
- Sjögren's syndrome
- Thyrotoxicosis
- Vitiligo

COMMON SYMPTOMS OF AN HC1 DEFICIENCY

- Acne
- A sense of fullness after eating
- Bloating, belching, burning, and flatulence immediately after meals
- Chronic candida infections
- Chronic intestinal parasites or abnormal flora
- Dilated blood vessels in the cheeks and nose (in nonalcoholics)
- Indigestion, diarrhea, or constipation
- Iron deficiency
- Itching around the rectum
- Multiple food allergies

- Nausea after taking supplements
- Undigested food in stool
- Upper digestive tract gassiness
- Weak, peeling, and cracked fingernails

If you suspect that you may have digestive symptoms—regardless if they are minor nagging ones or the more serious, such as heartburn or GERD—please don't fall for the standard "acid-blocker trap" without having your stomach acid tested. While I am a strong proponent of using medications when there is an identified need, there is a real danger in the shotgun approach of trying these drugs just to see if they will reduce your symptoms. There are so many side effects to this class of drugs—proton-pump inhibitors (PPIs)—taken over the long term. I'll give you a few: a 34 percent increased risk of heart attacks (with no other risk factors such as high cholesterol[8]), a 16 percent increased risk of osteoporosis in children under 18, and a 39 percent increased risk of osteoporosis in young adults ages 18 to 29.[9]

Very often, when patients come in to see us for a functional medicine overview and they have been prescribed a PPI for "acid stomach," they haven't been tested for high acid levels. Not once have these patients been tested before being given a drug that has serious side effects. PPIs are one of the top-10 selling categories of drugs in the world, with annual sales exceeding $6 billion. The most common PPIs prescribed are:

- Rabeprazole (AcipHex)
- Esomeprazole (Nexium)
- Lansoprazole (Prevacid)
- Omeprazole (Prilosec, Zegerid)
- Pantoprazole (Protonix)
- Dexlansoprazole (Dexilant)

If you suspect digestive problems and that an HCl deficiency may be a culprit, here's a safer approach: See a functional medicine practitioner who will check for biomarkers of an HCl deficiency. If that is not possible at the moment, here is a protocol that hundreds of functional medicine doctors use with minimal risk of side effects.

Begin by taking one 350-milligram to 750-milligram capsule of betaine HCl with a protein-containing meal. These pills can easily be found in a vitamin shop or health food store. A normal response in a healthy person would be heartburn. If you do not feel a burning sensation, this suggests that you're not "overloading" your system with too much HCl and that you may have an HCl deficiency and thus need this added digestion helper; your stomach may not be producing enough HCl on its own. To compensate, begin taking two capsules with each protein-containing meal. If there are no reactions after 2 days, increase the number of capsules with each meal to three. Continue increasing the number of capsules every 2 days, using up to eight capsules with each meal. These dosages may seem large, but a normally functioning stomach manufactures considerably more HCl. You'll know you've taken too much if you experience tingling, heartburn, diarrhea, or any type of discomfort, including a feeling of unease, digestive discomfort, neck ache, backache, headache, or any new odd symptom. Once you reach a state of tingling, burning, or any other type of discomfort, cut back by one capsule per meal. If the discomfort continues, discontinue the HCl and consult with your health-care professional. When you experience tingling, burning, or any symptom that is uncomfortable, you can neutralize the acid with 1 teaspoon baking soda in a glass of water or milk.

Whatever the dosage you can tolerate without symptoms, continue this dose with protein-containing meals. With smaller meals, you may require less HCl, so you may reduce the amount of capsules taken. Individuals with very moderate HCl deficiency generally show rapid improvement in symptoms and have early signs of intolerance to the dosage. In this case, cut down the dosage to below symptom level until you no longer require the extra supplement. This typically indicates a return to normal acid secretion. Individuals with low HCl/pepsin typically do not experience such quick improvement, so to maximize the absorption and benefits of the nutrients you take, it is important to be consistent with your HCl supplementation.

Intrinsic Factor

It is absolutely essential to absorb vitamin B_{12}. If you have antibodies to intrinsic factor, you may not absorb vitamin B_{12}. Data from the Framingham Offspring Study suggest that 40 percent of people between the ages of 26 and 83 have plasma B_{12} levels in the low normal range.[10] The result of that is often numbness, nerve degeneration for elders, memory loss that can mimic Alzheimer's disease, and atrophic gastritis, leading to pernicious anemia and a deficit of hydrochloric acid.

ASCA and ANCA

ASCA stands for anti-*Saccharomyces cerevisiae* antibodies, an accurate early marker of Crohn's disease. It's a common marker that's elevated in celiac disease patients as well. About 7 percent of people will have ASCA antibodies with celiac disease. ASCA antibodies appear to be gluten dependent and are associated with more severe manifestations of celiac disease: When you remove gluten from your diet, the ASCA antibodies often return to normal levels.[11] This is a classic example of removing the environmental trigger and calming down the autoimmune cascade. The positive predictive value with ASCA antibodies is up to 100 percent within 3 years for the development of Crohn's disease. That means that if you have elevated ASCA antibodies, you are likely to have the severe intestinal autoimmune disease Crohn's[12] within 3 years.

ANCA stands for antineutrophil cytoplasmic antibodies. These antibodies attack the inside of the most common white blood cells (neutrophils). When you have an elevated level of these antibodies, your immune system becomes compromised. We lost a great actor a few years ago: Harold Ramis, who onscreen and in real life, I read, had a heart of gold. He died from the most common disease associated with these antibodies—systemic vasculitis. I wished I had access to him in the years he was suffering with this autoimmune condition; I sincerely believe a functional medicine approach could have been of value. These antibodies are also associated with a common inflammatory bowel disease: ulcerative colitis.[13]

Tropomyosin

Imagine you are building a skyscraper. Imagine the steel beams that make the structure of the building, the inside "guts," if you will. Tropomyosins are the scaffolding inside our cells, called the cytoskeleton, that holds the cells together and helps them maintain their shape. When tropomyosin antibodies are elevated, the damage may affect any cell in the body. Mainly it's associated with the gut, where 95 percent of ulcerative colitis patients are found to have elevated antibodies to tropomyosins, but it can affect any system.[14] If you're losing the strength of the scaffolding inside that cell, it can't work the way it's supposed to. This may be why elevated levels of tropomyosin antibodies are directly associated with cancer development. Many studies have shown that there are specific changes to the repertoire of tropomyosins in cells that are undergoing cellular transformation into a cancer cell. These highly reproducible results suggest that during the process of cellular transformation, a process whereby a normal cell becomes malignant, the loss of tropomyosin is a critical step.[15]

Category 2: Thyroid

Thyroglobulin and Thyroid Peroxidase

These two distinct antibodies are related to the thyroid gland and thyroid autoimmune diseases. They are the most common of the five thyroid autoimmune diseases, which also include idiopathic myxedema, endocrine exophthalmos, and asymptomatic thyroiditis.[16] Thyroid autoimmune diseases are the third most common autoimmune condition behind diabetes and celiac disease.

If you can't lose that last 10 pounds, or are feeling sluggish or depressed, your doctor will often check your thyroid hormone levels. Even if your hormone levels are in the normal range, doctors usually prescribe thyroid hormone. While you might feel a little better, you won't feel great, because it's the wrong approach. Most doctors just don't look for antibodies to the thyroid because an elevation of antibodies will not change their treatment recommendations: They would still just prescribe thyroid hormone, and they wouldn't address the antibodies. Most doctors do not know that it's possible to reduce these elevated antibody levels by using a functional medicine approach.

Even if they look and see the elevated antibodies to the thyroid, almost every doc says, "Well, it looks like you've got a little autoimmune thing going on here, so let's give you some thyroid hormone and monitor you." The problem is that thyroid hormone has little to do with your immune system attacking your thyroid. This protocol is simply archaic. It's the same prescription that was given back in the 1960s, and they're still doing it today. A more modern approach would be to investigate why your immune system is attacking your thyroid: That's a functional medicine approach. By using this approach, a doctor might find that if you are on the celiac spectrum, producing celiac antibodies (transglutaminase), you are vulnerable to a molecular mimicry reaction and may begin producing antibodies to your thyroid.[17] That means you can develop a thyroid autoimmune disease from a sensitivity to gluten. Patients with Hashimoto's thyroid disease can reduce their dose of thyroid hormone medication (with their doctor's permission, of course) by 49 percent by eliminating gluten from their diet.[18]

There are chemicals in our environment that interfere with our thyroid hormone binding to and being escorted into the cells by the thyroid receptor sites. A receptor site is like a catcher's mitt. But if thyroid hormone can't get into the catcher's mitt (the receptor site), it can't get into the cell, and you have a "functional hypothyroid" situation. What does that look like? Have you suspected perhaps a sluggish thyroid, have had a blood test done and it came back normal, and your doctor prescribed thyroid hormone to you anyway (another shotgun approach here)? *Wait a minute*, you think. *My blood test says I have enough thyroid hormone, but you're going to give me more anyway. Why?* The doctor doesn't have a good explanation and might say, "Well, more thyroid hormone seems to help." But while the doctor is correct that the additional hormone does help with the symptoms, the prescription medication will not address the underlying mechanism of dysfunction, and the imbalance will likely continue. One common reason for this unaddressed dysfunction is related to environmental chemicals. When exposed, most people can eliminate these chemicals from their bodies naturally, but some people can't, and for those folks, the chemicals accumulate in the body. And if that accumulating chemical has a magnetic attraction to the catcher's mitt called your thyroid receptor sites (which it often does), there's no room for your thyroid hormone to get into the catcher's mitt, and the hormone cannot get into the cell. As a result, you'll have a "functional" low thyroid (hypothyroidism) with normal blood levels. The fancy Scrabble word for this condition is *euthyroidism*.

So what are the chemicals that can interfere with the function of your thyroid receptors? If you're on an elevator in a hotel, and the elevator door opens, can you immediately tell that the pool is on that floor? Do you smell it? Chlorine is the most common of the three chemicals that can interfere with thyroid receptor function. The other two are bromine and fluoride. If no one else on the elevator smells the chlorine like you do, it suggests your body may be hypersensitive to the chemical—

and you may have been accumulating higher levels in your system, possibly interfering with your thyroid receptor function. The most common way chlorine gets in our bodies is the shower—we inhale the steam right into our bloodstream through our lungs. If you install a chlorine-filtering showerhead for as little as $50, you might find your thyroid working better in a few months. A side benefit is that your hair will look shinier without the chlorine exposure. The common prescriptive approach in this example—shotgunning thyroid hormone without a deeper investigation—is one reason why the United States as a nation is ranked second from the bottom in overall quality of health care.[19]

Category 3: Adrenal Glands

21-Hydroxylase

This antibody is related to your adrenal glands. The more stress you're under, the harder your adrenals work making stress hormones. An autoimmune condition of the adrenal glands is called Addison's disease. You can also develop autoimmune endocrine disorders, meaning hormone imbalances. You start making antibodies to different hormones. You can get diabetes. You can get Graves' disease and Hashimoto's thyroid disease and vitiligo (white patches on the skin from loss of pigment), all from the elevated antibodies to your adrenal glands.

Category 4: The Heart

Myocardial Peptide and Alpha-Myosin

Cardiomyopathy, rheumatic heart disease, myasthenia gravis, autoimmune myocarditis, acute rheumatic fever, and rheumatic heart disease can all be related to having these two elevated antibodies. These were the antibodies that were elevated in Mark's story, page 117. Going on a gluten-free, dairy-free, sugar-free diet reversed his elevated levels.

Phospholipid and Platelet Glycoprotein

These antibodies are associated with cardiovascular dysfunction and endocrine dysfunction (hormone imbalances). These can manifest as antiphospholipid syndrome, like my patient Samantha had. Antiphospholipid antibodies (aPL) represent the most frequently acquired risk factor for a treatable cause of recurrent pregnancy loss and complications. Every woman of childbearing age with a family history of miscarriages (mother, aunts, sisters, etc.) should speak with the doctor about having this simple blood test done before attempting pregnancy. If you have elevated antibodies to phospholipids, you'll have a window of opportunity to reverse this situation, often with something as simple as following a gluten-free diet.

Kathy had two miscarriages (at ages 30 and 31) and began passing out for no known reason. She was at her wit's end when, after being admitted to the hospital, she was lucky to have a doctor who took the time to investigate all aspects of her health. He ran a battery of tests and identified that she had a number of problems.

- Recurrent iron-deficiency anemia that did not get better with iron supplements but did improve with intravenous iron therapy (that tells us immediately there is something not working right in her gut—she's not absorbing nutrients)
- High pancreatic enzymes
- Increased markers of inflammation
- Increased ANA antibodies (a sign of an autoimmune mechanism that could be occurring in many different tissues of the body)
- Positive markers of the autoimmune disease systemic lupus erythematosus
- Low levels of B vitamins
- Elevated antibodies to her thyroid
- Elevated antibodies that put her at great risk of pregnancy loss (anti-beta 2 glycoprotein 1)
- Blood and granular cysts in her urine

Because of the variety of symptoms with indicators of poor absorption of iron and B vitamins, she was checked for a gluten sensitivity. Sure enough, she had celiac disease. She was put on a gluten-free diet, and within 6 months, all of her autoimmune biomarkers were back to normal. Within 24 months, all of her abnormal markers putting her at risk of pregnancy loss were back to normal. No other treatment was administered: just a gluten-free diet and the proper testing.

You can also develop type 2 diabetes or lupus through the pathway of phospholipid antibodies being elevated, as well as autoimmune thrombocytopenia, cardiovascular disease, or coronary artery disease from the platelet glycoproteins being elevated. If your cardiologist suggests bypass surgery, it is imperative to get this test. To treat blocked arteries without addressing the underlying inflammation is an inefficient treatment protocol.

Category 5: Reproductive Health

Ovary and Testis

These are sex-specific antibodies that can lead to hypogonadism, premature menopause, premature ovarian failure (endometriosis), and other endocrine disorders.

Category 6: Musculoskeletal Health

Fibulin, Collagen Complex, and Arthritic Peptide

These antibodies are related to collagen production, muscles, tendons, ligaments, and joints, leading to lupus, sclerosis, osteoarthritis, or rheumatoid arthritis. These antibodies are also associated with atherosclerosis. Specifically, fibulin antibodies cause atherosclerosis (your pipes plugging up).

Osteocyte

This antibody is a biomarker for inflammation in the bones, the driving force in the development of osteoporosis.[20]

Category 7: Liver

Cytochrome P450 Hepatocyte

Your liver has more than 350 different functions. When you have elevated antibodies to your liver, creating inflammation, many different systems may be affected, producing diseases such as diabetes, hepatitis type 2, chronic hepatitis C, cancer, kidney disease, peptic ulcers, epilepsy, and congestive heart failure, among others.[21]

Category 8: Pancreas
Insulin + Islet Cell Antigen

These are the usual and customary antibodies doctors use to diagnose type 1 diabetes and unexplained hypoglycemia. In Chapter 2, we discussed that when infants are at high risk for type 1 diabetes (from a family history), parents are advised to avoid feeding their baby all cow's milk products for the first year of life. The reason is the vulnerability to produce islet cell antibodies if you are sensitive to milk.

Category 9: Brain
Glutamic-Acid Decarboxylase

These are antibodies to your brain that are also related to celiac disease, non-celiac gluten sensitivity, type 1 diabetes, stiff person syndrome, and cerebellar ataxia, which controls balance and muscle movement. These antibodies, when elevated, are also associated with insomnia and anxiety. A gluten-free diet has shown to be effective with these two conditions.

Myelin Basic Protein

These are antibodies to your brain associated with multiple sclerosis (MS), autism, lupus, and PANDAS (pediatric autoimmune neuropsychiatric disorders associated with Streptococcal infections, a childhood disease). In my practice, I did an informal study on my patients. I tested 316 consecutive patients between the ages of 2 and 90 for gluten, dairy, and brain antibodies, including myelin basic protein. If patients had elevated antibodies to dairy, 32 percent also had elevated antibodies to myelin basic protein. This is an example of an environmental trigger associated with an autoimmune mechanism.

Myelin is the Saran Wrap that coats your nerves in both the brain and the body. It's like the protective insulation around an electric wire.

Think of the wire that goes from the battery to the headlights in your car. If the insulation on that wire is frayed, so that the wire itself touches the frame of the car, the electrical current can short and your lights will flicker. When you develop an elevation of myelin antibodies, you destroy this coating around your nerves, and the messages that are being sent across them will flicker. This is what causes the symptoms of MS. Along with treating the symptoms (focusing on the headlights that are flickering), you must focus on stopping the damage to the wires.

Asialoganglioside GMI

The asialoganglioside cells function in many different nerves in your body. That's why many different symptoms are associated with these elevated antibodies. These are antibodies to your brain that can cause chronic inflammatory demyelinating polyneuropathy, cerebrovascular incidents (strokes), cranial trauma, Guillain-Barré syndrome, motor neuron disease, Alzheimer's, multifocal motor neuropathies, MS, myasthenia gravis, PANDAS, rheumatoid arthritis, and lupus.

Alpha + Beta Tubulin

Tubulin is a building-block protein and a major component of a cell's internal structure, called microtubules. These structures play key roles in many nerve functions. Elevated antibodies to tubulin appear in alcoholic liver disease, demyelinating diseases, recent-onset type 1 diabetes, Graves' disease, Hashimoto's, PANDAS, rheumatoid arthritis, and toxin exposures (including mercury and other heavy metals). This is another example of how an environmental trigger (excessive heavy metal exposure) can trigger a neurological autoimmune disease.

Cerebellar

The cerebellum is the part of the brain controlling movement and balance. Inside the cerebellar cortex there are large neurons called Purkinje cells. The cerebellar antibodies test measures antibodies against the cerebellum Purkinje cells. These antibodies are associated with autism, celiac disease, gluten ataxia, and paraneoplastic cerebellar degeneration syndrome.

Elevated levels of this antibody are often why people, as they begin aging, sometimes don't feel steady walking up and down stairs. The reason is not that they are getting old. Instead, their cerebellum, the part of the brain associated with balance, is shrinking because of years of elevated antibodies to the cerebellum slowly killing off the Purkinje cells. In my office study that I referred to earlier, if patients had elevated antibodies to gluten, 26 percent of them also had elevated antibodies to their cerebellum. That's one out of four people whose brains were shrinking from years of eating a food that may not have given them stomach pains when they ate it, so they thought there was no problem with consuming wheat, but the immune response was going after their cerebellum. This is an example of molecular mimicry: The immune system fights gluten, and in this case, brain tissue looks similar to gluten peptides, so it gets attacked.

My patient Sam came in one day and was feeling unsteady on his feet. We investigated and found that he had a gluten sensitivity manifesting as inflammation in his brain that was picked up with an MRI, yet there were no gut symptoms. His cerebellum looked normal on the MRI—just some inflammation. He refused to follow the recommendation to get off gluten. Seven years later, Sam came back, but this time he could hardly walk. You know what had happened: The increased level of antibodies to the weak link in his chain (his cerebellum) kept killing off his cerebellar cells, and his cerebellum had shrunk. It was no longer possible to arrest or reverse his condition.

Synapsin

Synapsin is a major immunoreactive protein found in most neurons of the central and peripheral nervous systems. It is a brain protein involved in the regulation of neurotransmitters (brain hormones). These antibodies to your brain cause demyelinating diseases (like MS) and numbness and tingling anywhere in your body. Synapsin also will inhibit the release of neurotransmitters and can cause lupus as well as mood disorders and depression.

HOW TO READ A RESULTS PANEL

Jerry was 16 when he came to see me. He had been to a number of doctors, the most recent being an endocrinologist (a hormone specialist) because Jerry wasn't growing. He was only 5 feet 2 inches tall and wanted to be on his high school wrestling team. The endocrinologist discovered that Jerry had celiac disease. There was a family history: His father had celiac disease, and his mother had a gluten sensitivity. The family immediately began following a strict gluten-free diet.

A few months later, Jerry had grown $3\frac{1}{2}$ inches, but then his growth abruptly stopped. His blood tests showed that his celiac antibodies were still 15 times above the acceptable limit. That's when he came to see me for my functional medicine approach. We drew the autoimmune panel and discovered that Jerry not only had elevated antibodies to celiac disease, but 18 out of 24 tissue antibodies were also elevated. This test result told me that Jerry had multiple autoimmune reactivity syndrome, even though he appeared to be a healthy young man. But with 18 different antibodies attacking his tissue, all over his body, I knew that his future wasn't bright.

Below is Jerry's first autoimmune test panel results. Just look at how many antibodies are marked in the "out of range" column. That tells the whole story—but because he was only 16, virile, and strong, he didn't have any noticeable symptoms other than the failure to thrive. There is no doubt in my mind that his future was going to be full of health complaints. Would it be his thyroid or his heart or his brain or his gut or his blood sugar? No one knew which weak link in his chain would show itself first.

TEST		RESULT		
Array 5 – Multiple Autoimmune Reactivity Screen	IN RANGE (Normal)	EQUIVOCAL	OUT OF RANGE	REFERENCE (ELISA Index)
Parietal Cell + ATPase			2.15	0.1-1.4
Intrinsic Factor	0.87			0.1-1.2
ASCA + ANCA			1.55	0.2-1.4
Tropomyosin	0.96			0.1-1.5
Thyroglobulin		1.12		0.1-1.3
Thyroid Peroxidase			1.36	0.1-1.3
21-Hydroxylase (Adrenal Cortex)	0.85			0.2-1.2
Myocardial Peptide	1.07			0.1-1.5
Alpha-Myosin		1.24		0.3-1.5
Phospholipid			2.44	0.2-1.3
Platelet Glycoprotein		1.30		0.1-1.3
Ovary/Testis ***		1.17		0.1-1.2
Fibulin		1.44		0.4-1.6
Collagen Complex	0.91			0.2-1.6
Arthritic Peptide		1.25		0.2-1.3
Osteocyte		1.34		0.1-1.4
Cytochrome P450 (Hepatocyte)	1.19			0.3-1.6
Insulin + Islet Cell			1.85	0.4-1.7
Glutamic Acid Decarboxylase 65		1.38		0.2-1.6
Myelin Basic Protein		1.37		0.1-1.4
Asialoganglioside		1.26		0.1-1.4
Alpha-Tubulin + Beta-Tubulin			1.93	0.4-1.4
Cerebellar			1.44	0.2-1.4
Synapsin			1.30	0.1-1.2

It took 4 years of vigilant work, including strengthening his microbiome, following a strict gluten-free diet, guarding against the most common cross-contaminations, and looking for other environmental triggers, until Jerry's immune system finally calmed down without any medications. His final blood test revealed a completely clean bill of health, and best of all, at age 20, Jerry was 5 foot 10. If you look at his last set of bloodwork, all of his biomarkers are in the normal range.

TEST	RESULT			
Array 5 – Multiple Autoimmune Reactivity Screen	IN RANGE (Normal)	EQUIVOCAL	OUT OF RANGE	REFERENCE (ELISA Index)
Parietal Cell + ATPase	0.56			0.1-1.4
Intrinsic Factor	0.54			0.1-1.2
ASCA + ANCA	0.84			0.2-1.4
Tropomyosin ****	0.54			0.1-1.5
Thyroglobulin	0.59			0.1-1.3
Thyroid Peroxidase	0.60			0.1-1.3
21-Hydroxylase (Adrenal Cortex)	0.57			0.2-1.2
Myocardial Peptide	0.68			0.1-1.5
Alpha-Myosin	0.73			0.3-1.5
Phospholipid	0.67			0.2-1.3
Platelet Glycoprotein	0.66			0.1-1.3
Ovary/Testis ***	0.57			0.1-1.2
Fibulin	0.65			0.4-1.6
Collagen Complex	0.67			0.2-1.6
Arthritic Peptide	0.64			0.2-1.3
Osteocyte	0.73			0.1-1.4
Cytochrome P450 (Hepatocyte)	0.81			0.3-1.6
Insulin + Islet Cell	1.07			0.4-1.7
Glutamic Acid Decarboxylase 65	0.73			0.2-1.6
Myelin Basic Protein	0.87			0.1-1.4
Asialoganglioside	0.85			0.1-1.4
Alpha-Tubulin + Beta-Tubulin	0.53			0.4-1.4
Cerebellar	0.76			0.2-1.4
Synapsin	0.78			0.1-1.2

SHOW THIS BOOK TO YOUR DOCTOR

I recommend that you do the Multiple Autoimmune Reactivity Screen at once to see if you have a problem. If you do have a problem, follow this program and track your progress by retaking the antibody test every year. If you would like to order this test from your doctor, you might be met with some resistance. He or she may say, "It's not possible to check all of these antibodies in one test." Explain that it is, and show your doctor this book. If the doc still doesn't believe you, it might be time to include another doctor on your health-care team. If your doctor refuses to do this test, you can learn more about ordering this test at my Web site (theDr.com).

I am on the teaching faculty of the Institute for Functional Medicine (functionalmedicine.org). To find a certified functional medicine practitioner like me in your area, visit that Web site. Most health insurance plans will cover services provided by a functional medicine practitioner. The type of practitioner (MD, DO, DC, acupuncturist) is not as important as the certified training in functional medicine that they have received.

The world of autoimmune disease is the best example of the limitations of conventional medicine. Just as a farm has individual silos to hold different grains, the silos of traditional medicine are referred to as specialties. Medical specialists in autoimmunity have their own silo, and few practitioners look for clues to solve a medical problem outside their training and expertise. For instance, there's an endocrinologist to examine hormonal output, and a rheumatologist for musculoskeletal diseases like arthritis. All know how to respond to autoimmune issues within their specialty, but few are trained to see the big picture. A traditional dermatologist focuses on the skin and treats the skin; a functional medicine practitioner looks at the skin but treats the whole body. The functional medicine doctor knows, for example, that many times skin issues from acne to psoriasis resolve completely when diet is addressed.

Traditional medical doctors usually treat only the symptoms (and usually through drugs and/or surgery) and rarely offer diet as either a solution or the initial problem of autoimmunity. Here's an example of how this can be a problem: Imagine that your child is suffering from seizures. You've been to three different doctors, and still the drugs are not controlling the seizures. This is called drug-resistant epilepsy. Fifty percent of children with drug-resistant epilepsy are found to go into complete remission on a gluten-free diet. Why don't our neurologists know this and test for it? The reason is that this research was not published in a neurology journal; it was published in a general medicine journal.[22]

The bottom line is that these tests exist, and the results are accurate. In today's modern era, new science is coming out exponentially quicker. Your doctor needs to get on board. It's not that these antibody tests are new. It's that we're measuring a large variety of antibodies to see where the inflammation is occurring.

By initiating the appropriate lifestyle interventions (diet, environmental exposures, stress reduction, exercise, and so on), you should be able to not only feel the difference but also demonstrate a reduction of antibody levels. It will take a minimum of 6 months before the antibody load reduces enough to show up in bloodwork. That's why you have to retest 6 months or a year after initiating a program. If the antibodies do not reduce, as in Jerry's case, it means that more investigative work needs to be done. Like peeling away the layers of an onion, it can take time to find the bottom-line trigger. Meanwhile, it's unlikely that your symptoms will go away completely. You might be able to mask the symptoms with a powerful drug, but the underlying pathology continues. Please don't get me wrong: I think that drugs for symptom relief can be very useful at times. However, the exclusive emphasis on symptom relief has produced the results that our current health-care system suffers from: shorter life spans for our children, terrible rankings by the World Health Organization for the quality of health care in the United States, and much more.

TESTING TELLS HOW COMMON GLUTEN SENSITIVITY IS

Bill goes to a doctor complaining that all of a sudden his thoughts are scattered, and he's finding it hard to concentrate. Bill tells his primary care doctor about his confusion and also about the fact that he's started to have headaches. The doctor recommends prescription-strength Tylenol for the headaches and sends him on his way.

Bill gives the medicine a shot, but it doesn't seem to help with the confusion, and it actually makes his headaches worse. The doctor, with nothing left in his arsenal, sends Bill to a neurologist, who recommends a stronger medication. It helps with the headaches, but it makes Bill feel queasy all the time. When he goes back to complain, the neurologist sends him to a research center where they see lots of people like Bill who have been suffering for quite a while. Like Bill, they've been to other doctors already and nothing has seemed to help.

The research center is on the cutting edge and knows to test for gluten sensitivities when the cause of a neurological disease is unknown. Why? When the cause of a neurological complaint at a research center is discovered, the number of patients with elevated antibodies to gluten is 5 percent. When the cause cannot be discovered, the number of patients with elevated antibodies to gluten is 57 percent.[23]

Like so many other patients with unexplained neurological complaints, Bill found that his headaches resolved on a gluten-free diet. We know that gluten is the most commonly recognized environmental trigger that sets off any autoimmune reaction. As no human can fully digest gluten, I recommend the following gluten sensitivity test, as well as a test for intestinal permeability, for everyone who has an unresolved health complaint. These blood tests, along with the Multiple Autoimmune Reactivity Screen, can be done from a single blood draw. Then you'll know what the most appropriate next steps should be for you to restore your health. Ideally, the following tests would be done before you begin my 3-week program and then again 3 to 6 months afterward.

Intestinal Antigenic Permeability Screen

This is the mother of all leaky gut tests. This blood test looks at just how leaky your gut is and how advanced the damage to your intestinal wall has become. It also shows you whether LPS is getting into

GENETIC TESTING IS NOT ACCURATE FOR CELIAC DISEASE

You may have heard that you can use genetic testing to diagnose celiac disease, but this is not true. The old school of thought was that genetic testing may be enough of an indicator to assume someone has celiac disease because research had shown that up to 95 percent of celiac patients have the HLA-DQ2 gene, and the other 5 percent will have the HLA-DQ8. However, in 2013, papers presented at the International Celiac Symposium showed that up to 7 percent of positively confirmed celiacs (through endoscopy) do not have either gene. What's more, research published in the *International Archives of Allergy and Immunology* in 2010 showed that up to 50 percent of patients with non-celiac gluten sensitivity carry the HLA-DQ2 or the DQ8 gene, so you could test positive genetically but not have full-blown celiac.

In the years to come, as more papers are published on this topic, we're going to find we are not really dealing with a "celiac gene" but possibly a "gluten gene," which to my mind gives credence to the idea of a spectrum of conditions that may be caused by a gluten-related disorder.

MEET CAMERON

My friend Pam's son Cameron, who is now 17, was classified in a *National Geographic* article as the poster child for food allergies when he was just 5 years old. He was breastfed but couldn't keep his food down, even though he continued to gain weight, and was covered with eczema. When he was still an infant, he was positively diagnosed as highly allergic to all of Pam's favorite foods, including fish, all nuts, peanuts, sesame, soy, and mustard. He also reacted to environmental triggers such as mold, pollen, hay, dogs, cats, trees, and grass. The allergist tested him for IgE reaction, but had he also checked for IgA, IgG, and IgM, they would have likely found that he had a sensitivity to gluten and dairy.

Over the next 15 years, Cameron was carefully watched by an allergist, and he eventually outgrew some of his food allergies and was treated with immunotherapy (allergy shots) for his environmental allergies. His skin cleared up immediately once the foods he was allergic to were avoided, so much so that when the *National Geographic* photographer arrived, they couldn't use his photo in the article because he looked "too healthy."

About 4 years ago, when Cameron was 13, even though he was feeling good, he put himself on a gluten- and dairy-free diet, mostly motivated by a favorite coach as a performance enhancer. But over this past summer, he started eating a lot of pizza, as only a teenage boy could. Seemingly out of nowhere, his entire back broke out with acne.

your bloodstream and triggering your inflammation and chronic symptoms. This is also a great follow-up test to measure the success of your program.

Wheat/Gluten Proteome Reactivity and Autoimmunity

Almost every lab in the country tests for just one component of poorly digested gluten. It's called alpha-gliadin, and 50 percent of people with celiac disease will have elevated antibodies to alpha-gliadin. That means that 50 percent don't. But if celiac disease is caused by a sensitivity to gluten, how can the test be 50 percent wrong? It's because there

When Pam told me the story, I suggested that his skin might be his weak link and that his acne might be related to his newfound love of pizza. Pam agreed and passed the information on to Cameron. Luckily he listened and eliminated the pizza, and the acne cleared up in less than a month.

Cameron is an excellent candidate for the predictive autoimmune testing given his background and health history. I explained to Pam that it would show exactly where the weak link in his chain is, and how it might manifest in his brain if it went unchecked. The reason is that a common mechanism triggering cognitive dysfunction is a sensitivity to gluten and dairy. The antibody transglutaminase 3 is a biomarker of a common auto-immune mechanism affecting the skin. This would be very useful information for Cameron in the long term, so he can see if he has elevated antibodies right now to his brain or any other tissue. If he does, he can watch his diet more closely to really cut down on inflammation. After following the diet for a year, he could repeat the testing again and confirm if his antibodies have reduced to normal levels. Would he have to follow this diet for a lifetime? The only food that has a lifetime restriction is gluten. Remember the memory B cells we talked about in Chapter 1? All other foods Cameron has the possibility of eating again. He is lucky enough to have biomarkers to check in the future if he tries reintroducing foods that he was sensitive to before.

are many components to poorly digested gluten, and alpha-gliadin is just one of them. Research shows that there are more than 62 different peptides of gluten that the immune system may react to. Why are all the laboratories checking only one? Believe me, I've asked; there is no answer to that question.

This test screens for sensitivity to 10 different peptides of gluten (not just alpha-gliadin). It also screens for the common celiac disease marker, transglutaminase antibodies. Other celiac tests screen for intestinal transglutaminase antibodies, and this test also screens for skin and neurological transglutaminase antibodies, making it a much more thorough, comprehensive gluten sensitivity screen. The value of looking for these antibodies (transglutaminase 6, or TG6) is that if they are elevated, they are a major component of brain tissue, and elevated antibodies to TG6 tell us your brain is on fire. This is one of the reasons why we now believe that Alzheimer's disease is a decades-long process: The brain is on fire, destroying cells for years, and you may not feel anything more than brain fog or an occasional headache.

THE NEXT STEP

Now that you understand the testing options and have identified where on the spectrum you might be, we're ready to start the program. In Chapter 6, you'll learn exactly what you can expect to achieve over the course of the next 3 weeks. Follow the protocol if you suspect that you have autoimmune issues, even if you are unable to have the tests done, or while you are waiting for their results. Tens of thousands of people are already following this protocol, and most of them did not have the opportunity to have testing done first. I hope that it will be your first step toward optimal healing.

> To watch a powerful video and learn more about gut health and how the microbiome works, go to GetYourGutTested.com.

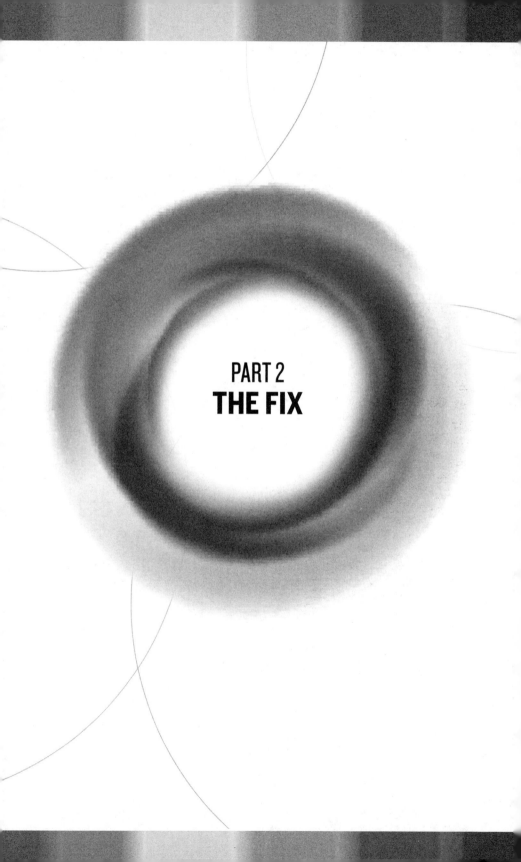

PART 2
THE FIX

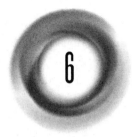

THE TRANSITION PROTOCOL:

WHAT YOU CAN EXPECT

I call my program the Transition Protocol because you will be transitioning to better health. You are now on a journey where you'll be introduced to new foods, new habits, and new ideas. Change is never black and white: We improve in increments, whether we take baby steps or big leaps. Along the way, you are going to move from a state of poor health to a state of optimal health. You will determine exactly how the foods you eat and the lifestyle choices you make are affecting how you think and feel.

You'll begin with a 3-week program I call Transition Phase 1, where you follow a strict gluten-free, dairy-free, sugar-free diet. During this time, you begin the work of creating a new, healthy environment that can lead to optimal healing. Most of us have a special place that we've been to more than once where we feel "right," a place where everything just seems to flow when we're there. Perhaps it's where you go for a walk to think. Perhaps it's a beach you can relax on. Perhaps it's a special chair in your home that just puts you in the right mood. The purpose of Phase 1 is to create an internal environment that allows you to be "in the flow" of your body function, where you can start feeling better and functioning better.

The latest brain science focuses on the process of neurogenesis, where the brain continues to create new cells and grow throughout our lives. This mechanism teaches us that it is rarely too late to change our habits or our health. But "rarely" does occur. Remember Sam, whom we talked about in Chapter 5? His cerebellar degeneration developed over 7 years after he refused to give up gluten. His MRIs had shown that when the elevated antibodies to his brain were first detected, he had a "normal" cerebellum. But 7 years later, his cerebellum was substantially smaller. You can't make lemonade out of prunes. You can't hope for enhanced brain function when you've killed off a major percentage of the tissue. Some actions will help, yes; but that level of degeneration is very difficult to reverse. That's why it is so important to identify these elevated antibodies killing off your tissue as early as possible. In this chapter, you will learn how to train your body so that it is in a constant "heal and repair" state that affects every cell of your body. We do this by creating the right internal environment, which then affects how we think and how we feel.

For example, your bloodstream is a highway with a lot of traffic. Our goal is to make sure there aren't traffic jams or lots of reckless drivers (free radicals) on your highway. Instead, you want to have a bloodstream of traffic where everyone is driving responsibly, not causing chaos: That's when you automatically stimulate your internal "heal and repair" mechanisms.

We can affect our internal environment in many different ways. This includes increasing our exercise and overall physical activity, pursuing lifelong learning for optimal brain function, learning lifestyle habits that reduce excessive stress, avoiding exposures to unnecessary chemicals and toxins, and changing our diet. In fact, one of the most far-reaching, impactful changes we can make to our environment is to both avoid foods that harm us and introduce foods that help us. As you begin to eliminate the foods that your body is sensitive to, you stop fueling the autoimmune fire. When this happens, the fire calms down. While it may not go away completely at first, when you stop throwing gasoline on the fire, you reduce the intensity of the inflammation and diminish the inflammatory cascade. Over time, your biomarkers of inflammation will reduce to a more normal range. This change can be quantified with simple blood tests any doctor can perform, including high-sensitivity C-reactive protein, ESR (erythrocyte sedimentation rate), a more balanced measure of your white blood cells called a "differential," or repeat stool analysis with reduced measures of the inflammatory markers calprotectin and eosinophil protein X.

In Chapter 2, we discussed the fact that from a cellular standpoint, we have an entirely new body every 7 years, because every cell in our body reproduces itself. Some cells (like the inside lining of our intestine) reproduce every 3 to 7 days. Others take much longer. The process of regeneration is going on 24/7 in our bodies. A basic premise in biology is that when a cell reproduces, it reproduces an exact duplicate of itself. Inside our cells, our DNA carries the blueprints for optimally healthy genetic expression, a "library of blueprints" for our perfect self. On a scale of 1 to 10, we have the potential to be a 10. This is the premise of using stem cells to stimulate new, healthier tissue. I'm not getting into politics here about using stem cells; I'm just saying what our anatomy contains. So why don't we reproduce perfect skin cells or brain cells or blood vessel cells on our own? Why aren't we already a 10? Here's why.

Let's say you're 35 years old. You're doing pretty well in life regarding your health—not quite what you were at 22, but doing fine. You lived through your late teens and early twenties with maybe a little too much partying, but you're not really the worse for wear or having any problems to complain about. Your blood tests are "normal" in your annual physical—there are no alarms going off. Perhaps your liver is functioning at a 7.6 on a scale where 10 is optimal. However, remember that when a cell reproduces itself, it reproduces an exact duplicate of itself. So a 7.6 functioning cell will replicate another 7.6 functioning cell, even though your DNA blueprint says that you can be a 10. Your cellular function is determined by what is happening around the cell, the "epi-cell," if you will. (I just made up a new word, but I hope the visual is clear for you.) Epigenetics means the environment around a gene determines whether that gene gets turned on or not. The epi-cell is the environment around the cell that determines how that cell functions and reproduces. So if the environment you created around this cell is full of inflammation, your cell is functioning as a 7.6 and you reproduce a 7.6 and life goes on.

But if you continue to live the same lifestyle, meaning eating foods that you have a sensitivity to, drinking too much, or eating junk foods, you are taxing your liver further. Pretty soon your liver will begin functioning as a 7.5. When that cell reproduces, you reproduce a 7.5. If your current lifestyle continues with the same or even greater inflammatory triggers, you begin functioning as a 7.4, and that cell reproduces as a 7.4. With the same lifestyle, you begin functioning as a 7.3, and that cell reproduces as a 7.3. The body continues to break down over the years and reproduce weaker cells determined by the function of those cells. This process of getting old is technically referred to as *catabolism*.

However, once you make the changes to create a healthier internal environment by applying the principles in this book, your liver function will improve. The damage to your mitochondria, the oxidative stress, and the inflammation that was affecting you on a cellular level are lessened and your body stops making elevated antibodies. Your body wants to be healthy, so it's trying to regenerate a healthier body by creating healthier cells. Your cells are now able to reproduce newer, healthier cells as long as you continue to provide a healthier environment by eating more nutrient-dense, less inflammatory foods. Instead of being a 7.3, you begin functioning as a 7.4. When that cell reproduces, it reproduces as a 7.4. You continue eating a more balanced, nutrient-rich diet as directed in this program, and you begin functioning as a 7.5. And that reproduces as a 7.5. You continue this program and begin functioning as a 7.6. When that cell reproduces, you reproduce a 7.6. And the body continues to rebuild over the months and reproduce stronger-functioning cells determined by the epi-cell (the environment that you

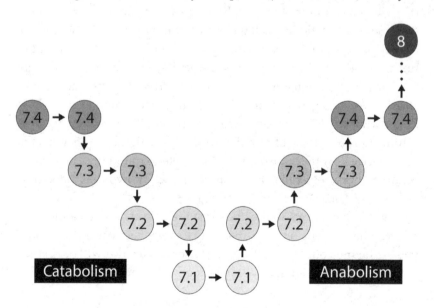

have supplied around the cell). This process of getting younger and stronger is technically referred to as *anabolism*.

My patients find that within about 3 to 6 months, other people start noticing how much better they look. Your friends or family members who may not have seen you in a few months say, "Wow, you look different. You look good," even if they can't quite put a finger on what the change is. It might be that your complexion is clearing up or 5 pounds have come off or your core energy is up so there's more life in your eyes. The reason is that by this point in time, your internal environment is replicating healthier cells. Now you're shifting from a catabolic state to an anabolic state, transitioning from the mechanism of getting older to one of youth, vibrancy, and better health.

WHAT YOU CAN EXPECT

There will be two subtle but impactful changes to your body in this Transition Phase 1: The first is that you are going to lower inflammation, and the second is that you will regenerate a healthier microbiome.

If you are like many of my patients, you'll find that after 3 weeks of following Transition Phase 1, you will notice that you start to feel better, no matter what condition you started with. When you're applying the principles that I recommend, by eliminating the most inflammatory foods, you will by default decrease inflammation immediately. It doesn't matter whether or not gluten or any other environmental toxin you have been exposed to is still in your system, because your symptoms are primarily related to the inflammation, not the toxin. That's why you start noticing a change in how you feel rather quickly. The stored toxins in your body are an emergency brake to getting healthier, but as the inflammation comes down, your body will naturally flush them out more easily. Depending on the type and levels of toxins in your body, you may need some help flushing them out. That's called detoxing, which you'll learn about starting on page 147.

Within 24 hours, you'll begin to balance your microbiome—the universe of bacteria in your intestines.[1] As your microbiome is rebalanced, your cravings will diminish, your energy comes up (if it's been low), and your brain hormones (the neurotransmitters) become more balanced, resulting in a range of good feelings from reduced anxiety to less depression. Your blood pressure calms down, your sleep improves, and the mechanism that causes hardening of your arteries (atherosclerosis) begins to reverse. Basically your entire outlook on life and your body functions improve. Your body now has a chance to address whatever imbalances you have been dealing with. There is no imbalance in your body, even cancer, that will not improve if you are successful in reducing systemic inflammation. The first step in reducing systemic inflammation, always, is to stop throwing gasoline on the fire.

All of these wonderful improvements will put you on the transition to better health. They don't mean you're necessarily cured or your symptoms will completely disappear. However, you certainly should notice that they're reducing, or that you are seeing benefits like weight loss or a decrease in brain fog. It's highly unlikely that you're going to be healed in 3 weeks: In Jerry's case, which we learned about in the last chapter, it took 4 years to completely restore his health. But you will notice better function. I tell my patients all the time that it's the small wins that accumulate to better health. Base hits, done repeatedly, win the ball game.

While you can change your microbiome in as little as 1 day, it will take a bit longer for the inflammation to subside completely and for your immune system to get the message to stop attacking you. When you start making changes, within 3 weeks you begin noticing the difference in how you feel because you're reducing the inflammatory cascade. Remember that even when you remove the offending invaders, which in this case are foods you may be sensitive to, the immune system continues to create antibodies for a couple of months. This means that while you may notice the beginnings of better health in as few as 3 weeks, you can expect to see even bigger changes to your health over the next 3 months.

In my office, I always use 3 weeks as a rule of thumb. I've found that it's the perfect amount of time for you to know if a program you're doing is working. If it's not, it means that we must have missed something, and we'll need to make an adjustment, possibly removing other potential irritants, which you'll learn about in Transition Phase 2.

Our society is based on quick responses, the "I want it now!" syndrome. But change takes time. This is the transition you're going through. You may not be able to see the change yourself on a daily basis because the base hits—the daily wins of food selection creating a healthier environment around your cells—are small. But the process is cumulative. And pretty soon you realize, "Wow, this is working."

Later, in Transition Phase 2, you'll build on your success. Over those second 3 weeks, you'll discover how easy it is to avoid other types of foods that many people are sensitive to. You'll continue following a gluten-free, dairy-free, sugar-free diet, but you'll also remove one specific exposure at a time and assess how you feel. Many people find that good habits build on each other, and even though the second phase is more comprehensive, it is easier to follow because you are already used to making changes to your diet and lifestyle, and you see that your changes in the first 3 weeks are working. You're on a roll!

Finally, you'll determine if you want to enhance your experience with supplements that both heal the gut and support your immune system. This is where the prebiotics and probiotics we mentioned in Chapter 3 come in, as well as specific supplements that enhance the rebuilding anabolic process and protect you against accidental exposures to gluten.

THE CONCEPT OF BODY BURDEN

The human body is confronted with toxic exposures every day, and it deals with them like a glass that is being continuously filled with water. Think of a glass that is already half full. If you continue pouring water into it, eventually the water will overflow. When toxic exposures are limited and the body can process them through its own mechanisms— the liver, skin, and digestive elimination—before the glass is full, the toxins won't cause health problems. But once the glass is completely full and water is spilling over the sides, it means the body's detoxification mechanisms are overwhelmed and we have crossed a threshold: the total toxic body burden. Now excessive amounts of toxic chemicals are circulating in your bloodstream.

According to a 2005 study from the Environmental Working Group, two major laboratories found an average of 200 industrial chemicals and pollutants in umbilical cord blood from 10 babies born in August and September 2004 in US hospitals. Tests revealed a total of 287 chemicals in the group. The umbilical cord blood of these 10 children, collected by the Red Cross, harbored pesticides, consumer product ingredients, and wastes from burning coal, gasoline, and garbage.[2] This is an overwhelming amount of toxins that the human body, especially at infancy, is not designed to deal with. These chemicals would then enter the infants' bloodstream and could interfere with both brain development and endocrine/hormone development.

The greatest fear of toxic exposure is its impact on the brain. The Centers for Disease Control and Prevention's Autism and Developmen-

TESTS SHOW 287 INDUSTRIAL CHEMICALS IN 10 NEWBORN BABIES

Pollutants include consumer product ingredients, banned industrial chemicals and pesticides, and waste by-products.

Sources and Uses of Chemicals in Newborn Blood	Chemical Family Name	Total Number of Chemicals Found in 10 Newborns (Range in Individual Babies)
Common Consumer Product Chemicals (and Their Breakdown Products)		47 Chemicals (23–38)
Pesticides actively used in the United States	Organochlorine pesticides (OCs)	7 chemicals (2–6)
Stain- and grease-resistant coatings for food wrap, carpet, furniture (Teflon, Scotchgard, Stainmaster, etc.)	Perfluorochemicals (PFCs)	8 chemicals (4–8)
Fire retardants in TVs, computers, furniture	Polybrominated diphenyl ethers (PBDEs)	32 chemicals (13–29)
Chemicals Banned or Severely Restricted in the United States (and Their Breakdown Products)		212 Chemicals (111–185)
Pesticides, phased out of use in United States	Organochlorine pesticides (OCs)	14 chemicals (7–14)
Stain- and grease-resistant coatings for food wrap, carpet, furniture (pre-2000 Scotchgard)	Perfluorochemicals (PFCs)	1 chemical (1)

tal Disabilities Monitoring Network reported in 2014 that approximately 1 in 68 children in the United States has an autism spectrum disorder. When I started my practice in 1980, autism prevalence was reported as 1 in 10,000. In the 1990s, prevalence was 1 in 2,500 and later 1 in 1,000. Today it's 1 in 68. Might chemical exposures that overtax the body's detoxification systems be a reason why the incidence of autism today is so incredibly high? Yes, it might be.

Sources and Uses of Chemicals in Newborn Blood	Chemical Family Name	Total Number of Chemicals Found in 10 Newborns (Range in Individual Babies)
Electrical insulators	Polychlorinated biphenyls (PCBs)	147 chemicals (65–134)
Broad-use industrial chemicals—flame retardants, pesticides, electrical insulators	Polychlorinated naphthalenes (PCNs)	50 chemicals (22–40)
Waste By-Products		28 Chemicals (6–21)
Garbage incineration and plastic production wastes	Polychlorinated and polybrominated dibenzo dioxins and furans (PCDD/F and PBDD/F)	18 chemicals (5–13)
Car emissions and other fossil fuel combustion	Polynuclear aromatic hydrocarbons (PAHs)	10 chemicals (1–10)
Power plants (coal burning)	Methylmercury	1 chemical (1)
All Chemicals Found		287 Chemicals (154–231)

THIS IS NOT YOUR MOTHER'S DIET OR DETOX

Just a few years ago, the new thing in health was to "detox." There were fasting cleanses, juice cleanses, cayenne pepper and honey cleanses, even banana cleanses. But detoxes are really not all that new: People have been talking about cleanses and detoxing since the days of Hippocrates more than 2,000 years ago. These programs are supposed to push toxins out of your body and restore equilibrium and better health. It's a valuable tool in cleaning up one's internal environment.

If a detox program creates an aha moment for you and gives you guidance for altering the food selections that created the toxic state that you needed to detox from, then that program has legs, or long-term value. I personally do a focused detox at least once per year. Some work, some don't. But even the detox programs that work are valuable only for a very short period. Once you go off your cleanse and back to your old habits, all the good work done to create a better internal environment goes down the drain. Literally.

My Transition Protocol is not a diet, and it's certainly not a one-off detox. You are not going to count a single calorie. You don't have to worry about nutrient ratios, serving sizes, or weighing yourself incessantly. The goal isn't weight loss, although that often happens when there are extra pounds to be shed. While you will be detoxing your body naturally because your liver begins functioning at a 7.8, then 7.9, then 8.0, and so on, by avoiding the foods you are sensitive to you, detoxification is only one of many benefits you will receive. Every cell in your body will function better, so your corresponding organs will function better. Your brain cells function better. Your liver cells function better. Your kidney cells, your muscle cells, your gallbladder cells, your reproductive system cells (yes, guys, that's right), every cell, every tissue in your body begins functioning better as you transition into an anabolic state. When you get the results you're looking for, as I expect you will, then you will know that you can't follow this program for 3 weeks and then go back to your old way of eating. Look at this as a chance to upgrade your ride: Treat your body like the Lamborghini you deserve instead of dragging it around like your dad's 20-year-old pickup truck.

Just as each of us is a unique and distinct individual, we each have our own threshold or body burden. Our genetics makes some of us better than others at detoxifying. It is possible to deal with toxic chemicals without overwhelming the detoxification capabilities of our body. But if you're exposed to all of these chemicals, plus daily exposure to foods that your body is sensitive to, you are more likely to fill the glass to overflowing and cross the line. And then inflammation begins to accumulate in response to the toxins you cannot eliminate. Now your body increases white fat cells to store the toxins your body can't shed and to keep them away from the brain. Here comes your spare tire.

One of the goals of this program is to lower your body burden so that you can better deal with the exposures that you have stored and continue to face. If you can modify your diet and eliminate the foods that are causing an immune response, then your body will have a chance to flush out the deposits of toxins it's storing.

When we cross the toxic threshold, minor toxins such as most food sensitivities can become major issues. For example, your body should be able to process exposures to mold or certain chemicals like pesticides, but when your detoxification system is overtaxed, things that your body normally could address easily now have "major toxic effects," including increased inflammation and increased white fat cell deposits. However, when you take out gluten, dairy, and sugar from your diet, you're lowering your body's toxic exposures (you stop pouring water into the glass), and you're better able to detoxify the unavoidable exposures you face every day, lowering your body burden. Then, when you are presented with other stressors, they will not respond as toxic. If you have 100 toxins coming in and you reduce 80 of them, then your body can handle the other 20 much easier.

This is why some people can actually return to eating dairy or sugar once their body has completely healed. Their immune response can completely reset, and the body will no longer mistake these foods as offending invaders. I've seen it happen frequently.

A WORD ABOUT YOUR WEIGHT

The dieting world is full of speculation and not a lot of hard science. That's why fad diets are constantly changing. It's also why people have difficulty not only losing weight but maintaining weight loss: There is no one answer that works for everyone. Part of the problem is that weight gain is associated with everything—including aging, the foods we eat, hormonal changes that affect metabolism, emotional stress, and current health status. Calorie restriction by itself is doomed to have a high-percentage failure rate. Weight-loss programs are well intentioned, but they often result in yo-yo dieting: You lose 20 pounds in 2 months, but within a year, you're back to your old habits and you gain the weight back. The Transition Protocol is different because the target here is reducing the volume of inflammatory triggers and building a healthier microbiome instead of focusing on weight loss. I've found that most often, people have difficulty losing weight because the foods they are eating are actually toxic to their system. There are two major ways your food selections can be toxic to your body.

If your armed forces (the immune system) says, "We've got a problem," it does not matter what you "think" about the food, your body is saying no and will create an inflammatory response, which by itself is associated with obesity.

The food directly impacts your microbiome, which will change within 24 hours, and is now recognized as a primary modulator (the control center) for resistant weight loss.[3]

The relationship between weight gain and inflammatory food exposure is straightforward: The more environmental toxins you are exposed to in your food selections, the more weight-retaining microbiota you feed, the more inflammation your body responds with, and the more weight you gain. When you're exposed day after day to foods your body treats as toxins (like gluten, dairy, and sugar), there are a number of consequences.

First, these foods overwhelm your response system, triggering and feeding the "survival bacteria" in the gut. Decades of less-than-ideal food choices have created a microbiome that has a will of its own, and it wants to survive. If you have a calorie-hoarding microbiome, it will send out chemical messengers to your brain that say, "I want more . . ." whatever the food is that feeds the obesity bacteria (such as high volumes of bad fats or sugar or allergenic foods or simple, processed carbohydrates).

Remember the Pima Indians we introduced in Chapter 3? When we compare the US Pima Indian diet with that of the genetically similar Pima Indians of Northern Mexico, who eat a more traditional, less processed diet, the US Pima have five times more diabetes than their genetic cousins, even though both groups have similar genetically derived, calorically hoarding microbiomes. The mechanism we identified for the US Pima having such a high rate of diabetes (50 percent have type 2 diabetes by age 35) was the introduction of abundant low-quality, high-calorie foods onto a majority gut bacteria that was designed to support their save-every-calorie-you-can type of microbiome. The Mexican Pima are still eating the traditional diet of their ancestors, and even with the same microbiome, they are not faced with an epidemic of diabetes.[4]

Second, with excessive inflammation, in this case from poor food selections, you increase the storage capacity of fat cells, specifically white fat, the "spare tire" around the waist that is difficult to get rid of through dieting alone. White fat is important to our survival but becomes a problem in excess amounts and because of where it's located. You don't increase your white fat simply from eating too many calories. The body also produces excessive white fat cells as a protective mechanism to keep toxins that you've been exposed to away from the brain, things such as heavy metals, toxic chemicals, and foods that we can't fully digest. If your detoxification capabilities are overburdened and you can't eliminate these toxins through your liver, bowel movements, urine, and skin, then in order to protect the brain, these chemicals get stored in the body and can create more white fat cells. Excessive amounts of white fat create more inflammation, which manifests as fluid retention (edema). In addition to the inflammatory response, a primary cause of edema is the increased levels of salt in prepared or processed foods, even in "healthy" options such as ready-to-eat bran and oat cereals, instant hot cereals, microwave popcorn, crackers, and pretzels.

If you pull your socks or underwear down and you have marks on your skin from the elastic, it's possible that your clothes are too tight, but for the vast majority of people it's a sign of water retention or mild edema. Other signs of water retention include dark rings under the eyes (also called allergic shiners) and lines underneath the eyes that aren't wrinkles (Dennie's lines).

Once the body has created these toxic fat cells and swelling, it's not so willing to release them. A toxic body may intentionally hold on to excess body fat or fluid to prevent being reexposed to the same toxins during elimination. In other words, your body may be protecting you from toxic exposure by keeping these toxins out of circulation so they cannot get to the brain, in effect forcing you to hold on to excess weight. When you improve your detoxification capabilities by reducing inflammation and by drinking enough water (½ ounce per pound of body weight daily at a minimum), you increase your ability to eliminate, with better bowel movements and more frequent urination, which is the safest and easiest way for your body to let go of stored toxins.

When you end your exposure to the foods you are sensitive to, your body is better able to focus on getting rid of the excess fluid it has been retaining and burning the fat where the toxins are stored. And because you will be avoiding the most undesirable calorie-dense, nutrient-poor foods and replacing them with more desirable nutrient-rich options, you're likely to drop more than a few pounds if you need to. This is one reason why thousands of people have reported losing as much as 15 to 30 pounds within 60 to 90 days on a gluten-free diet.[5]

LIFTING THE VEIL OF PERVASIVE SICKNESS

As you learned in Chapter 1, there are more than 300 conditions that are related to just a gluten sensitivity, let alone sugar or dairy. The ways you may begin to feel better are too many to list. What's more, each person's health is directly determined by pulling on the weak link in the chain: The results from taking part in the Transition Protocol will be as individual as you are. I truly believe that almost everyone will benefit and see positive changes in their body function and how they feel by implementing this Transition Protocol. Regardless of whether or not you are sensitive to gluten, dairy, or sugar, these are toxic foods that take you closer to your threshold or body burden.

I've found that the majority of people notice a difference in their health profile in a few days and certainly within the first 3 weeks. My patients often report that their skin begins to look better, and they have less severe seasonal allergies. Usually the difference is quite noticeable, though sometimes the difference is subtle, but rarely can you not discern a difference. But if you have a reintroduction exposure, like Cameron, the boy we met in Chapter 5 with extreme food allergies, you may have a setback. Cameron didn't know he had a problem with dairy and gluten until he reintroduced them into his diet, and his acne flared.

You might find that some of your symptoms will go away, yet new

Samantha's Story, Part 4

Remember my patient Samantha, who had one of the worst cases of lupus that the UCLA Rheumatology lupus research center had seen in 20 years, whose total health was so compromised because of autoimmunity? As I have with thousands of my patients, I started her on the Transition Phase 1 protocol. She removed wheat, dairy, and sugar from her diet and then came back to see me about a month later.

Samantha's story is a good example of the autoimmune spectrum wearing down many different systems of the body and becoming dysfunctional. Once healing began, Samantha noticed that her energy went up, but she still had some physical complaints. The years of damage could not turn around immediately, but the healing and improved function continued incrementally.

I asked her how she felt after she began the program. She told me, "I'm getting stronger every day. All of my weakened systems are improving, some faster than others. Some days I have constipation, but nowhere near as often as in the past. Some days I'm still fatigued, but nowhere near as often as before. I think my thyroid is working better, because I'm rarely cold anymore. The program has made a difference in my being able to bounce back from my most egregious symptoms."

In 2 years of remaining on this protocol, Samantha has regained 2 inches of height that she lost from her collapsed vertebrae. She told me recently, "I know my entire body is on its way to coming back to normal function."

ones might emerge. This is because most of us have more than one weak link, and very few individuals on the autoimmune spectrum are suffering from only one autoimmune disease (in other words, they have comorbidities). For example, if your presenting autoimmune disease was celiac or non-celiac wheat sensitivity with gut-related symptoms, and you follow the Transition Protocol and remove gluten from your diet, your gut pain may diminish, but you may suddenly notice that you have constipation. In the past, every time you ate gluten, your immune system in the gut was called into action and you'd suffer with stomach cramps (your stomach was functioning at a 5.6 out of 10). Without gluten, your primary weak link was resolved and the cramps went away, but it's possible that another weak link was simultaneously being pulled on but that symptom wasn't as dominant (constipation was a 7 out of 10). However, by resolving the cramps, you now notice the constipation. In time, the constipation will also resolve as long as you stay on a gluten-free diet (improving from a 7.0 to 7.1 to 7.2, and so on).

Earlier in life, I had participated in many marathons, running 26.2 miles in a race. I can assure you that when the demand I put on my body was over (crossing the finish line), I was not feeling like a 10 (quite honestly, I felt like a 5.5). I wasn't immediately able to go out and live my day-to-day life with my customary levels of energy and function. It took a few days to get back to normal. My brain wasn't functioning as it normally would, even though my brain wasn't taxed during the marathon. However, my whole body and brain needed to rest and reset. When you have systemic inflammation with food sensitivities, a number of systems are affected, whether you realize it or not. So your cramps go away, but the constipation shows up.

THE NEXT STEP

Let's take the first plunge. In the next chapter, you'll learn exactly what you can and cannot eat during Transition Phase 1. Good luck: I know you'll do great!

7

TRANSITION PHASE I:

WEEKS I–3

You can begin the process of optimal healing by eliminating the primary foods that your immune system may recognize as toxic. When you remove the three most common inflammatory foods at once—gluten, dairy, and sugar—both your digestive and immune systems have a chance to calm down, heal, and reset. But remember, when you stop pouring gasoline on the fire, you still have a fire to deal with. No matter where you are on the spectrum, along with reducing inflammation, we need to rebuild the damaged tissue so that we can create a better, healthier intestinal environment for good bacterial growth and heal a leaky gut.

Combined with Phase 2, the Transition Protocol is the beginning step to a full autoimmune diet: an eating style featuring food selections and vital nutrients meant to calm down inflammation and reverse the autoimmune cascade. A full autoimmune diet is a highly restricted food plan that eliminates all potential triggers. But clinically, I've seen that not everyone requires a full autoimmune diet. Instead, I've found that by eliminating the three primary triggers—gluten, sugar, and dairy— more than 80 percent of my patients feel dramatically better and begin reversing the autoimmune cascade. Another 10 percent require the investigation of other common food sensitivities, which is what Phase 2 is all about. The last 10 percent of autoimmune patients require a highly restrictive, full autoimmune diet. I want you to explore your health in baby steps so that you can continue eating the foods you love that don't affect your health. I've also found that the fewer foods I restrict, especially at the beginning of a program, the better the compliance.

Phase 1 of the Transition Protocol begins what is known as a classic elimination diet, where we eliminate specific foods for a specific time and notice the physical impact on our bodies and how we feel. If for any reason state-of-the-art food sensitivity testing is not available, this protocol is considered to be the best way to determine which foods are causing sensitivities. For the next 3 weeks, I will help you go completely dairy-free, gluten-free, and sugar-free. Instead of eating harmful foods that make you forgetful, sick, fat, and tired, you'll be enjoying all types of fruits and vegetables; clean meats, fish, and poultry; and healthy fats. The goal is simple. Take away the bad stuff, including highly processed foods, and add in the good stuff: whole, real foods that are easy to find and prepare.

The first thing people always ask me is what they *can* eat. The truth is, there's plenty to choose from, and as you'll see soon, I've listed all of the acceptable options. I don't want you to feel that this program is limiting in any way. In reality, you can select from hundreds of options every day. And just wait until you try some of the recipes!

Because this program leans in the direction of being Paleo-inspired, you'll be eating the way people ate for most of human history. Plants (vegetables, fruits, nuts, seeds, and herbs and spices) and animals (meat, fish, poultry, and eggs) will represent the vast majority of your foods. Plants will be your main source of healthy carbohydrates and micronutrients (vitamins, minerals, antioxidants, and anti-inflammatory agents). Raw nuts, seeds, their derivative butters, and animal foods offer quality forms of healthy protein and fat. In Phase 1, you can add in rice and corn, unless you've already identified a sensitivity to those grains.

MORE THAN A WORD ABOUT GMOS

One of my primary concerns when it comes to the health of our food supply is the prevalence of genetically modified foods and organisms, otherwise known as GMOs. These plants or animals are created in laboratories where their genetic makeup has been altered to create versions that cannot occur in nature or through traditional crossbreeding. Large-scale commercialization of genetically modified foods began in 1994. According to the FDA and the USDA, today there are more than 40 GMO plant varieties, the three most prevalent being grains like rice, soy, and corn, with 89 percent of US corn acreage now considered GMO.[1] There are nine genetically modified (GM) food crops currently on the market: soy, corn, cotton (oil), canola (oil), sugar from sugar beets, zucchini, yellow squash, Hawaiian papaya, and alfalfa. GM grains are fed to the animals we eat and therefore affect dairy products, eggs, beef, chicken, pork, and other animal products. Some of these raw ingredients are also added to even the most "natural" of processed foods, like tomato sauce, ice cream, and peanut butter. GM corn or soy is added to some spices and seasoning mixes, and to soft drinks (in the form of corn syrup or the artificial sweetener aspartame, or the glucose, citric acid, and colorings such as beta-carotene and riboflavin). The ubiquity of soybean and corn derivatives as food additives virtually ensures that all of us have been exposed to GM food products. In fact, more than 80 percent of all processed foods, such as vegetable oils and breakfast cereals, contain some genetically modified ingredients.

Notice that wheat is not listed above as genetically modified. That doesn't mean that wheat is safe to eat. Wheat has been hybridized through natural breeding techniques over the years. However, like most GMO crops, it has been engineered to tolerate a weed killer called Roundup, whose active ingredient glyphosate is now authoritatively classified as a probable human carcinogen.[2] The majority of US wheat crops are sprayed with Roundup a few weeks before harvest to kill the plant. A dead field of wheat is easier to harvest. Therefore, the majority of wheat products in the United States contain cancer-initiating glyphosate traces.

Animal studies have suggested that GMOs might cause damage to the immune system, liver, and kidneys. Roundup has also been shown to alter the microbiota and create an environment of increased intestinal permeability. Scientists are studying the interaction of this chemical with the detoxification capabilities of the liver, going as far as to say this is a "textbook example" of environmental triggers disrupting homeostasis and leading to many autoimmune diseases, including gastrointestinal disorders, obesity, diabetes, heart disease, depression, autism, infertility, cancer, and Alzheimer's disease.[3]

I know this information is both shocking and upsetting, but it helps to explain the dramatic increase in so many diseases in the last 30 years. The graphs on page 160 represent a world of concern regarding the impact of GM foods and organisms on our long-term health. These are just two of many conditions graphed in a referenced article associating the increase of GM foods on the market and specific disease. For more information, you can read the 13-page authoritative report I

Hospital discharge diagnoses (any) of Inflammatory Bowel disease
(Crohn's and Ulcerative Colitis ICD 555 & 556)

plotted against glyphosate applied to corn & soy (R = 0.9378, p <= 7.068e-08)
Sources: USDA & CDC

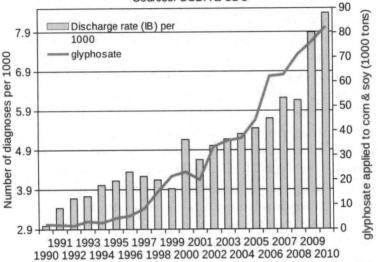

Prevalence of Diabetes in US (age adjusted)

plotted against glyphosate applied to corn & soy (R = 0.971, p <= 9.24e-09)
along with %GE corn & soy grown in US (R=0.9826, p <= 5.169e-07)
sources: USDA:NASS; CDC

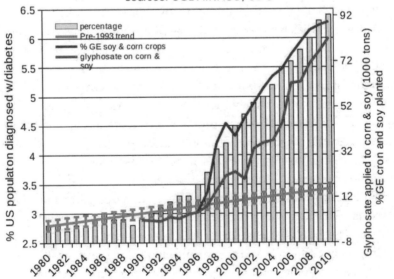

Reprinted with permission from Nancy L. Swanson.

helped write: *Can Genetically Engineered Foods Explain the Exploding Gluten Sensitivity?* (available on my Web site, theDr.com).

The scariest part about GMOs is that consumers don't know what they're eating, because GMO labeling is prohibited in the United States. Although most developed nations do not consider them safe, and labeling of GM food products is required in 64 countries, no labeling or restrictions are required in the United States. The only way you can avoid GMOs is by following these three simple rules:

1. Buy local produce. The simplest way to steer clear of GM crops is to join a local food co-op or CSA (community supported agriculture) or shop at local farmers' markets. Buy foods in their raw, whole, unprocessed state. You are more likely to find truthful answers from a local farmer or co-op compared to a major corporation.

2. Buy organic. Certified organic products cannot include GM ingredients. This includes both produce and meats, because if cattle have eaten GM feed, it alters the bacteria in their guts, which then affects both their meat and their milk.

3. Look for "Non-GMO Project Verified" or "USDA Organic" seals on single-ingredient packaged goods like flours, seeds, and nuts. And while you are doing that, make sure they all are marked as "gluten-free" somewhere on the label to reduce your risk of cross-contamination.

ENJOY YOUR FAVORITE FRESH FOODS

During Phase 1, you can eat all forms of fruits, vegetables, and nuts, especially when they are fresh and in season. I always recommend fresh fruits and vegetables when available, but for many, this isn't always possible. Frozen fruits and vegetables are acceptable because they are harvested when ripe and have had the opportunity to build a full repertoire of antioxidants and polyphenols. Choose organic produce whenever possible and, if you can, find locally sourced varieties. Avoid canned fruits or vegetables that may have been preserved with sugar or salt.

A number of foods are known to heal the gut. These are foods that are anti-inflammatory by nature, and you can alternate among these choices every day.

- Cinnamon ($\frac{1}{10}$ teaspoon daily is a safe and effective dosage)
- Cruciferous vegetables (broccoli, Brussels sprouts, cauliflower, cabbage, bok choy) contain a family of vital nutrients called glucosinolates that are potent polyphenols particularly useful for lowering inflammation in the intestines
- Dark-colored fruits with a high concentration of polyphenols, such as berries, cherries, and red grapes
- Green tea (1 to 3 cups a day), which is also a prebiotic
- Omega-3 fatty acids must be acquired through diet, because the body cannot produce them. Among so many other benefits they bring us, they turn on the genes that lower inflammation in the gut. Foods high in omega-3s include grass-fed beef, cold-water fish, seafood, black walnuts, pecans, pine nuts, chia seeds, flaxseeds, basil, oregano, cloves, marjoram, and tarragon
- Parsley
- Tomato juice (5 ounces)

There is a class of carbohydrates called fructan, which acts like fertilizer to support the good bacteria in our intestines. The best-known fructans are in the family called inulin. Inulin is a natural storage carbohydrate present in more than 36,000 species of plants. Inulin is also considered to be a prebiotic used as an energy reserve and for regulating cold resistance. Chicory root is a prebiotic that contains the highest concentration of inulin (our New Orleans readers will be happy to hear this, as it's a cultural addition to their regional cuisine). Other plants that contain this healthy bacterial fertilizer include wheat, sugar beets, leeks, asparagus, artichokes, onions, garlic, dandelion root, bananas, and plantains.

One of the potential pitfalls of a gluten-free diet is that most of us get more than 70 percent of our inulin from wheat. When we lose the wheat, whatever level of good bacteria we have in our gut, which has grown dependent on wheat as the major source of its fertilizer, begins to starve. Gluten-free products often are much lower in inulin. So in our efforts to fix intestinal permeability, we create a worse environment in our microbiome than we had before. This is why we must be sure to include inulin-rich foods as part of our daily diet. Fermented foods, which we discussed in Chapter 3, will both inoculate and encourage the growth of gut-protecting families of bacteria. Other high-fiber vegetables are equally important. Remember, the fastest-growing cells in the body are the inside lining of the intestines: We have an entire new lining every 3 to 7 days, and we need butyrate to make this lining strong. Vegetables, especially root vegetables, contain insoluble fiber, which produces butyrate in the gut.

Fruits

Fruits can be abundant in Phase 1, unless:

1. You have a known allergy or sensitivity to a particular fruit.
2. The volume of fruit you're eating is over your personal threshold of what your blood sugar regulating mechanisms can handle.

Fruits are higher in sugar than vegetables, and some are very high on the glycemic index, which we discussed in Chapter 2. Fruits that are considered "low glycemic" (apricots, plums, apples, peaches, pears, cherries, and berries) are excellent choices. Other fruits, although they have significant health benefits, have to be eaten in moderation. For example, have you ever heard the phrase "No one wants to go bananas in life"? A ripe banana is a healthy fruit, and its glycemic index is 51 (that's a good number). But if we eat bananas every day, along with other medium to high glycemic index foods, the impact of too much sugar eventually sends our bodies down the path of roller-coaster blood sugar levels that lead to high-anxiety states (going bananas) and potentially to diabetes.

- Acai berries
- Apple
- Apricot
- Avocado
- Banana
- Blackberries
- Black raspberries
- Blueberries
- Boysenberries
- Cantaloupe
- Cherries
- Coconut
- Cranberries
- Fig
- Goji berries
- Gooseberries
- Grapefruit
- Guava
- Honeydew
- Huckleberries
- Juniper berries
- Kiwifruit
- Kumquat
- Lemon
- Lime
- Loquat
- Lychee
- Mango

- Nectarine
- Olive
- Orange
- Papaya
- Passionfruit
- Peach
- Pear
- Persimmon

- Pineapple
- Plum
- Pomegranate
- Pomelo
- Quince
- Star fruit
- Strawberries
- Watermelon

Nuts and Seeds

Nuts and seeds are excellent sources of protein. Many of them are now ground into flours and butters that you can use instead of traditional wheat flour or butter (for toast). There are no nuts or seeds that are off-limits in Phase 1, unless you have a known allergy or sensitivity. Peanuts and coconut are both acceptable (I treat coconut as a super-food), although neither are technically nuts or seeds: Peanuts are in the legume family, and coconut is a fruit.

However, this is not an open invitation to eat every nut bar on the shelves. You must read ingredients and labels carefully and avoid the bars made with sugar or dairy and those not labeled gluten-free. Organic and gluten-free processed foods are often made with unhealthy ingredients. Good seed and nut choices for Phase 1 include:

- Almond
- Australian nut
- Beech
- Black walnut
- Brazil nut
- Butternut
- Cashew
- Chestnut
- Chia seeds
- Chinese almond
- Chinese chestnut
- Filbert

- Flaxseeds
- Hazelnut
- Hemp seeds
- Indian beech
- Kola nut
- Macadamia
- Pecan
- Pine nut
- Pistachio
- Poppy seeds
- Pumpkin seeds
- Safflower

- Sesame seeds
- Sunflower

- Walnut

Vegetables

Vegetables are extremely adaptable. There are so many different ways to prepare them. You can eat most of them raw, lightly steamed, baked, or sautéed and enjoy them as a snack, side dish, or main dish. You can also add them to soups, chilies, stews, roasts, salads, stir-fries, and casseroles. Aim for buying the highest quality you can find, meaning organic, local, and farm fresh whenever possible.

The more vegetables you eat every day, the better. Remember the "pound a day" guideline from the Polymeal in Chapter 3: The best way to achieve this goal is to eat some vegetables at every meal. I always recommend you include five different colors of vegetables per day. Each color provides a different family of antioxidants and polyphenols, which activate different genes that will keep you strong and healthy.

I know it can be a challenge to work vegetables into every meal, especially when you are cooking for children. My advice is to prepare vegetables in a way that your kids will eat them, which is more important than if they did not eat any vegetables at all. Strive for the least-altered way possible. It's a stretch to see the health benefits in deep-fried vegetables.

The type of vegetables matters, too. The glycemic index of a yam is 37, a sweet potato 44, new potatoes 57, white-skin mashed potatoes 70, French fries 75, baked Idaho potato 85, instant mashed potatoes 86, and red-skin boiled potatoes 88. Given that the glycemic index plays a significant role in the development of weight gain and obesity, we always want to choose the foods with the lowest glycemic index that our children will eat. The glycemic load of food plays a subtle but determining role in the effects on our body of the foods we choose, so choose carefully.

There are no vegetables that are off-limits in Phase 1, unless you have a known allergy or sensitivity. The only caveat is nonorganic soy or corn. Practically all the soy and corn grown in this country is genetically modified, and that in itself can cause intestinal permeability: You need to read labels carefully and look for organic, which is always GMO-free.

Good vegetable choices for Phase 1 include:

- Artichoke, globe
- Artichoke, hearts

- Artichoke, Jerusalem
- Arugula

- Asparagus
- Avocado
- Beans (all varieties)
- Beets and beet greens
- Bok choy
- Broccoli
- Broccoli rabe
- Brussels sprouts
- Cabbage
- Carrots
- Cauliflower
- Celery
- Collard greens
- Corn—organic only!
- Cucumbers
- Eggplant
- Fennel
- Fiddlehead ferns
- Garlic
- Jicama
- Kale
- Leeks
- Lettuce
- Mushrooms
- Mustard greens
- Onions
- Parsnips
- Peas
- Peppers (all varieties)
- Potatoes
- Pumpkin
- Radishes
- Rhubarb
- Romaine lettuce
- Rutabaga
- Sea vegetables
- Shallots
- Soy (edamame, tofu, etc.)—organic only!
- Spinach
- Squash
- Sugar snap peas
- Sweet potato (yams)
- Swiss chard
- Tomatoes
- Turnips and turnip greens
- Watercress
- Zucchini

Animal Proteins

Our first priority when choosing protein sources is to avoid eating animals that have been grain-fed. The best option comes from animals that have been grass-fed and pastured that you can buy directly from a local farm; the second best choice is organic. For example, grass-fed beef has four times more omega-3s than corn-fed beef. For a source of good meat near you, contact a Weston A. Price Foundation chapter leader, or visit your local farmers' market. Another great resource for information is americangrassfed.org.

When choosing proteins, a critical concept is the biological value (BV), the proportion of absorbed protein from a food that becomes incorporated into the proteins of our body. There is a reason why eggs are called "the perfect food"—their BV is 100 percent. That means that our bodies can use all of the protein in an egg (as long as we do not have an allergy or sensitivity to them). Cow's milk has a biological value of 91 percent—that's why it has always been considered a healthy option for children, as protein is the essential building block for growth. The problem, of course, is that the immune system can recognize milk as a toxin; it may be easy to use the protein, but it's not a food we are supposed to be eating. Fish has a BV of 83 percent. Casein (one of the proteins in milk often found in protein powders) has a BV of 80 percent. Beef is 80 percent. Soy is 74 percent. Chicken is 79 percent. Wheat is 54 percent. The BV of beans is below 50 percent.

These numbers point out how hard it is to get enough usable protein by following a vegetarian diet. This is one reason why vegetarians are often the sickest patients I see. They are typically protein deficient. However, the European Food Information Council has found that when two vegetable proteins are combined in one meal, the amino acids of one protein can compensate for the limitations of the other, resulting in a combination of a higher biological value. That is why many different cultures serve nonmeat sources of protein together. Mexican beans and corn, Japanese soybeans and rice, Cajun red beans and rice, or Indian dal and rice combine legumes with grains to provide a meal that is high in all essential amino acids.

Whenever possible, avoid factory-farmed meats and fish that contains antibiotics and hormones. We've all heard how valuable fish is to eat. It has a high biological value, is loaded with the good fats that feed our brain exactly what it needs for optimum growth and function, and reduces our risk of cardiovascular disease. As a matter of fact, of all of the vitamins and minerals that you can take, nutritionists worldwide agree that it is the omega-3s found in high concentrations in cold-water fish that are the most ideal. They are cardioprotective, reduce high cholesterol, and are a primary raw material for healthy brain cells.

The healthiest choices are wild-caught fish; avoid the farm-raised varieties. In one study, scientists analyzed two metric tons of farmed and wild salmon, looking for toxic PCBs, dieldrins, toxaphenes, dioxins, and chlorinated pesticides. Almost all of the contaminants that were found in farmed salmon (13) are known as probable or possible human carcinogens, according to the Environmental Protection Agency (EPA)[4]. Farm-raised salmon has six times the omega-6s fats. We need a little, but not too much of the omega-6s. In excess, they may be linked to coronary artery disease. The studies suggest we lose about two-thirds of the cardioprotective benefits of healthy fats with farm-raised salmon.[5]

Just take a look at the summary statement from another study published in the *Journal of Nutrition*: "Young children, women of child-bearing age, pregnant women, and nursing mothers concerned with health impairments such as reduction in IQ and other cognitive and behavioral effects can minimize contaminant exposure by choosing the least contaminated wild salmon or by selecting other sources of (n-3) fatty acids."[6] Again, eat wild-caught fish or look for other sources of omega-3s—avoid the farm-raised fish.

I had the privilege of meeting Randy Hartnell a number of years ago. Randy was a salmon fisher in Alaska who decided to make the highest-quality seafood possible available to the world. He's put together a group of fishermen in Alaska who sell their catch through one company, Vital Choice Wild Seafoods and Organics (vitalchoice.com). You really can taste the difference. And they have the safest canned tuna that is almost free of mercury contamination I've ever found—it's great for kids' tuna fish sandwiches on gluten-free bread.

Unless you can make them yourself, avoid processed meats like hot dogs, bacon, sausage, jerky, or luncheon meats. Often these foods are flavored with sugar, contain gluten as a binding agent, and are laced with preservatives.

Eggs can be used for a wide variety of quick and healthy meals. Look for ones that are marked "free range and organic." Not only are these eggs healthier, they taste better and look a little different: The yolk has an orange tinge instead of a pure yellow color.

Good protein choices for meats, poultry, and fish for Phase 1 include:

- Beef
- Bison/buffalo
- Boar
- Chicken
- Duck
- Eggs (any variety)
- Goose
- Lamb
- Pork
- Turkey
- Veal
- Venison

THE TRUTH ABOUT FISH

Fish, which is an extremely beneficial food source because of its good fats, is another casualty of environmental pollution. The majority of scientists, the EPA, and the FDA are in agreement that pregnant women, women who might become pregnant, breastfeeding women, infants, and young children need to be extremely cautious in their fish selection and volume consumed. There is convincing evidence of serious problems for a baby's in utero developing brain from mercury exposure (methyl mercury, to be exact), which continues after birth. The same type of brain and nerve development problems occur in infants and young children exposed to fish high in mercury. Dioxins and polychlorinated biphenyls present in contaminated and farm-raised fish may also present a risk for both infants and adults.

In 1988, my 5-year-old son suffered from a resistant anemia that couldn't be addressed through the usual protocols. I researched extensively and discovered that mercury toxicity could produce these symptoms. But I couldn't imagine how my son could have high mercury levels. We lived in a good neighborhood, and his food was always the highest quality. I checked anyway, and sure enough, his mercury levels were sky-high. Where was he getting this from? Well, even back in 1988, early studies were showing that tuna was measuring higher levels of mercury, and he had a tuna fish sandwich every day in kindergarten! Once we eliminated the tuna and chelated the mercury from his system, his resistant anemia was gone.

The National Resources Defense Council (NRDC) has put together "The Smart Seafood Buying Guide," which details five ways to ensure the fish you eat is healthy for you and good for the environment. The guidelines include: think small, buy American, diversify your choices, eat local, and be vigilant. It's an excellent publication to read.[7] And below are some general rules that I believe will help protect you and your family.

In general, fish is a good source of food, especially if you make smart choices. The majority of epidemiological studies have proven that the benefits of fish intake exceed the potential risks with the exception of a few selected species in sensitive populations.

Whenever possible, use the best sources you can find. Choose these types of fish identified by the NRDC as the "least mercury" fish types.

Low Mercury: Enjoy These Fish Often

Anchovies
Butterfish
Catfish
Clam
Crab (domestic)
Crawfish/crayfish
Croaker (Atlantic)
Flounder*
Haddock (Atlantic)*
Hake
Herring
Mackerel (North Atlantic, chub)
Mullet
Oyster

Perch (ocean)
Plaice
Pollock
Salmon (canned)**
Salmon (fresh)**
Sardine
Scallop*
Shad (American)
Shrimp*
Sole (Pacific)
Squid (calamari)
Tilapia
Trout (freshwater)
Whitefish
Whiting

Moderate Mercury: Eat Six Servings or Fewer per Month

Bass (striped, black)
Carp
Cod (Alaskan)*
Croaker (white Pacific)
Halibut (Atlantic)*
Halibut (Pacific)
Jacksmelt (silverside)
Lobster
Mahi mahi

Monkfish*
Perch (freshwater)
Sablefish
Skate*
Snapper*
Tuna (canned chunk light)
Tuna (skipjack)*
Weakfish (sea trout)

High Mercury: Eat Three Servings or Fewer per Month

Bluefish
Grouper*
Mackerel (Spanish, gulf)

Sea bass (Chilean)*
Tuna (canned albacore)
Tuna (yellowfin)*

Highest Mercury: Avoid Eating

Mackerel (king)

Marlin*

Orange roughy*

Shark*

Swordfish*

Tilefish*

Tuna (bigeye, ahi)*

*Fish in trouble! These fish are perilously low in numbers or are caught using environmentally destructive methods. To learn more, see the Monterey Bay Aquarium and the Safina Center (formerly Blue Ocean Institute) Web sites, both of which provide guides to fish to enjoy or avoid on the basis of environmental factors.

**Farmed salmon may contain PCBs, chemicals with serious long-term health effects.

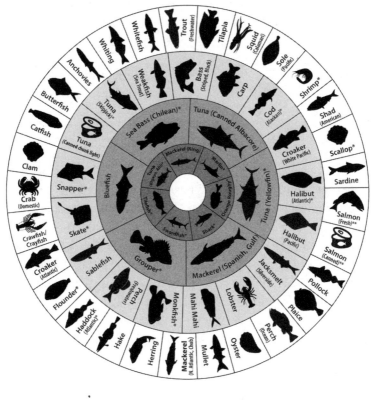

☐ **Enjoy these fish**

☐ **MODERATE MERCURY**
Eat six servings or less per month

▨ **HIGH MERCURY**
Eat three servings or less per month

■ **HIGHEST MERCURY**
Avoid eating

Healthy Fats

Coconut and coconut products have become synonymous with Paleo diets, for good reason. Coconut oil, coconut butter, coconut milk, coconut cream, and so on are loaded with healthy fats and are shelf stable. Coconut's creamy texture is great for dairy-free cooking. Because of its high fat content, you can substitute coconut milk in any recipe that calls for a dairy equivalent.

The least processed options for cooking oils are clearly labeled as extra-virgin or cold-pressed. Look for oils sold in UV-protected bottles so they won't go rancid quickly. One of the primary cautions for cooking with oils is to make sure you do not heat them to smoking levels. When oils begin to smoke, they are becoming oxidized and produce high amounts of free radicals. So you want healthy oils that have a higher heating point before they smoke. Good choices for Phase 1 include:

- Avocado oil
- Coconut oil
- Ghee
- Macadamia oil
- Olive oil

Flours for Baking

Once you get comfortable with Phase 1, you can explore lots of home baking to replicate some of your old favorites. You can make your own gluten-free breads and muffins that taste exactly like the muffins you used to eat—and are better for you. The following flours are allowed on a gluten-free diet (unless you have a sensitivity to them) as long as the packaging is clearly marked as "gluten-free" and there are no added sugar or dairy ingredients (as in a pancake mix):

- Amaranth flour
- Arrowroot flour
- Bean flour
- Brown rice flour
- Buckwheat
- Corn flour or meal
- Millet flour
- Plaintain flour
- Potato flour and starch
- Quinoa flour

- Sweet potato flour
- Sweet rice flour

- Tapioca starch

Fermented Foods

You benefit from eating a forkful of fermented foods every day. This is an excellent strategy for rebuilding and maintaining healthy gut bacteria: The foods themselves supply and produce probiotic bacteria that are then introduced into your digestive tract.

In Chapter 10, you will find recipes and instructions that show how easy it is to make your own fermented vegetables. The typical sauerkraut that we purchase at the supermarket has sodium benzoate in it, which stops the fermentation. A few brands available at your grocer are genuinely fermented and free of sugars or additives. Look for some of my favorites, like Gold Mine Natural Food, Farmhouse Culture, Divina Organic, Eden Foods, Wildbrine, and Bubbie.

Fermented foods should be sold in airtight containers or purchased fresh at an olive bar in the grocery store. This type of storage allows the vegetables to ferment without producing mold that can trigger histamines that some people react to (including rashes, digestive upset, and inflammation). Good choices include:

- Coconut kefir
- Naturally fermented pickles (which are different from pickles, which are made with malt vinegar that may contain gluten)
- Kimchi
- Kombucha
- Olives
- Pickled ginger
- Sauerkraut

GETTING GLUTEN OUT OF YOUR DIET

A critical component of the Transition Protocol is being completely gluten-free. A gluten-free diet avoids the grains that contain gluten: primarily wheat, along with rye, barley, spelt, and kamut. There's no reason why you can't have rice or other gluten-free grains during this 3-week period, unless you know you have a sensitivity to them. You may have already been told by a doctor, or figured out yourself, that you are sensitive to rice, corn, or even quinoa. If so, add those to the "no" list.

Oats do not contain toxic gluten. However, when you purchase oats off the shelf, it's very likely there is gluten in them because of cross-contamination. Either the fields where they are grown are contaminated (the farmer grew wheat in that same field in previous years), the trucks that transport the oats to the manufacturing facility transported wheat the previous week and the trucks weren't cleaned between deliveries, or the manufacturing facility processes both wheat and oats on their assembly lines. In a study published in the *New England Journal of Medicine* that looked at four different samples of oats from three different companies (one organic, one where the oats were manufactured in an oats-only facility so there was no chance of cross-contamination, and one very famous large manufacturer), only 2 of 12 samples were free from toxic levels of gluten.[8] There are companies that take pride in the fact that their oats are gluten-free: They take the extra step. Bob's Red Mill, GF Harvest (glutenfreeoats.com), and Trader Joe's whole grain gluten-free rolled oats are some of my favorites.

I'm not going to lie: Going gluten-free is a challenge at first. Wheat is everywhere in our Western diet, including pasta, snack foods, breakfast cereals, most breads, condiments, sauces, thickeners and stabilizers used in soups, frozen foods, and processed meats. The following lists, and the meal plans and recipes in Chapter 10, will make the transition easier. It just takes a bit of planning.

My friend Melinda Dennis is the nutrition coordinator of the Celiac Center at Beth Israel Deaconess Medical Center, a division of Harvard Medical School. She reminded me that it's important to replace the wheat you are leaving out of your diet with lots of healthy proteins and fiber-rich vegetables, as we listed on pages 165 to 168. She believes, as I do, that if you completely pull wheat out of your diet, you lose a tremendous amount of prebiotic fiber, B vitamins, and iron. If you move from wheat to a gluten-free diet and you don't pay particular attention to what you are substituting, you're setting yourself up for failure with potential nutrient deficiencies and development of an unhealthy microbiome. You might even gain weight, depending on the gluten-free foods you choose to modify your diet with.

Avoid These Foods Entirely *Unless* Labeled Gluten-Free, Dairy-Free, and Sugar-Free

Food manufacturers have jumped on the bandwagon with hundreds of gluten-free products. The problem is that they are usually just as bad as their gluten-containing counterparts, but for different reasons. These foods are often made with highly refined carbohydrates, sugar, and various chemicals. As is the case with fat-free foods, once the manufacturers take out one ingredient, they have to replace it with something else that offers the similar flavor, consistency, or mouthfeel. Gluten-free products often contain a ton of filler in an effort to add flavor. So as tempting as gluten-free pastries sound, we have to avoid them due to their high sugar content. Here are other gluten-containing store-bought foods you should avoid:

- Beer
- Bouillon cubes
- Bread
- Cake
- Candy
- Cereal
- Cookies
- Couscous
- Crackers
- Croutons
- Gravy
- Imitation meats or seafood
- Oats not labeled as gluten-free
- Pasta
- Pie
- Salad dressing
- Soy sauce

Always Look for a Gluten-Free Label

The majority of packaged foods with a gluten-free label are in fact safe for you to eat. In a 2014 study appearing in the journal *Food Chemistry*, three FDA scientists demonstrated that 97.3 percent of gluten-free foods were correctly labeled.[9] This means that the guidelines are working at the industry level and the requirements by the FDA are being met. That sounds great. But if you're a person with celiac disease and you eat one of the 3 percent of products that are contaminated with toxic levels of gluten, you may experience an immune reaction that you think comes out of the blue, and you will never know why you're having a relapse because you've been working extra hard at eating gluten-free.

According to a directive by the FDA, all packaged foods labeled as gluten-free must contain fewer than 20 parts per million (ppm) of gluten. However, in the same 2014 study referenced on page 175, researchers found that among the foods that should naturally be gluten-free (not those labeled gluten-free), such as rice pasta, for which the ingredients are only rice, salt, and water, 24.7 percent still had toxic levels of gluten. That's one out of four foods that you may think are safe choices, yet aren't. This inadvertent exposure is a primary reason that some people don't heal even when they follow a strict gluten-free diet. In fact, only 8 percent of people with celiac disease heal completely on a gluten-free diet; another 65 percent will heal the shags but will still have inflammation causing intestinal permeability. The likely culprit is these types of inadvertent exposures to gluten. That's what makes this topic of hidden gluten so critical for those with a sensitivity—with every exposure, you run the risk of months of elevated antibodies destroying tissue wherever your weak link is.

Last, when a product has been labeled as gluten-free, the equipment used tests only for alpha-gliadin, the most common peptide fragment of poorly digested wheat. Yet elevated alpha-gliadin antibodies are present in only 50 percent of those diagnosed with celiac disease; the other celiac patients are reacting to other peptides. But the equipment only tests for alpha-gliadin. Thus the term "gluten-free" is a misnomer in the industry. The accurate term would be alpha-gliadin–free. This makes food labeled as gluten-free more than slightly suspect for at least 50 percent of those with a non-alpha-gliadin sensitivity to wheat.

For all of these reasons, I highly recommend that you avoid as much processed foods as possible during Phase 1. For the next 3 weeks, you are better off preparing your own foods by using ingredients as they occur in nature, like fresh vegetables, fruit, and animal proteins.

REVIEW INGREDIENTS CAREFULLY

The following list contains some of the tricky ingredients people don't always know to look for. All of these ingredients are wheat in disguise.

- Abyssinian hard wheat (*Triticum durum*)
- Ale
- Atta flour
- Barley (*Hordeum vulgare*)
- Barley enzymes
- Barley flakes
- Barley grass

- Barley groats
- Barley malt
- Barley malt extract
- Barley malt flavoring
- Barley pearls
- Beer
- Bleached flour
- Bran
- Bread crumbs
- Bread flour
- Breading
- Brewer's yeast
- Brown flour
- Bulgur
- Bulgur wheat
- Cereal binding
- Cereal extract
- Chilton
- Club wheat (*Triticum aestivum* subspecies *compactum*)
- Couscous
- Croutons
- Dinkel wheat
- Disodium wheatgermamido peg-2 sulfosuccinate
- Durum wheat (*Triticum durum*)
- Edible coatings
- Edible films
- Edible starch
- Einkorn (*Triticum monococcum*)
- Emmer (*Triticum dicoccon*)
- Enriched bleached flour
- Enriched bleached wheat flour
- Enriched flour
- Farina
- Farina graham
- Farro
- Filler
- Flour (normally this is wheat)
- Fu (dried wheat gluten)
- Germ
- Gluten
- Glutenin
- Graham flour
- Granary flour
- Hard wheat
- *Hordeum vulgare* extract
- Hydrolyzed wheat gluten
- Hydrolyzed wheat protein
- Hydrolyzed wheat starch
- Kamut (Khorasan)
- Kluski pasta
- Lager
- Macaroni wheat
- Macha wheat
- Maida (Indian wheat flour)
- Malt
- Malted barley flour
- Malted milk
- Malt extract
- Malt flavoring
- Malt syrup

- Malt vinegar
- Matzah meal
- Matzo
- Meripro 711
- Mir
- Nishasta
- Oriental wheat (*Triticum turanicum*)
- Orzo pasta
- Pasta
- Persian wheat (*Triticum carthlicum*)
- Perungayam
- Polish wheat (*Triticum polonicum*)
- Poulard wheat (*Triticum turgidum*)
- Roux
- Rusk
- Rye
- Rye flour
- Secale
- Seitan
- Self-rising flour
- Semolina
- Shot wheat (*Triticum aestivum sphaerococcum*)
- Sooji
- Spelt
- Sprouted barley
- Sprouted wheat
- Steel-ground flour
- Stone-ground flour
- Stout
- Strong flour
- Tabbouleh/tabouli
- Teriyaki sauce
- Timopheevi wheat (*Triticum timopheevii*)
- Triticale x triticosecale
- *Triticum aestivam*
- *Triticum vulgare*
- *Triticum vulgare* (wheat) flour lipids
- *Triticum vulgare* germ oil
- Udon noodles
- Unbleached flour
- Vavilovi wheat (*Triticum aestivum*)
- Vital wheat gluten
- Wheat (Abyssinian hard *Triticum durum*)
- Wheat amino acids
- Wheat atta
- Wheat bran extract
- Wheat durum triticum
- Wheat germ extract
- Wheat germ glycerides
- Wheat germ oil
- Wheatgrass
- Wheat groats
- Wheat nuts
- Wheat protein
- Wheat sprouts
- Wheat starch
- Whole-meal flour

WHAT ABOUT WHEATGRASS JUICE?

There has been much written about the healing benefits of wheatgrass juice. To me, it is indisputable that for some people, the high-antioxidant and healing qualities of wheatgrass juice are real. But is it safe during Phase 1? The answer is yes and no.

At about day 17 of the wheat sprout's life, the genes for protein synthesis are activated, and the plant will start producing gluten and other proteins. If you harvest your own wheatgrass between days 11 to 14, it should be safe for those with a gluten sensitivity. But with commercial wheatgrass juice, there is no way of telling when the wheatgrass was harvested. So if you want the healing benefits of wheatgrass juice, it is safer to grow your own.

- Whole wheat berries
- Whole wheat couscous
- Whole wheat flour
- Whole wheat pasta

COOKING INGREDIENTS THAT MAY CONTAIN GLUTEN

Manufacturers introduce gluten to lots of foods you wouldn't think twice about cooking with on a gluten-free diet. These are the type of questions we get all the time (i.e., "Is vanilla extract okay?"). The answer: Some brands contain gluten—you have to check. Some of these ingredients are used in the recipes in Chapter 10, so be sure to purchase versions clearly marked as gluten-free on the label. If you have to eat or use gluten-free packaged foods, avoid those with long lists of unfamiliar ingredients, especially if they contain any of the following terms:

Avena sativa	Additionally may have been contaminated by other grains
Baking powder	May contain wheat starch

Bicarbonate of soda	May contain wheat starch
Bouillon	May contain gluten
Broth	May contain gluten
Brown rice syrup	May contain barley
Caramel color	May be derived from highly processed wheat or barley, usually gluten-free in North America
Caramel flavoring	May contain gluten depending on manufacturing, usually gluten-free in North America
Carob	May contain barley
Cellulose	May be derived from gluten-containing grain
Cereal	May consist of gluten-containing grain
Cider	May utilize barley in production
Citric acid	May be derived from wheat (or corn/beet sugar/molasses)
Clarifying agents	May contain a gluten-containing grain or by-product
Codex wheat starch	A highly processed wheat starch with gluten removed
Crisped rice cereals	May contain barley
Curry powder	May contain wheat starch
Dextrimaltose	A highly processed starch that can be derived from barley
Dextrin	A highly processed starch that can be derived from wheat (or other starch)
Dextrose	A highly processed starch that can be derived from wheat or barley (or other starch). Gluten source does not need to be labeled in Europe
Edible food coatings and films	May contain wheat starch
Edible paper	May contain wheat starch
Emulsifier	May be derived from gluten-containing grain
Fat replacer	May be derived from wheat
Flavored liquors	May contain gluten
Flavoring	May be derived from gluten-containing grain

Gin	Derived from a combination of distilled grains
Glucose syrup	A highly processed sweetener that can be derived from wheat (or other starch). Is usually derived from corn in North America. Gluten source does not need to be labeled in Europe
Grain alcohol	May be derived from distilled gluten grain
Grain-based vodka	May be derived from distilled rye or wheat
Heeng/Hhng	Usually mixed with wheat flour
Herbal tea	May contain gluten in flavoring, such as barley
Hydrogenated starch hydrolysate	May be derived from wheat
Hydrolyzed plant protein (HPP)	May be derived from wheat
Hydrolyzed protein	May be derived from wheat
Hydrolyzed vegetable protein (HVP)	May be derived from wheat
Hydroxypropylated starch	May be derived from wheat
Kecap/ketjap manis (soy sauce)	May contain wheat
Maltodextrin	May be derived from highly processed wheat
Maltose	May be derived from barley or wheat
Malt vinegar	Derived from barley, contains only traces of gluten due to fermentation process
Miso	May be made from barley
Mixed tocopherols	Commonly derived from wheat germ (or soy)
Modified (food) starch	May be derived from highly processed wheat
Mono- and diglycerides	Wheat may be used as a carrier during processing
Monosodium glutamate (MSG)	May be derived from wheat
Mustard powder	May contain wheat starch
Natural flavoring	May be derived from gluten-containing grain

Perungayam	Usually sold mixed with wheat flour
Pregelatinized starch	May be derived from a gluten-containing grain
Protein hydrolysates	May be derived from a gluten-containing grain
Rice malt	May contain barley
Rice syrup	May contain barley enzymes
Sake	May be derived from distilled wheat, rye, barley
Scotch	May be made from a gluten-containing grain
Seasoning	May contain wheat starch
Smoke flavoring	May contain barley
Soy sauce/shoyu	May contain wheat
Soy sauce solids	May contain wheat
Spice and herb blends	May contain wheat starch
Stabilizers/stabilizing agents	May be derived from gluten-containing grain
Starch	May contain barley
Suet	Suet from a packet contains wheat flour
Tamari	May contain wheat
Textured vegetable protein	May be derived from a gluten-containing grain
Tocopherols	Commonly derived from wheat germ (or soy)
Vanilla extract	May contain grain alcohol
Vanilla flavoring	May contain grain alcohol
Vegetable gum	May be derived from a gluten-containing grain
Vegetable protein	May be derived from a gluten-containing grain
Vegetable starch	May be manufactured using gluten-containing grain
Whiskey	May be derived from distilled wheat, rye, barley (or corn)
Xanthan gum	May be derived from wheat
Yeast extract	May be manufactured using gluten-containing grain

HOW TO GO DAIRY-FREE

The protein structure of cow's milk is eight times the size of the proteins found in human breast milk, which is why so many people have a hard time digesting cow's milk. The protein structure of goat's milk is six times human breast milk.[10] It's not as bad, but it's still not easy to digest. However, some types of animal dairy may be acceptable, if you can find them. According to a 2007 study published in the *Journal of Allergy and Clinical Immunology*, if the milk of an animal has a protein structure that's more than 62 percent similar to human tissue, that milk is more likely to be nonallergenic.[11] These options really do exist. Some ethnic-specialty stores carry good alternatives to cow's milk: camel milk,[12] reindeer milk,[13] and donkey milk.[14]

There are also plenty of animal milk substitutes. I'm not a fan of soy milk, even in its organic form. Although there are studies that show the pros and cons of soy, there is no question of its phytoestrogen impact. These plant-based, estrogen-like molecules from soy bind on receptor sites in the body and act like a weak form of the hormone estrogen. If you have an estrogen deficiency, consuming additional soy may be a good thing. Yet if you have adequate levels of estrogen, or excess levels of estrogen, this may be a bad thing, for both men and women. What's more, the studies that show the benefits of soy come from Asian institutes, where participants ate foods made from whole soybeans. In the process of creating soy milk, key nutrients are lost, and sweeteners including barley malt (which may contain gluten) are added to enhance the taste.

My favorite milk substitute is coconut milk, which is rich in lauric acid, a heart-healthy saturated fat that improves HDL (good) cholesterol. You can also try nut or rice milks, but as a rule of thumb, always choose the unsweetened variety. Flavored milk substitutes labeled "plain" actually have 6 grams (1.5 teaspoons) of added sugar per cup. Flavored varieties can have anywhere from 12 grams (3 teaspoons) to 20 grams (5 teaspoons) per cup. You can get vanilla flavor without the added sugar if you look for the "unsweetened" marker on the label.

The Food Allergen Labeling and Consumer Protection Act requires that all packaged food products that contain milk as an ingredient must list the word *milk* on the label. However, you will still need to read all product labels carefully. Milk is sometimes found in products even if they are labeled as "nondairy." Many nondairy products contain casein (a milk protein that would be listed on a label), including some brands of canned tuna. And some processed meats may contain casein as a binder. Exposure to casein has been linked to migraine headaches.[15] I've seen remarkable improvements when patients with migraines go gluten- and dairy-free. Many times these patients, who may have suffered for years, will become migraine-free inside of a month or two.

Shellfish is sometimes dipped in milk to reduce the fishy odor. Many restaurants put butter on grilled steaks to add flavor. Some medications contain milk protein, so always ask your pharmacist when filling prescriptions and discuss with your doctor before you stop taking any medications.

Most people are not sensitive to the fat molecules in dairy but rather the proteins. If you've ever had lobster or crab legs served in a restaurant, it comes with clarified butter (also called ghee). Ghee is the fats of butter with all of the proteins removed, which is why it is usually okay for someone with a dairy sensitivity and why we allow it in Phase 1.

Avoid foods that contain milk or any of these ingredients:

- Artificial butter flavor
- Au gratin dishes and white sauces
- Baked goods
- Butter, butter fat, butter oil, butter acid, butter ester(s)
- Buttermilk
- Cake mixes
- Caramel candies
- Casein
- Caseinates
- Casein hydrolysate
- Cereals
- Cheese
- Chewing gum
- Chocolate milk

- Cottage cheese
- Cream
- Curds
- Custard
- Diacetyl
- Gelato
- Half-and-half
- Ice cream
- Lactalbumin, lactalbumin phosphate
- Lactic acid starter culture and other bacterial cultures
- Lactoferrin
- Lactose
- Lactulose
- Margarine
- Milk (in all forms: condensed, derivative, dry, evaporated, goat's milk, low-fat, malted, milk fat, nonfat, powdered, protein, skimmed, solids, whole)
- Milk protein hydrolysate
- Nisin
- Nougat
- Pudding
- Recaldent
- Rennet
- Salad dressing
- Sherbet
- Sour cream, sour cream solids
- Sour milk solids
- Tagatose
- Whey
- Whey protein hydrolysate
- Yogurt

THESE INGREDIENTS SOUND LIKE MILK, BUT AREN'T

These ingredients do not contain milk protein and are therefore safe to eat:

- Calcium lactate
- Calcium stearoyl lactylate
- Cocoa butter
- Cream of tartar
- Lactic acid (however, lactic acid starter culture may contain milk)
- Oleoresin
- Sodium lactate
- Sodium stearoyl lactylate

HOW TO GO SUGAR-FREE

We are a sugar-crazed society: Seventy-four percent of food products contain caloric or low-calorie sweeteners, or both. Of all packaged foods and beverages purchased in the United States in 2013, 68 percent (by proportion of calories) contained caloric sweeteners and 2 percent contained low-calorie sweeteners.[16] In my Gluten Summit online interview with Liz Lipski, PhD, academic director of nutrition and integrative health programs at Maryland University of Integrative Health in Laurel, she told me that the average American is eating somewhere between 130 and 145 pounds of sugar in the form of table sugar and high fructose corn syrup every single year. That's more than many adults weigh. When I looked into this topic a little deeper, I discovered that the USDA states that each American consumes an average of 152 pounds of caloric sweeteners per year, which amounts to more than two-fifths of a pound—or 52 teaspoons—per day![17]

With all of the detrimental side effects of refined sugar, and its inclusion in most of the processed foods we eat, it begins to make sense where the unbelievable increased rates of obesity and diabetes come from in our country today.

Raw sugarcane actually has health benefits ranging from protecting the liver from toxic substances to lowering cholesterol to stabilizing blood sugar.[18] Yet when we take this plant with its many antioxidants and flavonoids, and we extract just the crystalline white powder we call sugar, we lose all the protection the plant could give us.

With only a few medical exceptions, we need a little sugar in our diet. But those sugars are supposed to come in the form that they're found in nature, called complex carbohydrates. Refined carbohydrates are the sugars that feed cancer cells. As a matter of fact, there's an entire branch of chemotherapy devoted to reducing sugar's ability to get into cancer cells. Sugar is also a scrub-brush irritant to the intestinal lining, causing a great deal of inflammation (more gasoline on the fire). Excess sugar feeds the wrong kinds of yeast in our bodies and encourages the excessive growth of bad bacteria (dysbiosis), all of which increases gut inflammation, creating the leaky gut.

On Phase 1, you will be avoiding all sugars, including zero-calorie sweeteners, which can be just as damaging as sugar. In a 2014 study published in *Cell Metabolism*, researchers found that the artificial sweetener Splenda dramatically increases the growth of the calorie-hoarding bacteria that trigger weight gain, kills beneficial intestinal bacteria, and blocks the absorption of prescription drugs.[19]

Sugar is as difficult to remove from your diet as gluten because it's as pervasive. To avoid sugar, you have to be diligent about reading ingredient labels on packaged goods: Even spice mixes and rubs sometimes contain sugar. Every fast-food item that I've ever checked includes refined sugar as a primary ingredient—even the salt. This is just another reason why I strongly suggest you use the recipes and meal plans in Chapter 10 and focus on eating only whole foods during Phase 1.

Beverages are one of the biggest hidden sources of sugar. It is loaded into sodas, fruit juices, and milk substitutes (pages 184 to 185), so they must be avoided. A school education program for 7- to 11-year-old children that emphasized drinking more water over sweetened beverages produced a 7.7 percent reduction in the number of kids overweight or obese in 1 year.[20] Diet sodas are no better because of the artificial sweeteners that alter the gut bacteria and encourage more obesity.

Alcoholic beverages are basically liquid sugar—carbohydrates that are either derivatives of wheat (starting on page 179) or sugar (like wine or rum). Alcohol, even fine wines, damages the intestines, leads to intestinal permeability (the leaky gut), and unfavorably alters gut bacteria. If you are on a leaky gut repair protocol, it is important to completely avoid alcohol while your intestinal lining is healing. I recommend that you stay off the hard stuff for the first 3 weeks so you can give your body a break. Afterward, you can experiment with some of the gluten-free wines, beers, and distilled liquors. Or you might realize that you haven't missed them all that much. Now, I'm half Italian. And my grandfather would turn over in his grave if I said no to vino. But we all have to take a realistic evaluation of what are the triggers that take us over the edge. If after the 3-week Phase 1 program you add a glass of wine per day back into your routine and you notice your "feeling good" result is reversing because of the sugar in these drinks, you have to reevaluate the importance of that glass of wine.

Registered dietician Erica Kasuli, director of nutrition for the world-famous Amen Clinics, taught me to think differently about this journey of tweaking what you eat. She gave me a great line that I use with my patients: "Don't erase. Replace." In this case, instead of using sugar-filled mayonnaise, ketchup, or barbecue sauces, switch to homemade guacamole or salsa or hummus. Little changes can lead to big results. So if you want to do some gluten-free baking, replace sugar with raw honey, which is very different from refined honey. Raw honey contains an entire family of nutrients and compounds: It's a whole food. Local raw honey is always preferred, as it has preventive characteristics to the local pollens you may be sensitive to.

Hidden Sources of Sugar

Beware of these ingredients.

- Agave syrup
- All-natural sweetener
- Amulet
- Aspartame
- Auamiel
- Barbados molasses
- Barbados sugar
- Beet sugar
- Brown sugar
- Cane sugar
- Cane syrup
- Caramel
- Caramel color
- Clarified grape juice
- Concentrated fruit juice
- Confectioners' sugar
- Cornstarch
- Corn sweetener
- Corn syrup
- Dark brown sugar
- Date sugar
- Date syrup
- Dextrine
- Dextrose

- Disaccharides
- Evaporated cane juice
- Fig syrup
- Filtered honey
- Fructose
- Fruit juice concentrate
- Fruit sugar
- Fruit sweetener
- Galactose
- Glucose
- Glycerine
- Granulated sugar
- Grape sugar
- Guar gum
- Heavy syrup
- High fructose corn syrup
- Hydrogenated glucose syrup
- Invert sugar
- Invert sugar syrup
- Jaggery
- Lactose
- Levulose
- Light brown sugar

- Light sugar
- Light syrup
- Lite sugar
- Lite syrup
- Mannitol
- Modified food starch
- Monosaccharides
- Natural syrup
- Nectars
- Polysaccharides
- Powdered sugar
- Raisin syrup
- Raw sugar
- Ribbon cane syrup
- Ribose
- Rice malt
- Rice syrup
- Saccharine
- Sorbitol
- Sorghum molasses
- Sorghum syrup
- Soy
- Splenda
- Succanat
- Sucrose
- Turbinado sugar
- White sugar
- Xylitol

Watch Out for Withdrawal Symptoms

People occasionally report that they experience withdrawal symptoms during the first few days or so of Phase 1, feeling tired, depressed, or nauseated. Some don't want to exercise, and some have headaches (just like with coffee withdrawal). This is especially true of those who in their blood tests have elevated levels of the peptide in wheat called gluteomorphin or elevated levels of the peptide in dairy called casomorphin. These poorly digested peptides can stimulate the opiate receptors in the gut and brain. Opiate receptors trigger the production of hormones called endorphins and enkephalins that produce that feel-good response. Remember the last time you laughed out loud in a movie or with your friends? Perhaps you even had belly laughter—when you laugh so hard your belly hurts? Remember how good you felt after that? It's because your opiate receptors were stimulated and you now have a little more endorphins circulating in your bloodstream. Well, gluten and dairy can mildly stimulate these same receptors. And just as an addict may have withdrawal symptoms when they stop their drug of choice, such may be the case with gluten and dairy withdrawal. My friend William Davis, MD, author of *Wheat Belly*, even came up with a name for it: wheat withdrawal. The same may be true for removing dairy or sugar.

If this happens to you, don't be surprised. First of all, this may be the first time you had to give up some of your favorite comfort foods cold turkey. And these favorite foods become comfort foods for a reason: Sugar-laden foods, especially refined carbohydrates, are highly addictive. Your body is actually going through a gliadin-casein-sugar–derived opiate withdrawal.

I've found that a small percentage of people might feel tired, depressed, or even nauseated for about 2 to 5 days after they stop eating wheat, dairy, and sugar. They can't exercise and often have headaches. It's the same mechanism as the 2- to 3-day withdrawals that so many folks experience when they give up coffee. That's why the comprehensiveness of the 3-week transition is so important and why I made sure the recipes taste great. I want everyone to stay on the program and notice how much better they feel.

Dr. Davis believes that wheat withdrawal can be quite unpleasant for close to 40 percent of the population. That has not been my clinical experience. Our number has been closer to 10 percent, which is still a substantial number. You may have a friend or family member who has tried to go gluten-free and has told you, "My body must need wheat. It's been 3 days since I've had anything made of wheat, and I feel awful!" This response can be scary. But remember, it's not that the body needs wheat; it *craves* it. This is just the body craving a toxic substance that it has gotten accustomed to. Don't worry: The symptoms will disappear quickly. And best of all, the cravings for sugar and wheat will subside, and then you feel wonderful!

To lessen withdrawal symptoms:

- Stay well hydrated. There is a diuretic effect when you stop eating wheat, dairy, and sugar. If you lose weight the first week, about half that will be water from excess inflammation.
- Season your food with a little more salt than usual. A few people develop leg cramps during Phase 1, and a bit of sea salt can prevent this. Nothing major: Just an extra pinch of salt per day will do the trick (unless your doctor has told you otherwise). Try putting the salt directly on your tongue. If you are sodium deficient and can get past the belief that "any salt is bad for you" (which is the furthest thing from true), you may notice that it tastes really good and you'd like a little more. Body language never lies.

And it won't take long before you can tell the difference between a message from your body to fill a true nutrient insufficiency (need for a little salt), and a craving for a stimulatory toxin (gluten).

- Stay calm. Start this program when life is not at the peak of stressfulness. Don't begin this new routine the same day you start a new job or end a relationship. Giving yourself permission to launch this new program when you feel comfortable can lessen your body burden and reduce your withdrawal symptoms.

- Keep moving. Exercise will take your mind off your symptoms and create the endorphins you are looking for in a much healthier way.

FAQS ABOUT PHASE I FOODS

Here are some of the most common questions I receive from my patients about Phase 1 and autoimmunity diets in general.

Q. I've already tried Paleo. What's the difference between Paleo and this program?

A. Even though the Transition Protocol shares some of the same properties as Paleo, it's a dramatically different approach. One of the primary differences is that the Paleo diet is strictly no grains. During Phase 1, you can enjoy rice and other grains. Just avoid wheat, rye, and barley.

Q. Can't I have just a little bit of wheat or dairy or sugar?

A. You're not going to like the answer, but it's a firm no. There is no such thing as being mostly good during this transition. It is an all-or-nothing experiment. Little mistakes or cheats can sabotage your chances at feeling better, as all it takes is the tiniest speck of gluten, sugar, or dairy to keep the immune system on red alert and inflammation raging. Less than $\frac{1}{8}$ thumbnail of a toxin like gluten has the ability to activate the inflammatory cascade, which will last for 2 to 6 months.

I want to share one of my favorite patient stories from the medical literature. A 34-year-old woman had been diagnosed with celiac disease. Her blood markers for both celiac disease and gluten sensitivity were sky-high, and an endoscopy showed that her microvilli were completely worn down. Her health history revealed that she was always the shortest girl in the class growing up and was one of the last to start her period (all factors that are lumped together by doctors as *failure to thrive*). More recently, she had recurrent hair loss and anemia, chronic fatigue, and early-onset osteoporosis. Her doctors put her on a gluten-free diet, but when she came back to check in a year later, she wasn't feeling any better. The examination revealed no improvement in either her bloodwork or a new endoscopy. The doctors asked if she was adhering to the diet, and the woman reported, "Absolutely. I've been meticulous about what I eat." Everyone was completely baffled, and they were about to label her with refractory sprue, meaning celiac disease that doesn't heal, which is connected to a very high risk of fatal cancer.

Finally, one doctor asked, "Are you a religious woman?" It turns out that this woman was in fact a nun dressed in street clothes. Even though she was following a gluten-free diet, she was still taking the communion wafer, and she refused to give up taking this sacrament.

The doctors got hold of a communion wafer and analyzed its gluten content. When they broke it up into a typical serving, each piece contained just a milligram of gluten, approximately ⅛ a thumbnail in size. That tiny amount of gluten was all it took to keep this woman feeling sick and tired.

Unbeknownst to the scientists, the bishop made the nun give up communion. Eighteen months later, she returned to the clinic, and she was in radiant health. Her hair was rich and full, and her energy was better than ever. The osteoporosis was gone, and upon examination, the doctors were thrilled to see that her microvilli were completely healed. Her blood values were normal.[21]

Hopefully you can now see why I'm so adamant about going completely gluten-free. There is no "cheat day" on this program. However, chances are very good that you will feel so much better that you'll wonder why you were eating the foods that clearly made you sick all along.

Q. How will I know which of these three foods I'm sensitive to?

A. After week 6, you will reintroduce a sample of one of these foods all by itself. A good place to start would be a packet of sugar in your tea, a glass of milk, or a handful of croutons. Once you clean up your diet and start functioning more as the body that you're designed to have or the brain that you're designed to think with, and you have an exposure, you may feel the symptoms more dramatically and quickly.

If you can add back a type of food and do not experience any symptoms, then you are not sensitive to that food and can probably go back to eating it without any problems. However, if you add a food type back and you begin to notice symptoms, such as fatigue, achiness, fluid retention (sock marks), stuffy nose, rash, or whatever symptom you had before, then that food will have to be eliminated for at least 3 to 6 months, if not longer, in an attempt to fully reset your immune system to that particular type of food. You'll learn more about how to add foods back to your diet in Chapter 11.

Hopefully you will be among the majority of people for whom this diet makes them feel permanently fabulous. Nothing makes me happier than when a patient says, "I followed the Transition Program and felt great. Then I had a piece of pizza and felt terrible!" That's when I congratulate patients on their success and remind them that no one can argue with the body's language: It never lies. Now they understand how to listen to their body when it is exposed to a toxic food. Usually this leads to a stronger resolve to follow the plan. You may also find that after a while, you'll become so in tune with your body that you will notice even the slightest degree of dysfunction. You won't have to be knocked overboard with a symptom before you recognize when your body starts speaking to you.

There is a caveat here. If you have not had the opportunity to do a comprehensive blood test for gluten sensitivity (with or without celiac disease), there is no scientific basis upon which I can say that your avoidance of gluten needs to be lifelong. It is when you have elevated antibodies to gluten that you make memory B cells to gluten that never forget—that's when you have a lifelong sensitivity. But if you haven't done the test, we can't say it's a permanent avoidance.

Q. How am I supposed to drink my morning coffee?

A. First, I don't want you to overdo caffeine, which can contribute to gut inflammation, leaky gut, and bacterial infections. I'm not saying give up coffee entirely, but if you're one of those people who are drinking it all day, you are damaging your gut. Studies showing that

1 cup of coffee per day is a problem are rare. After 1 cup, the risk for illness caused by inflammation is higher as you drink more.

Start by looking at your choice of coffee: Some brands of instant coffee are contaminated with gluten. If you don't like to drink black coffee, try it with one of the acceptable milk substitutes listed above. My personal preference is Native Forest unsweetened organic coconut cream (which can also be whipped for whipped cream). If you must sweeten your coffee, try it with a bit of raw honey.

Q. What if I'm hungry all the time?

A. First, rule out a parasite. Then focus on food selections. The type of food that lasts the longest in your digestive tract, releasing energy into your bloodstream, is healthy fats—they last for hours. That's why I personally like Dave Asprey's Bulletproof Coffee recipe, featured on his Web site (bulletproofexec.com/bulletproof-coffee-recipe/). Once you start filling your day with satisfying proteins, colorful vegetables and fruits, and healthy fats, you'll see that this program is "feel-good satisfying." In Chapter 10, you'll find plenty of meal ideas and easy recipes so you won't be caught off guard without anything substantial to eat. And because your choices will all be healthy ones, you can snack throughout the day if you're feeling hungry.

I also want you to think about the difference between hunger and deprivation. Hunger can easily be solved with a piece of fruit or a handful of nuts, but deprivation is a mind game. As Erica Kasuli told me, "Instead of thinking that my life was over because I can't eat wheat or dairy, I feel so blessed that I have figured out what the triggers are that are contributing to my symptoms." I'm hoping that you'll discover the same thing. Your symptoms were depriving you of living a full life. Wouldn't you want to know if something as simple as making different food choices could make you feel better?

During an interview on the Gluten Summit (theglutensummit .com), Erica also taught me a great trick for dealing with cravings. She told me, "When I'm working with patients at the Amen Clinics who complain about cravings, I tell them to say in their minds, 'Pause. Take a HALT.' HALT stands for Hungry, Angry, Lonely, or Tired. Ask yourself, 'Why am I eating? Am I going to eat because I'm hungry? Or am I eating because I'm angry at somebody or something? Am I lonely? Am I tired?'

"If you're really hungry, then have some protein because it will give you energy to help stabilize your blood sugar versus having a carbohydrate. If you're angry, maybe write in a journal. If you're lonely, call a friend. If you're tired, take a nap. We don't have to eat to fulfill our body of all these other feelings that we have. It's okay to feel those feelings. And it's better to feel the feelings. Otherwise, we're just eating those feelings. And then it's going to be harder on the digestion because we cannot process the food."

Q. I think I'm gaining weight. What am I doing wrong?

A. Because celiac patients have an inability to absorb nutrients, studies have shown that these people often have an innate preference for a high-fat diet (they crave fat) coupled with a high intake of sweets and soft drinks (they crave energy) and a low intake of vegetables, iron, calcium, and folate.[22] Researchers believe, as I do, that their bodies crave fats and sweets. While you're following this transition phase, you might be experiencing those cravings, and replacing the foods you can't eat with others that are acceptable is a key component to being successful on this plan. I say, "Long live the avocado!" It's going to be your best friend.

However, you have to make good choices in terms of quantity and quality. For example, if in the past you would stop at a coffee shop on your way to work and grab a blueberry muffin, you know you can't continue that habit. But if you start making gluten-free muffins, or see them on display at your coffee shop, you might try one, or even two, because they're technically allowed on the protocol. Unfortunately, these muffins aren't really healthy at all, especially if you don't know all the ingredients they are made with. While they might not contain gluten, they're probably still made with some form of low-nutrition white-paste flour. Gluten-free products are usually not enriched like wheat flours are, so they are of less value to you in terms of being healthy and nutrient dense. That's the primary reason why people gain weight on a gluten-free diet: They mistake gluten-free products for healthy options. A gluten-free muffin is still a muffin.

Even if you aren't celiac, as you avoid sugar, wheat, and dairy, your body may still crave fat. It's okay to listen to your body and eat healthy fats, like avocado. Fat isn't bad for you; bad fats are bad for you. Use good judgment and stay away from obvious unhealthy fats like deep-fried foods, artificial butter used in movie theaters, margarines, and so on.

Q. Since there is a genetic component to autoimmunity, should I have my kids follow this program?

A. Absolutely! The earlier people can clean up their diets, the better. You'll have much better luck being compliant to the plan if everyone in your family is on board. This way, you won't have to prepare separate meals.

Rodney Ford, MD, is a pediatrician, gastroenterologist, and allergist, and he puts children on this type of Phase 1 eating plan all the time. He told me during a Gluten Summit interview that for kids, "going gluten-free is not such a biggie. Children who come to my clinic are sick, tired, and grumpy. They've got sore tummies, acid reflux, migraine, other headaches, maybe vomiting, diarrhea, constipation, eczema, rashes, and more. They are predominantly irritable children, lethargic, lacking energy, and had poor sleep. Some were hyperactive and diagnosed already with attention-deficit disorder or ADHD. Most of them don't test positive for celiac disease. But when I put them on a gluten-free diet, most of them got better."

Even if the symptoms your child may be experiencing are vastly different than your own, the source of the problem may still be one of these three inflammatory foods: gluten, dairy, or sugar. The difference again is where the weak link in your chain is. Your child may have a different weak link than yours, but you can both reverse the damage of autoimmunity by following this program.

> Go to theDr.com/autoimmune for my personal invitation to learn more about living gluten-free and recovering from autoimmune conditions.

THE TRANSITION PROTOCOL CHEAT SHEET: PHASE 1

	Allowed	Not Allowed
Grains	Plain brown and white rice Grains and flours that are packaged and labeled as gluten-free	Nonorganic corn Nonorganic soy
Fruits/Vegetables	All fresh fruits/vegetables Fermented vegetables	Canned or dried fruits or vegetables
Proteins	Fresh meats, poultry, eggs, fish, shellfish Dried beans Unseasoned nuts (in their shell) and seeds packaged and labeled as gluten-free Vital Choice canned tuna	Lunchmeats Breakfast ham, bacon, or sausage Self-basted or cured meat products Canned tuna or chicken Nuts and seeds that are not packaged and labeled as gluten-free
Condiments	Coconut, olive, avocado oils Vinegar Honey Salt	Generic "vegetable" oil Flavored and malt vinegars
Beverages	Water Tea, coffee (unsweetened, no milk added) Unsweetened coconut, hemp, almond, or rice milk Unsweetened fruit juices Kombucha	All sodas, including diet sodas Cow's, goat's, or soy milk Sweetened milk substitutes Sweetened fruit juices Sports drinks

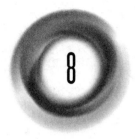

SUPPORTING YOUR TRANSITION

The ultimate goal of the Transition Protocol is to reduce inflammation throughout the body, especially in the intestinal tract, which will set the stage to heal intestinal permeability. Remember, a leaky gut is the gateway for developing autoimmune disease. According to research published in the *Nature Clinical Practices: Gastroenterology and Hepatology*, "The autoimmune process can be arrested if the interplay between genes and environmental triggers is prevented by reestablishing intestinal barrier function."[1] By healing a leaky gut, you are minimizing the passage of toxic bacteria and large food molecules into the body, which is what's causing the immune protective response that creates systemic inflammation.

In this chapter, you'll learn what else you can do, besides making good food choices, to help heal the gut and protect your overall health. By focusing on replenishing the intestinal environment while we reduce the toxic load that is triggering the immune system (stop throwing gasoline on the fire), we will begin to reverse illness. Remember, the fastest-growing cells in the body make up the inside lining of the intestines. That's why it takes only 3 weeks to see improvements: Once the leaky gut begins to heal, you begin your path back to better health. Best of all, these are some of the easiest strategies to put into place to improve your health.

Now that you know what to eat, the next step is to literally put out the fire of inflammation. Even when you stop throwing gasoline on a fire, you still have a fire to extinguish. The nutrients we'll discuss in this

chapter will help lower inflammation and then heal the gut by supporting cellular regrowth.

The right nutrients can help reduce the probability of developing autoimmune diseases, regardless of where you are on the spectrum. So many
people believe they're "feeling fine," even though they have a raging fire
inside. It's just that the condition hasn't destroyed enough tissue yet to
produce obvious symptoms. Yet once you begin healing the gut, even
those who aren't currently experiencing symptoms will feel a lot better.

I'm sure you've read in other books or on the Internet that we are
supposed to "boost" the immune system with nutrients such as antioxidants. That's not entirely correct. The truth is, immune *balancing* is
more important than immune boosting. You don't want to boost the
immune system if you already have an autoimmune disease. You don't
want to suppress the immune system either. You want to balance
immune function so it can protect but not overreact.

When our immune system detects a threat and activates the inflammation response, it produces different chemical bullets known as
cytokines that create the fire to address the threat. One problem in our
medical system today is that the drugs that are often prescribed as
anti-inflammatories typically target one of these specific cytokines, like
nuclear factor–kappaB, or tumor necrosis factor, and they terminate the
production of that cytokine completely. When this happens, we no
longer have the required adequate protection from that cytokine to any
other perceived threat that comes along. In response, the immune system
backup will create more inflammation using a different cytokine or bullet.
This means that while the medication will reduce the progression of
inflammation along the pathway that is connected to that specific cytokine,
excessive systemic inflammation may (and often does) still occur.

If you are in severe crippling pain or a life-threatening autoimmune
cascade, the standard pharmaceutical approach for dealing with autoimmune diseases is to suppress the immune system entirely. While
there is a time and place for these prescription medications, too often the
long-term use of these drugs will suppress the immune system so completely that you end up with an underperforming immune system, which
then cannot protect you from other triggers or irritants that come your
way. Worse, there can be significant side effects to these drugs that affect
other tissues in the body. This is one reason that these powerful medications, which can be helpful in the short term, may have long-term side

effects like cancer or serious bacterial and fungal infections. My counsel has always been, "Ms. or Mr. Patient, let's continue the medications that your previous doctor prescribed because they are helping. *And* let's see if we can reduce the need for these medications."

MEDICATIONS CAN INCREASE YOUR AUTOIMMUNE DISEASE DEVELOPMENT

Some medications can actually accelerate the development of gluten sensitivity and the development of autoimmune diseases. The worst offenders are the category of drugs that suppress acids, ranging from simple, over-the-counter antacids like Maalox to H_2 receptor antagonists, including Zantac, Tagamet, and Pepcid, to the proton pump inhibitors like Prilosec, Prevacid, Nexium, AcipHex, the long-lasting gastric acid suppressors. All of these medications raise our pH and reduce hydrochloric acid. This result increases the likelihood of developing food intolerances and food sensitivities more than one-hundredfold.

Hydrochloric acid is a critically important digestive enzyme. The production of acid in our stomach is supposed to break down foods and activate many signals farther down the intestinal tract. We're designed to house hydrochloric acid in the stomach. If you were to take hydrochloric acid produced in our stomach and put it on a wood table, it would start breaking down the wood. But that same acid can sit in your stomach all day without ever causing a problem. When we interfere with the mucus-producing cells of the stomach (by food exposures, coffee consumption for those who are sensitive to it, phosphoric acid in soda pop, etc.), we start causing stomach damage (like ulcers, heartburn). Instead of treating the stomach with acid suppressors, we can bring balance to this tissue by eliminating the triggers causing the stomach inflammation and loss of mucus cell production and function.

When we interfere with the body's production of digestive enzymes, and couple that with malabsorption from intestinal permeability, it is not possible to get the vitamins and minerals out of our foods in a high enough percentage. It is critical to speak with your doctor about how you are going to ensure good digestion when they recommend antacids, PPIs, or H_2 receptor antagonists.

Our goal in creating a balanced immune system is to allow it to function as it was intended so that you can stay healthy. Remember, to bring balance to an overactive or underperforming immune system, we cannot just take a pill. We must address the lifestyle habits that caused this imbalance (a food sensitivity, an environmental toxin, etc.). It can take months to do this. But once you balance the immune system by continually hitting base hits, your symptoms begin diminishing, your vitality comes back, your sleep improves, and you'll be better equipped to handle the challenges and stresses of everyday life.

NUTRIENTS THAT ATTACK INFLAMMATION AND HEAL AND SEAL THE GUT

The development of inflammation involves the activation of a highly coordinated gene expression program that includes more than 1,100 genes. Remember, inflammation is not bad for you; excess inflammation is bad for you. To address an excessive inflammatory response, you need to modulate your inflammatory genetic expression by turning off as many genes as you can that are inflammatory activators and turning on as many genes as you can that are anti-inflammatory activators. This is the remarkable world of epigenetics—what we do in our environment influences our genes.

The safest way to modulate your genetic expression with the fewest side effects or long-term problems is twofold. First and most important, eat the highest-quality food, preferably organic. Second, supplement your diet with the right nutrients. Natural vitamin and mineral anti-inflammatories are nowhere near as powerful or dangerous as pharmaceutical anti-inflammatories. It's not even on the same scale. It's David to Goliath, bicycles to Ferraris, rowboats to speedboats . . . you get the picture.

Natural anti-inflammatory substances in the form of vitamins, antioxidants, polyphenols, and nutrient supplements—like the epigallocatechin gallate (EGCG) antioxidant polyphenol found mostly in green tea, the lycopene in tomatoes, the curcumin in turmeric, or vitamin C—activate some of the 1,100 genes associated with the inflammatory cascade by either dimming the inflammatory genes or activating the anti-inflammatory genes. They do not shut down the gene activity as completely as pharmaceuticals. Even though they're much weaker, they are still a critical part of a more effective strategy: The team that keeps making base hits wins the ball game. None of them are 90-pound weaklings either—they all hold their own. They're just not overwhelming bullies that come into the body and take over one pathway the way pharmaceuticals can.

Remember the old adage "All roads lead to Rome"? The best course of action to rid the body of chronic inflammation is to take a *pleiotropic approach*: Greek *pleio,* meaning "many," and *trepein,* meaning "to turn, to convert"; thus, many that convert. With an approach that uses many safe, natural substances that activate multiple genes and provide multiple weak benefits, you not only reduce excess inflammation, you also activate the genes to begin the healing process. With this approach, we use multiple natural anti-inflammatories. You just can't use one natural product and expect it to achieve similar results as a pharmaceutical in putting the fire out.

Here's an example—only one of hundreds, but this one has always stuck in my mind. Green tea has been shown to modulate genes to heal intestinal permeability,[2] to protect from the damage of a powerful pharmaceutical that shuts down TNF production (a powerful anti-inflammatory),[3] and to protect the elasticity of your blood vessels (a very important feature).[4] Green tea can protect our thinking capabilities[5] and stabilize our blood sugar levels by protecting our liver.[6] I could go on and on. Green tea, and its active polyphenol EGCG, is a beneficial food/nutrient because it modulates so many genes to produce an anti-inflammatory effect.

Now, quite honestly, I read all of these studies and started to drink green tea once in a while. But one study was the game changer for me. In a 2006 article published in the *Journal of the American Medical Association,* researchers looked at the effect of green tea consumption on the risk of dying from cardiovascular disease and on the risk of dying from anything (known as all-cause mortality). For 11 years, they followed 40,530 adults ages 40 to 79 without history of stroke, coronary heart disease, or cancer at baseline. In terms of all-cause mortality (dying from cancer, heart disease, brain disease, etc.), if men drank 1 to 2 cups of green tea per day, they had a 7 percent reduced risk of dying. Three to 4 cups per day was a 5 percent reduction, and 5 or more cups per day was a 12 percent reduced risk. For women, those who drank 1 to 2 cups of green tea per day had a 2 percent reduced risk of mortality, 3 to 4 cups per day was an 18 percent reduced risk, and 5 or more cups was a 23 percent reduced risk of dying. And when the researchers looked specifically at dying from cardiovascular disease, if men drank 1 to 2 cups per day, they had an 8 percent reduced risk, 3 to 4 cups per day was a 21 percent reduction, and 5 or more cups per day was a 27 percent reduced risk. For women, those who drank 1 to 2 cups of green tea per day had a 26 percentreduced risk of mortality, 3 to 4 cups per day was a 39 percent reduced risk, and 5 or more cups was a 38 percent reduced risk of dying from cardiovascular disease.[7] Those are dramatic numbers, but what do they really mean? Is green tea *the* answer to all of our health concerns? While we don't know for sure, we do know that it activates many genes for an anti-inflammatory net effect. Since reading this study in 2006, I have been trying to drink a little green tea every day. It's a base hit.

A pleiotropic approach (using a number of weak natural products) to addressing intestinal permeability will win the ball game for you. Remember the Polymeal? Pleiotropism is the basis of the Polymeal approach. No single component of the diet by itself will produce that 75 percent risk reduction of heart disease, but the synergy of all the ingredients (a pound of vegetables, dark chocolate, almonds, garlic, fish, and red wine) cumulatively creates that result.

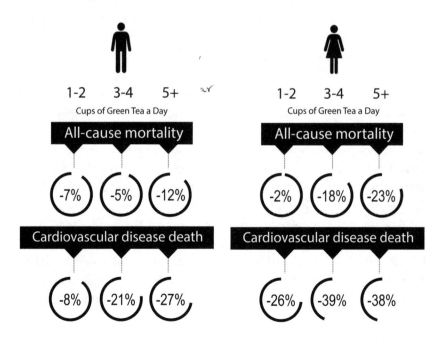

Americans easily take more than 60 billion doses of nutritional supplements every year, and with zero related deaths, this is an outstanding safety record. The most recent data come from the US National Poison Data System's annual report, which tracked data from 57 US poison centers and showed vitamin and mineral supplements caused zero deaths.[8]

There are naysayers who focus on the facts that nutrition is an unregulated field and that some products do not contain what they say they do or the amounts claimed on the label. These complaints are valid. There are crooks in every discipline who will squeeze a profit any way they can. That's why you want to turn to trusted sources for your supplements. Your doctor may know which brands are the highest quality and the safest. But before you ask a doctor that question, you must clarify if that practitioner is the right person to ask.

First, ask your docs how many courses in nutrition they've taken or what was the last nutrition postgraduate seminar they attended. It's an awkward question to ask someone who hasn't taken any courses and really is not qualified to give advice on this topic. We think our doctors are supposed to know everything about our health. That is not a fair expectation. Almost all doctors have an expertise, an area of study they are passionate about and in which they are extremely knowledgeable. But if they do not have a passion for nutrition, unfortunately in the medical field, their training is quite poor.

For example, an article in the journal *Academic Medicine* stated that in 2010, only 28 (27 percent) of the 105 medical schools in the United States met the minimum 25 required nutrition education hours set by the National Academy of Sciences. Six years earlier, in 2004, 40 (38 percent) of 104 schools did so.[9] What does that tell us? First, only one-quarter of medical doctors receive the *minimum* required nutrition education hours set forth by the National Academy of Sciences (and I can guarantee that your doctor does not know if his or her education met the minimum). Second, the trend is going the wrong way.

After reading hundreds of studies showing the benefits of nutrients influencing the genes of inflammation and healing, I have identified 22 different anti-inflammatory nutrients that work together synergistically to lower inflammation and restore the intestinal lining. I have taught this nutrient model to many doctors, who have used it with more than 10,000 patients. There are no side effects to this approach that I'm aware of.

The Gluten Sensitivity Support Packs are a powerful combination of six pills that contain these 22 different nutrients. My formula promotes the creation of healthy tissue in the intestines, the skin, the brain, the joints, the entire digestive system, and nearly every other organ system in the body, and it does not contain any wheat or gluten. You can find these one-of-a-kind packs on my Web site (theDr.com).

There are no contraindications to take this protocol for people who are currently on prescription medications. I recommend taking the GS Pack, or your own version, for a minimum of 6 months, and then retest through the bloodwork described in Chapter 5 to confirm if the abnormal biomarkers have returned to normal. You can also complete the Medical Symptoms Quiz in Chapter 4 once again to see if you can quantify a change.

Although it's very likely that you will begin feeling better almost right away on the Transition Protocol, it takes a while to stop the production of the antibodies, calm down the inflammatory cascade, activate the anti-inflammatory genes, and stimulate the genes for healing. Without the retesting, it is very easy to assume you're "fine" when your symptoms dramatically reduce. Remember, in the spectrum of autoimmune development, there are years of tissue destruction with no symptoms. In autoimmune tissue regeneration, there is also a spectrum of healing that takes time. That's why the minimum is 6 months to a year for you to see noticeable improvements in laboratory testing.[10]

FOCUSING ON KEY NUTRIENTS

Six key nutrients are critical for reversing intestinal permeability. The first three (vitamin D, glutamine, and fish oil) can be found in the GS Packs. The rest are additional supplements you should consider.

1. VITAMIN D: A primary reason why vitamin D is exceptional for healing intestinal permeability is that it supervises the function of the tight junctions, the spaces between the cells in your gut that could allow large, undigested molecules to pass into the bloodstream if you have intestinal permeability. The protein family called zonulin that holds our cells tightly together in the gut works like shoelaces that are supposed to be tied tightly most of the time. The usual mechanism is that the shoelaces loosen a little to let small molecules slide down between the cells to be screened and cleared by security (our immune system) before being allowed into the bloodstream. This is how we're supposed to absorb the vitamins and minerals from our food. However, when the shoelaces are untied, larger food particles called macromolecules slide through the tight junctions into our bloodstream—this is referred to as *pathogenic intestinal permeability*. Macromolecules aren't supposed to get into the bloodstream. That activates the immune system, and in turn you make antibodies to that macromolecule. If it's a macromolecule from chicken, you may become allergic to chicken. If it's a macromolecule from tomato, you may become allergic to tomato. This is why some people do a full IgG panel and come back sensitive to 20-plus foods and say, "Oh no, I'm sensitive to everything I eat!" Of course you are—your immune system is doing exactly what it's supposed to do to protect you. Once you heal the intestinal permeability and do the test again, you'll find that you are sensitive to far fewer foods.

Vitamin D plays a critical role in the tying and untying of the intestinal shoelaces. Without enough vitamin D, the laces won't tie tightly, leading to intestinal permeability. That's one reason why so many autoimmune diseases are more prevalent in countries far from the equator— people in those areas have less exposure to the sun, thus their bodies make less vitamin D. We also know that vitamin D can halt and in many situations reverse the production of deleterious antibodies that might influence some immune-mediated disorders, including dermatitis and asthma.[11]

2. GLUTAMINE: The gastrointestinal tract is by far the greatest user of the amino acid glutamine in the body: The epithelium cells (those fastest-growing cells in the body) use glutamine as their principal metabolic fuel. Glutamine is known to help shield damaged intestines. It has been successfully used with HIV and cancer patients to help them absorb nutrients better and thus gain needed weight. Glutamine turns on a number of genes allowing the gut to heal.

However, if you have a history of yeast infections, you need to carefully monitor the amount of glutamine you take because this amino acid may increase yeast growth. Glutamine is also a raw material for the immune cells that produce a healthy amount of inflammation in our intestines. But if you are already inflamed, glutamine may increase the inflammation (rarely, but it can happen). That is why I always tell my patients, "Ms. or Mr. Patient, rarely, but on occasion, someone will have a sensitivity to the GS Packs. If you don't feel well taking the GS Packs, take the glutamine out for a couple of weeks, keep taking everything else to turn on genes and produce the anti-inflammatory effect, and after a few weeks, reintroduce the glutamine." You can do the same if you are creating your own supplement packs.

3. FISH OILS: Fish oils are remarkably useful because they contain omega-3 fatty acids that turn on or off many genes to produce an anti-inflammatory effect. Fish oils are also known to reduce your risk of cardiovascular disease (mainly stroke and acute myocardial infarction), lower high blood pressure, and enhance brain function because they modulate the genes for inflammation in many different areas of your body.

The primary ingredients in fish oils are EPA and DHA. EPA has anti-inflammatory properties. It is able to turn on the genes for anti-inflammation in the gut and turn off other inflammatory genes. DHA plays a major role in fetal brain development and the retina of the eye during the first 2 years of life. About 35 percent of the walls of your brain cells are made of omega-3 fats. If there is not enough of these good fats available to make good strong brain cells, the body will use whatever raw material it can find as a fat resource. If you eat French fries, or deep-fried foods, the body will use that as the raw material for your brain cells. And those fats are much thicker and gooier and don't allow for easy transmembrane passage.

I'm dating myself here, but it used to be that if you were going to give a urine sample in a doctor's office, you'd go into the bathroom, fill the container they gave you, and put the container on the lazy Susan built into the wall. The nurse stationed on the other side of the wall would spin the lazy Susan, and your sample would come into the other room. That's how your brain cells communicate to each other—chemical messengers produced in one brain cell go right through the walls of the brain cell into the neighbor brain cell. But if your diet is full of the wrong kinds of fats, your lazy Susan will get rusty and won't spin well, interfering with the message from one brain cell to another. That is why when you supplement with fish oils rich in omega-3s, you can raise a child's IQ by more than three points (that's substantial). Your brain will push out the bad fats in the cell walls and replace them with the good fats, and your lazy Susan starts working better.

Omega-3s can be acquired only through diet, as the body cannot produce them. Fish have high omega-3 values, but because so many are not safe to eat, high-quality fish oil supplements (tested for heavy metals and chemical contaminants) provide a perfect way to get these essential nutrients. Therapeutic dosages up to 3 grams for adults have been shown to be remarkably effective and safe.[12] I typically prescribe the following for my patients:

Therapeutic dosages:

30–75 pounds = at least 1 gram per day (total omega-3s)
76–125 pounds = at least 2 grams per day (total omega-3s)
125 pounds = 3+ grams per day (total omega-3s)

4. PROBIOTICS: Probiotic supplementation supports the microbiome in the same way that fermented foods do: They introduce beneficial bacteria. The microbiome has a direct impact on practically every function of our bodies, from conversion of inactive thyroid hormone T4 to active hormone T3, to directing the production of brain hormones (called neurotransmitters), to reducing our cardiovascular risk factors, including body mass index, waist circumference, blood pressure, and triglyceride levels.[13] As the science continues to expand on the benefits of working with the microbiome, I believe we'll see more sophisticated protocols for taking probiotics.

Thirty years ago, we knew it was important to give probiotics to our patients, but we were all working with limited scientific data. The best recommendation we could give was to "take some probiotics, the more the better." Today we know there are thousands of different strains of good bacteria in the microbiome that can positively react with probiotics, yet there are currently still many unanswered questions about what happens if you give a large amount of one or two types. Until we know more, it seems rational to have a moderate dosage of a number of different probiotics than a larger dose of one or two.

This is one reason why I strongly suggest that you get your probiotics from whole fermented foods rather than supplements. Try to vary the fermented vegetables, because each vegetable can host different cultures and families of good bacteria. I also recommend taking a mixed probiotic capsule along with your fermented vegetables. The families of bacteria I look for in a probiotic supplement include *Lactobacillus*, *Bifidobacterium* (they're the most common), *Bacillus subtilis* (which will increase the *Bifidobacterium* count by more than 500 percent), and *Saccharomyces boulardii*.

5. **ZINC CARNOSINE:** There are 18 different types of zinc, and each has a specific function. Zinc carnosine has long been identified as having properties that heal the GI tract. It has been used in treating ulcers because it is known to promote a 75 percent increase in proliferation and migration of new cells to heal damage in the stomach. Recent research has shown that it also promotes a 50 percent increase in proliferation and migration of new cells to heal damage in the small intestines.[14] This mechanism is crucial for healing a leaky gut because much of the damage of intestinal permeability occurs in the small intestine.

Zinc carnosine can also help reverse damage caused by taking NSAIDs (nonsteroidal anti-inflammatory drugs) like aspirin and ibuprofen. In 1998, the health world was rocked when a landmark study showed that 16,000-plus people per year were dying, and more than 100,000 people per year were hospitalized, just from taking NSAIDs.[15] It is now well known that NSAIDs increase intestinal permeability, leading to inflammation, erosions, ulcers, bleeding, perforation, and obstruction.[16] Ironically, these medications, which are designed to be anti-inflammatory, can cause inflammatory damage in the gut. One-third of the deaths caused by NSAIDs are linked to low-dose daily aspirin.[17] Even a dose as small as 10 milligrams of aspirin per day causes gastric ulcers[18] (a baby aspirin is typically 81 milligrams).

Please consider these statistics every time you reach for one of these medications. Culturally, we rely too heavily on them. In fact, studies show that 44 percent of patients consume more than the recommended dosage of NSAIDs.[19] If you choose to use NSAIDs and aspirin, it certainly makes sense to use a little nutritional protection to heal the gut. I recommend to my patients that if they are going to take NSAIDs, they take one GS Pack per day as a protective feature, along with one tablet per day of zinc carnosine (at 75 milligrams per tablet) if you weigh 125 pounds or less, and one tablet twice per day if you weigh more.

6. **COLOSTRUM:** At childbirth, the first 3 to 5 days' worth of breast milk is not milk at all—it's colostrum. Colostrum is produced by the

mammary glands of all mammals during late pregnancy. Colostrum contains antibodies newborns need to be protected against disease. Colostrum modulates genes like no other substance on the planet, and we now know that it is the best remedy for all-around gut health. It contains growth factors and hormones designed to close the tight junctions for newborn babies (who are all permeable in utero). In adults, it turns the same genes on to help repair damage to the intestinal lining, restore gut integrity, close the tight junctions, and serve as a primary modulator of inflammatory genes in the gut. It also promotes recolonization of the bowel with good bacteria.

Roughly one-quarter of the total solids in colostrum are antibodies (IgG, IgE, IgA, IgD), which newborns need to colonize their microbiome. The IgGs in colostrum provide a baby with immediate protection from bugs, bacteria, viruses, mold, fungus, and parasites. For adults, colostrum will also provide protection from these same invaders. It also activates the genes that repair the microvilli, so that you can regrow the shags that have been worn down if you have celiac disease. As Andrew Keech, PhD, a world-renowned authority on colostrum, said on my Gluten Summit, "There are many one-note players on the health food store shelves that can help heal damaged intestines; only colostrum plays the entire symphony."

We can supplement with colostrum from cows to help heal our guts. The structure of colostrum is identical between cows and humans. In fact, the immunological part of the colostrum—these peptides—is exactly the same in every mammal. However, there is a difference in the quality of colostrums on the market. The product I promote on our Web site is exactly the same product licensed by six governments in Africa as the first treatment of choice for HIV. That's how beneficial colostrum can be. Look for colostrum made by grass-fed cows that haven't been given antibiotics or bovine growth hormone. For most adults, one scoop per day of the powder is the recommended dosage.

Even though colostrum can be considered a dairy product, it is typically low in allergenic proteins and is extremely low in casein. However, if you have a dairy sensitivity, speak with your doctor before taking this supplement. Together, you can determine whether or not it's a good idea to try the colostrum and see if you notice any symptoms.

Whenever I discover a patient who has a true dairy sensitivity, I will suggest trying the colostrum for at least 2 months, because it will turn on more genes to reduce inflammation and heal the intestines than anything else I could recommend. At the same time, take all other dairy out of the diet. If you find that you are having any symptoms of gas, bloating, abdominal pain, etc., then discontinue the colostrum. Clinically, I have found that 7 or 8 out of 10 patients with a dairy sensitivity will thrive on this protocol.

READ ALL SUPPLEMENT AND MEDICATION LABELS: AVOID THESE INGREDIENTS

Inside supplements, and even medicines, can be small, hidden exposures to gluten, dairy, or sugar. As with everything you put in your mouth, read labels carefully and look for clues that signal gluten contamination—current labeling regulations do not require gluten to be labeled in vitamins or medications. While supplements and medications are usually gluten-free, gluten can be added as a binding agent or as another inactive ingredient. Often they are the starches used to absorb water in the pills so they have a longer shelf life. When a product contains the word "starch," the source needs to be identified. The primary offender is maltodextrin, a starch typically derived from corn, but it can also be extracted from wheat, potato, or rice.

Tablets and capsules are the most likely potential source of gluten contamination, as they often contain excipients, absorbents, protectants, binders, coloring agents, lubricators, and bulking agents that may contain gluten. Each of these additives can be made from synthetic materials or natural sources that are derived from plants or animals. While they are considered inactive and safe for human use by the FDA, they can still be a potential source of contamination. Pharmacists tell us that some of these agents are safe while you are following Phase 1, and some of them are not. Mannitol or xylitol would be considered safe. These are sugar alcohols that are refined to the point where they're no problem for most people, even though some of them may be derived from wheat. Other safe additives that you might find in medication are titanium dioxide, lactose (unless you have a lactose sensitivity), gelatin, dextrin, and magnesium stearate.

A good rule of thumb is to always ask your pharmacist to make sure whatever prescription you are filling is gluten-free. Pharmacists will be able to review the patient package insert and let you know what's included in the medicine, or they can give you the paperwork so you can read the ingredients. They can also go online and check for you, or teach you how to contact the pharmaceutical manufacturer.

Unfortunately, it's not as easy to find the hidden sources of gluten with supplements. Although there are some health food store employees who are brilliant at what they do, the majority have no formal training in the composition of and additives to nutritional products. If you are lucky enough to have health-care practitioners who recommend nutritional supplements to you, they will be able to answer your questions as a pharmacist would. And if they do not know the answer to the question about ingredients, they have the channels to find out. You can be assured that any products I recommend have been vetted more than once to ensure they're safe.

Treat every refill of a nutritional supplement or medication as if it's a brand-new product for you. Companies often change their formulations, and generics do not have to be exact duplicates of brand-name medicines when it comes to the inactive ingredients. The same is true for over-the-counter medications. Read all labels carefully and avoid the following ingredients:

- Alcohol
- Alpha tocopherol
- Alpha tocotrienols
- Avena
- *Avena sativa*
- Barley
- Barley beta glucans
- Barley bran
- Barley grass
- Barley leaf
- Barley powder
- Beta glucans
- Beta glycans
- Beta tocopherol
- Beta tocotrienol
- Brewer's yeast
- Caramel color
- Cereal fiber
- Cernilton (rye grass)
- Citric acid
- Cross linked starch
- D-alpha-tocopherol
- D-beta-tocopherol
- Delta tocotrienol
- Dextrate
- Dextrimaltose
- Dextrin (if source is not specified, the source is usually corn or potato, which is acceptable, but wheat is sometimes used)
- D-gamma-tocopherol

- Dietary fiber
- Gamma tocopherol
- Gamma tocotrienols
- *Hordeum distichon*
- *Hordeum vulgare*
- Maltodextrin
- Maltose
- Mixed tocopherols
- Mixed tocotrienols
- Modified starch
- Oat beta glucan
- Oat bran
- Oat extract
- Oat fiber
- Oat grass
- Pregelatinized modified starch
- Pregelatinized starch
- Rye grass
- Rye grass pollen extract
- *Secale cereale*
- Sodium starch glycolate
- Starch
- Tocopherol
- Tocopherol acetate
- Tocopheryl succinate
- *Triticum aestivum*
- Vitamin E
- Wheat bran
- Wheat germ extract
- Wheat germ oil
- Wheatgrass
- Wheat protein
- Wheat starch
- Wild oats
- Xanthan gum
- Yeast

PROTECT YOURSELF FROM INADVERTENT FOOD EXPOSURES

Inadvertent exposures—mistakenly eating gluten, dairy, sugar, or anything else you have a sensitivity toward—are a very real concern and can stand in the way of your success on the Transition Protocol. Sadly, inadvertent exposure is the primary reason why so many people don't feel better even when they are "strictly" following a gluten-free diet. It's not that people are cheating and eating gluten foods every so often. Most of my patients with food sensitivities are trying hard to live a clean life, yet they are still suffering from symptoms because they are ingesting gluten, often without knowing it. That's why I listed every possible ingredient that contains gluten in the last chapter. However, we are not always able to read ingredient lists, especially when we eat outside of our homes.

Toxic gluten exposure (from wheat, rye, and barley) triggers intestinal permeability—the gateway into development of autoimmune diseases in everyone. Americans average 132½ pounds of wheat consumption per year. Now, I don't eat any. That means someone else is eating 265 pounds of wheat per year. And every forkful triggers a tear in the lining of our intestines. For some people, those tears easily heal. But when you've crossed the line and created enough intestinal permeability that it cannot heal, if the weak link in your chain is your intestines, you will develop celiac disease. That is why a family member of someone with confirmed celiac disease can be tested and come back negative, but if they're retested 7 years later, they may now have celiac disease. Their body could no longer heal the tears in the cheesecloth that developed from gluten exposure. The truth is, only a small number of celiac patients ever completely heal. According to a 2012 article published in the *American Journal of Gastroenterology*, even after 12 years following a gluten-free diet, 31 percent of the patients in the study still had the same symptoms they were originally faced with: increased inflammation in their intestines.[20] It turns out that only 8 percent of people with celiac disease fully heal on a gluten-free diet, leading these researchers to write, "A gluten-free diet alone may be insufficient to fully control the disease in some patients."

Worse, as we learned in Chapter 1, having one autoimmune condition puts you at greater risk for developing others. A second study from the *American Journal of Gastroenterology* looked at 7,600 celiac patients following a gluten-free diet, of whom 43 percent continued to have persistent villous atrophy: the worn-down shags in their intestines. For those people, the overall risk for cancer in the intestines was almost threefold higher than the general population.[21]

For you, this may mean that even when your headaches go away, or your poor digestion resolves after following Phase 1 for 3 weeks, the underlying inflammation may remain. You may still have some intestinal permeability caused by inadvertent exposures. That's why you can't base your success on this program with simply the resolution of your symptoms and go back to your old lifestyle. You have to be more vigilant. Going gluten-free is critical but only one part of the solution. Unless you tackle the other causes of intestinal permeability, you will still have inflammation. That is why it is helpful to measure the biomarkers of inflammation with blood or urine tests after your symptoms are gone. This is the only way to make sure inflammation is no longer causing intestinal permeability.

In order for you to heal more completely, you have to protect yourself from hidden sources of gluten. We need to give the body extra ammunition, and the most effective way to do this that I know of is by supplementing your diet with additional digestive enzymes. Digestive enzymes are naturally produced in the pancreas and small intestine. They break down our food into nutrients so that our body can absorb them. You can also supplement with additional, specific enzymes that will more fully digest inadvertent gluten. These enzymes protect you from the effects of an inadvertent exposure to any of the top eight allergens (wheat, dairy, soy, egg, nuts, fish, hemp, pea).

Take gluten-assisting digestive enzymes before every meal to make sure no traces of poorly digested gluten leave the stomach. That includes any time you're eating a meal that contains anything other than simply prepared meats and vegetables (because gluten, dairy, or sugar are often added to soups, sauces, seasonings, dressings, etc.).

While there are many gluten digestive enzymes on the market, I wasn't happy with their results. Over the years, a number of my patients were not responding as well as they should have from this extra step of taking enzymes. The research showed that these enzymes worked in the laboratory but not always in clinical practice. I started looking into why this approach wasn't completely effective. I found researchers who had spent 11 years developing an enzyme to help digest gluten more completely and quickly. We spent 2 more years collaborating, figuring out what the unknown factor was. Then it hit us.

We realized that the immune system's sentries, designed to protect you, are standing guard in the first part of the small intestine (the duodenum) right where it connects to the stomach. This area contains dendritic cells and antigen-presenting cells (the sentries). If any poorly digested protein molecules come out of the stomach, the sentries send out an alarm message activating our defense mechanisms. The immune system response produces a great deal of inflammation in the places we absorb vitamins and minerals. That's why people with adverse reactions to food have symptoms in so many different areas of the body—it depends on two things: how your immune system responds and which nutrient deficiencies develop from the poor absorption.

Remember, once the immune system turns itself on, it can be active for 3 to 6 months from any one exposure. Realizing that the alarm gets pulled just as food comes out of the stomach, we determined that we need to make sure these foods are completely digested *before* they get into the small intestine. We needed to create a digestive enzyme that would produce full digestion of all eight major food sensitivity offenders within 60 to 90 minutes, before the food you eat moves out of the stomach and into the small intestine. These digestive enzymes are called E3 Advanced Plus and are available on my Web site (theDr.com). Your health-care practitioner can order them from the nutrition company NuMedica. Every other gluten-assisting digestive enzyme on the market may work, but they take 3 to 4 hours to digest gluten, which still allows partially digested peptides to come out of the stomach, activating the sentries standing guard and starting the entire autoimmune cascade.

These three enzymes support a healthy microbiome because they contain prebiotics that support our beneficial bacteria. This creates a balanced environment specifically in your small intestine, which is very difficult to do with any supplements. They also contain specially selected probiotics that have the dual result of reinoculation and assisting in digesting gluten.

You can achieve a similar result by including varied fermented vegetables and prebiotics in your diet daily.

STOPPING LEAKY GUT RIGHT IN YOUR MOUTH

The main bacteria that cause gum disease, *Porphyromonas gingivalis*, release an extremely potent toxin that disrupts gut flora and has been shown to cause leaky gut. These bacteria can cause a little permeability in the mouth, allowing the bacteria to move from the mouth into the bloodstream. Today, researchers are connecting these bacteria to a number of chronic conditions, including heart disease, dementia, diabetes, and infertility. Dentists now prescribe antibiotics to their patients who have heart problems before they work on their mouths, in case they create gum permeability during a cleaning. But we already know that antibiotics on their own can disrupt gut bacteria and cause intestinal permeability.[22]

One simple thing you can do to ensure that you have healthy flora in your mouth, in addition to brushing and flossing your teeth, is to swish

SAMANTHA'S STORY, PART 5

Remember my patient Samantha? After taking Glutenza for just a few months, she wrote this letter that I have to share with you.

Dr. Tom, thank you for changing my life! Since we started working together, I've survived the worst case of CNS lupus vasculitis UCLA Medical Center has seen in 20 years. I also had antiphospholipid syndrome as well as a slew of other conditions stemming from high doses of prednisone, two types of chemotherapy for 1½ years, and a variety of other medicines used to treat the diseases. In my journey to heal and reverse all of the damage done to my body from the diseases and drugs, hidden exposures to my sensitive foods have caused setbacks time and again. But now, I NO LONGER have those setbacks if I'm exposed to hidden sources of gluten, soy, dairy, or corn. I no longer experience 2 weeks of exposure symptoms and a 4- to 6-month balancing act of detoxing my body and balancing my immune system after an assault! I'm actually seeing a much more rapid immune system rebuilding progress, and I know that the secret to making all the protocols you recommend actually work is because now I'm protected from unknown exposures to gluten!

I can now travel, have a social life, and still stay on my path to rebuild my immune system and GI tract. Thank you for creating Glutenza!

around a bit of coconut oil in your mouth every day, even for just 30 seconds. This is referred to as *oil pulling*. In one 30-day study using coconut oil swished in the mouth, a statistically significant reduction in plaque was noticed after 7 days. The researchers also pointed out that the health of the gingiva was greatly improved. These two markers kept improving as the study went on.[23]

I've learned to make coconut oil my friend. Coconut oil is a useful cooking oil that is solid at room temperature. It is a staple in diets in many tropical countries, including India, and is also used for cosmetic properties. Coconut oil contains medium-chain triglycerides that have proven anti-inflammatory and antimicrobial effects. And it is a natural antibiotic filled with beneficial prebiotic bacteria.

I keep a small amount of coconut oil in a container in my shower, and I swish around about a teaspoon in my mouth for a few minutes and then spit it out. At first, the taste and the consistency are a little hard to get used to. Now I look forward to it because my mouth feels so fresh afterward.

TOXIC FOOD EXPOSURES OCCUR IN THE MOST UNLIKELY PLACES

While we are doing our absolute best to keep our bodies clean from the inside out, we also have to examine our environment and how we take care of our outer selves. Unfortunately, there are other hidden sources of gluten that we can come in contact with just by using everyday commercial products. It could be in your shampoo, your laundry detergent, or anything that you are inhaling.

The science behind the effect of gluten in commercial products is real and well documented.[24] That said, some researchers argue that gluten molecules cannot penetrate the skin. They say that gluten-filled household products, including cleaners, shampoos, lipsticks, and even eye makeup, cannot penetrate the skin or scalp and should not pose a problem. However, for some people, they do. It is possible that these molecules enter our bodies through our respiratory system when we smell them. The respiratory route of delivery of a food toxin is well referenced in the scientific literature. When you are using any of these gluten-containing products, you're breathing in the tiniest particles, and they can activate an immune response.[25] Even if you don't experience symptoms, you could be doing damage to your internal tissue.

Cosmetics and Body-Care Products

Gluten proteins found in cosmetics can be a problem for some highly sensitive individuals. At the annual meeting of the American College of Gastroenterology in 2013, researchers presented a case study of a 28-year-old woman who successfully managed her celiac disease through diet. After trying a new body lotion, however, she developed an itchy, blistering rash on her arms, along with stomach bloating and diarrhea. Once she stopped using the lotion, her symptoms disappeared. In a 2014 scientific article "Food Allergen in Cosmetics," the authors reported a meta-analysis of eight different studies on more than 1,900 patients who suffered with symptoms from severe wheat allergies, yet these patients were not eating wheat. The authors found it was a facial soap containing wheat protein that caused this reaction. Once the patients stopped using the soap, their symptoms disappeared.[26]

The most common symptom of a wheat-sensitive reaction to body-care products is hives. Other reported symptoms include asthma and atopic dermatitis, a chronic inflammatory skin condition including severe itching, dry skin, and visible lesions. The estimated prevalence of atopic dermatitis has dramatically increased over the past 30 years, especially in urban areas, emphasizing the prevalence of environmental exposures like cosmetics in triggering the disease.[27]

Wheat is not the only culprit that can cause a problem in cosmetics—it's just a common one. For example, sunscreen—which is crucial for preventing sunburn, early skin aging, and skin cancer—contains more than 20 chemicals that are not approved for use by the US Food and Drug Administration. The benzophenones and dibenzoyl methanes are the most commonly implicated chemicals in sunscreens causing allergic and photoallergic contact dermatitis.[28]

Luckily, specialty manufacturers have created entire lines of organic, gluten-free, dairy-free, sugar-free beauty products. Annmarie Skin Care (annmariegianni.com) is one company my patients rave about.

Watch for the following ingredients in cosmetics and body-care products because they may contain gluten:

- Alcohol
- Amino peptide complex
- Amp-isostearoyl hydrolyzed wheat protein
- Amp-isostearoyl wheat amino acids
- Aspergillus/saccharomyces/ barley seed ferment filtrate

- Avenanthramides
- *Avena sativa*
- *Avena sativa* (oat) bran
- *Avena sativa* (oat) bran extract
- *Avena sativa* (oat) kernel meal
- *Avena sativa* (oat) kernel oil
- *Avena sativa* (oat) kernel protein
- *Avena sativa* (oat) meal extract
- *Avena sativa* (oat) peptide
- *Avena sativa* (oat) protein extract
- *Avena sativa* (oat) starch
- Barley (*Hordeum distichim*) extract
- Barley (*Hordeum vulgare*) powder
- Barley lipids
- Cetearyl wheat bran glycosides
- Citric acid
- Cocodimonium hydroxy-propyl hydrolyzed wheat protein
- Cocoyl hydrolyzed wheat protein
- Colloidal oat flour
- Cyclodextrin
- Denat alcohol
- Dextrin
- Dextrin palmitate
- Disodium wheatgermamido MEA-sulfosuccinate
- Disodium wheatgermamido PEG-2 sulfosuccinate
- Disodium wheatgermamphodiacetate
- Ethanol
- Ethyl wheat germate
- Fermented grain extract
- Grain alcohol
- *Hordeum distichon* (barley) extract
- *Hordeum vulgare* (barley) extract
- *Hordeum vulgare* phytosphin-gosine extract
- Hydrogenated wheat germ oil
- Hydrolyzed barley protein
- Hydrolyzed malt extract
- Hydrolyzed oat flour
- Hydrolyzed oat protein
- Hydrolyzed rye phytopla-centa extract
- Hydrolyzed wheat gluten
- Hydrolyzed wheat protein hydroxypropyl polysiloxane
- Hydrolyzed wheat protein/ PEG-20 acetate copolymer
- Hydrolyzed wheat protein PG-propyl methylsilanediol
- Hydrolyzed wheat protein PG-propyl silanetriol
- Hydrolyzed wheat protein/ dimethicone PEG-7 acetate
- Hydrolyzed wheat protein/ dimethicone PEG-7 phos-phate copolymer

- Hydrolyzed wheat protein/ PVP crosspolymer
- Hydrolyzed wheat starch
- Hydroxypropyltrimonium corn/wheat/soy amino acids
- Hydroxypropyltrimonium hydrolyzed wheat protein
- Hydroxypropyltrimonium hydrolyzed wheat protein/ siloxysilicate
- Hydroxypropyltrimonium hydrolyzed wheat starch
- Lactic acid
- Lactobacillus/rye flour ferment filtrate
- Laurdimonium hydroxypropyl hydrolyzed wheat protein
- Laurdimonium hydroxypropyl hydrolyzed wheat starch
- Malt extract
- Oat amino acids
- Oat beta glucan
- Oat bran
- Oat bran extract
- Oat extract
- Oat fiber
- Oat flour
- Oat kernel extract
- Oat kernel flour
- Oat kernel meal
- Oat kernel oil
- Oat kernel protein
- Oatmeal extract
- Oat peptide
- Oat protein extract
- Oat starch
- Oat straw extract
- Olivoyl hydrolyzed wheat protein
- Palmitoyl hydrolyzed wheat protein
- PG-hydrolyzed wheat protein
- Potassium cocoyl hydrolyzed oat protein
- Potassium cocoyl hydrolyzed wheat protein
- Potassium lauroyl wheat amino acids
- Potassium olivoyl hydrolyzed wheat protein
- Potassium olivoyl wheat amino acids
- Potassium palmitoyl hydrolyzed oat protein
- Potassium palmitoyl hydrolyzed wheat protein
- Potassium undecylenoyl hydrolyzed wheat protein
- Prolamine
- Propyltrimonium hydrolyzed wheat protein
- Protein hydrolysate
- Quaternium-79 hydrolyzed wheat protein
- Rye extract
- Rye seed extract
- Secale cereale
- Secale cereale (rye) extract
- Secale cereale (rye) seed extract

- Secale cereale (rye) seed flour
- Secale seed extract
- Sodium C8-16 isoalkylsuccinyl wheat protein sulfonate
- Sodium cocoyl hydrolyzed wheat protein
- Sodium cocoyl oat amino acids
- Sodium lauroyl oat amino acids
- Sodium lauroyl wheat amino acids
- Sodium palmitoyl hydrolyzed wheat protein
- Sodium/TEA-undecylenoyl hydrolyzed wheat protein
- Sodium wheat germamphoacetate
- Soyamidoethyldimonium hydroxypropyl hydrolyzed wheat protein
- Soydimonium hydroxypropyl hydrolyzed wheat protein
- Spent grain wax
- Steardimoniumhydroxypropyl hydrolyzed wheat protein
- Stearyldimoniumhydroxypropyl
- Stearyldimonium hydroxypropyl hydrolyzed wheat protein
- Tocopherol
- Tocopherol acetate
- Tocopherol/wheat polypeptides
- Trimethylsilyl hydrolyzed wheat protein PG-propyl methylsilanediol crosspolymer
- *Triticum aestivum*
- *Triticum aestivum* (wheat) bran
- *Triticum aestivum* (wheat) bran extract
- *Triticum aestivum* (wheat) bran lipids
- *Triticum aestivum* (wheat) flour lipids
- *Triticum aestivum* (wheat) germ extract
- *Triticum aestivum* (wheat) germ oil
- *Triticum aestivum* (wheat) leaf extract
- *Triticum aestivum* (wheat) peptide
- *Triticum aestivum* (wheat) seed extract
- *Triticum turgidum* (wheat) seed extract
- *Triticum vulgare*
- *Triticum vulgare* (wheat) bran
- *Triticum vulgare* (wheat) bran extract
- *Triticum vulgare* (wheat) bran lipids
- *Triticum vulgare* (wheat) flour lipids
- *Triticum vulgare* (wheat) germ extract
- *Triticum vulgare* (wheat) germ oil

- *Triticum vulgare* (wheat) germ oil unsaponifiables
- *Triticum vulgare* (wheat) germ powder
- *Triticum vulgare* (wheat) germ protein
- *Triticum vulgare* (wheat) gluten
- *Triticum vulgare* (wheat) gluten extract
- *Triticum vulgare* (wheat) kernel flour
- *Triticum vulgare* (wheat) protein
- *Triticum vulgare* (wheat) seed extract
- *Triticum vulgare* (wheat) sprout extract
- *Triticum vulgare* (wheat) starch
- Undecylenoyl wheat amino acids
- Vitamin E
- Wheat amino acids
- Wheat bran
- Wheat bran extract
- Wheat bran lipids
- Wheat ceramides
- Wheat flour lipids
- Wheat germamide DEA
- Wheat germamidopropalkonium chloride
- Wheat germamidopropyl betaine
- Wheat germamidopropyl dimethylamine
- Wheat germamidopropyl dimethylamine lactate
- Wheat germamidopropyl epoxypropyldimonium chloride
- Wheat germamidopropyl ethyldimonium ethosulfate
- Wheat germamidopropylamine oxide
- Wheat germamidopropyldimonium hydroxypropyl
- Wheat germ extract
- Wheat germ glycerides
- Wheat germ oil
- Wheat germ oil/palm oil aminopropanediol esters
- Wheat germ oil PEG-8 esters
- Wheat germ oil PEG-40 butyloctanol esters
- Wheat germ powder
- Wheat germ protein
- Wheat gluten
- Wheat gluten extract
- Wheat hydrolysate
- Wheat peptides
- Wheat protein
- Wheat protein hydrolysates
- Wheat sphingolipids
- Wheat starch
- Xanthan gum
- Yeast extract

Household Products

Household products may trigger intestinal permeability and cause inflammation due to a direct inflammatory response or indirectly from one of the hidden ingredients (such as gluten).

Symptoms may or may not be obvious. For some people, it's obvious. If they're exposed to a particular product or chemical, they have a reaction. Yet for most, it's not so clear-cut. The symptom might be low energy levels or joint pains that come and go.

One difficulty in isolating a product that may cause symptoms is that for most products, there is no government oversight. For example, the Environmental Protection Agency (EPA) governs the labeling of laundry detergents, and it does not adhere to the labeling requirements set forth by the FDA. The EPA's concern is whether a laundry detergent is "environmentally friendly," not whether the detergent contains gluten as a filler, and so it does not require labels on household products to list all ingredients.

For those of us who need to avoid gluten or have other chemical sensitivities, it's buyer beware. Look for the same list of ingredients above on product labels. If they are not included, or if there is no label, and you believe that you are reacting to a household product, stop using it immediately and see if your symptoms resolve.

Some manufacturers produce nontoxic cleaners by using natural ingredients that do not release harmful fumes or contain gluten. Their formulas are based on the same tried-and-true ingredients used for generations, and I've found that it's easy enough just to make your own. The formulas are easy to mix, and the ingredients are inexpensive. The only downside is they often require a little more elbow grease.

The following formulas are some of my favorites:

All-purpose cleaner—Mix together in a spray bottle:

1 cup water

¼ teaspoon organic, gluten-free liquid dishwashing soap

1 tablespoon baking soda

½ teaspoon borax

All-purpose scouring powder—Mix in a can with a perforated lid:

1 cup baking soda

10 drops rosemary essential oil

All-purpose disinfectant—Mix together in a spray bottle:

1 cup water

2 tablespoons Castile soap

1 teaspoon tea tree oil

8 drops eucalyptus essential oil

Glass cleaner—Mix together in a spray bottle:

1 cup water

1 cup vinegar

10 drops lemon essential oil

Porcelain polish—Mix together in a small bowl:

2 tablespoons cream of tartar

½ cup hydrogen peroxide

Wood floor cleaner—Mix in a large bucket:

3 tablespoons Castile soap

½ cup vinegar

½ cup black tea

2 gallons water

Wood cabinet cleaner—mix in a squirt bottle:

2 cups water

2 tablespoons vinegar

1 tablespoon lemon oil

THE NEXT STEP

In Phase 2, we'll explore some of the most common food offenders beyond gluten, dairy, and sugar that can be easily eliminated. When you have been reacting to gluten for years or possibly even decades, it can damage the gut considerably, triggering reactions to other foods. Even if you are feeling remarkable after Phase 1, I recommend that you try Phase 2 anyway. The more you know about your body and what it's trying to tell you, the better off you'll be.

HOUSEHOLD ITEMS THAT MAY CONTAIN GLUTEN

Product	Reason to Avoid	Solution
Charcoal briquettes	May contain wheat as a binding agent.	Replace with natural wood charcoal.
Disinfectant	May contain alcohol from a gluten-containing grain.	See recipe on page 225.
Dish soap/ washing-up liquid	May contain proteins from gluten grains.	Look for organic, gluten-free options.
Drywall/ plasterboard	Starch from gluten-containing grain may be used in the manufacture of drywall.	If you feel better when you're away from home for a few days, it might be your home that is the toxin.
Envelopes	Envelope glue is primarily derived from cornstarch or gum arabic. However, it can also be produced from other starches, including dextrin.	Use a wet sponge to seal envelopes instead of licking them.
Glue	Some household glues may contain wheat starch.	Wear cotton gloves when applying glue.
Hand soap	May contain ingredients derived from gluten grains.	Look for organic, gluten-free options.
Household cleaning products	May contain proteins or starches from gluten grains.	See recipes on pages 224 to 225.
Laundry detergent/ washing powder/ washing liquid/ fabric softeners/ stain removers	May contain proteins from gluten grains.	Look for organic, gluten-free options.
Paste for craft purposes	Wheat paste may be used for papier-mâché, decoupage, book binding, and collage. Wheat paste may also be used to glue posters or flyers.	Wear cotton gloves when applying pastes.

Product	Reason to Avoid	Solution
Pet food	May contain gluten grains.	Look for an organic, gluten-free brand.
Pet litter	May contain wheat.	Look for an organic, gluten-free brand.
Play dough	Contains wheat.	Choose organic clays, or follow this recipe from the Celiac Disease Foundation for a safe option your kids will love: *½ cup rice flour* *½ cup cornstarch* *½ cup salt* *2 teaspoons cream of tartar* *1 cup water* *1 teaspoon cooking oil* *Gluten-free food coloring, if desired* In a medium pan, combine the ingredients. Cook and stir over low heat for 3 minutes, or until a ball forms. Cool completely before storing in a resealable plastic bag.
Plywood glue	May be made from wheat flour.	Wear cotton gloves when applying glue.
Wallpaper paste	May contain wheat starch: In Poland, wheat plus water is used as wallpaper paste.	Remove wallpaper from your home.

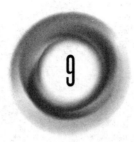

TRANSITION PHASE 2:

WEEKS 4–6

If you have been seeing improvements to your health during the first transition phase, you might not want to make further changes to your diet. It's quite likely that by simply removing sugar, dairy, and gluten, you are decreasing inflammation to such a large extent and reducing the need for your immune system to protect you from these invasive foods that you are already feeling better than you've felt in a long time. If so, you're on the right track. Keep going—ride this wave as long as you can. There is no need to make the transition any more complicated.

However, if you have been following Phase 1 for 3 weeks and have not recognized a discernable difference in your health, it is likely that there are other culprits. That's why I put a 3-week limit on the Phase 1 food plan: If you don't know within 3 weeks that you're on the right path, other types of environmental triggers may be fueling an immune response.

In Phase 2, I want you to continue avoiding gluten, dairy, and sugar. Even if these are not the only culprits that cause your symptoms, they are still highly inflammatory foods. I want you to avoid them until we can correctly identify your triggers. While you stay gluten-, dairy-, and sugar-free, we can determine if there are other offenders affecting your health by either doing a comprehensive food sensitivity test or by eliminating the next most common irritants from your diet.

In this chapter, you'll learn how specific foods beyond the three main inflammatory choices are particularly worrisome for people on the autoimmune spectrum. Earlier, in Chapter 2, we learned that intestinal permeability is one of the three factors that must be present for autoimmunity to occur. When poorly digested fragments of certain foods leak out of the gut into the bloodstream, the immune system, in an effort to protect you, attacks these fragments and begins the cascade reaction. As a result, you may develop an allergy or sensitivity to various foods that most people can easily tolerate or that you were able to tolerate before.

According to Natasha Campbell-McBride, MD, these food sensitivities can manifest as any symptom, from a skin rash to chronic cystitis, from a headache to a lapse in memory or drop in blood sugar, or from lagging energy to an asthmatic attack. The reaction can be immediate or delayed: It can happen immediately, 2 hours later, or even 2 days later. I have found in my clinical practice that the "unexplained symptoms" we occasionally experience are often associated with a prior exposure to an irritant. That's why sometimes it's close to impossible to correlate how you feel with what you've eaten. On any given day, you may have no idea what exactly you're reacting to. You might actually be reacting to several overlapping irritants: It might be the gluten, tomatoes, and even emotional stress all pushing the inflammatory cascade. By removing the gluten and tomatoes, you'll have more bandwidth available to better address the emotional stress.

In Phase 2, we will eliminate all of the most likely foods that trigger inflammation until we notice a positive response, which means you're feeling better. At the same time, you'll be restoring the gut lining with "heal and seal" nutrition so that these same foods have the chance to be digested properly. Then, once the gut is fully restored, you may be able to reintroduce some of these foods without difficulty.

TRANSITION PHASE 2: FOODS TO AVOID

If you need to explore other food culprits, the next 3 weeks might seem more challenging. But in this time, you'll finally be able to determine if what you are eating is making you sick, fat, or tired. It makes sense to begin by avoiding the most common food allergens. As many as 8 million Americans, or 2½ percent of the population, have food allergies—an IgE reaction that may produce life-threatening anaphylaxis but could also cause any immune-related symptoms.

The most frequent allergy-causing foods are in the list below. You are already avoiding cow's milk and wheat from Phase 1. In the next 3 weeks, avoid:

- Cow's milk
- Eggs
- Peanuts
- Soy

- Tree nuts (such as walnuts, pecans, and cashews)
- Wheat

Many millions more people have food sensitivities (IgG, IgA, IgM reactions) to these same foods and a host of others. Clinically, I've found that there are tiers of food sensitivities (foods that are most likely to be problems).

- Tier 1: Gluten, dairy, sugar
- Tier 2: Soy, other grains, and nightshade vegetables (such as eggplant, peppers, potatoes, tomatoes)

Soy

There are two main reasons why soy is a common irritant. The first is the fact that soy is almost always genetically modified (unless labeled as organic). According to the USDA, 93 percent of soy grown in the United States is genetically modified.[1] The second reason is that soy is one of the top eight allergens that also cause food sensitivities for many people.

In Transition Phase 1, it was acceptable to eat organic soy, but in Phase 2, you will avoid all soy products. Soy is a staple of processed foods under various names, including hydrogenated oils, lecithin, and emulsifiers. It is frequently found as an ingredient in cereals, salad dressings, meat alternatives, and baked goods, even gluten-free ones. Look out for the following when you read labels:

- Edamame
- Miso
- Mono-diglycerides
- Soy lecithin
- Soy milk

- Soy oil
- Soy protein isolate
- Soy protein powder
- Soy sauce
- Tamari

- Tempeh
- Tofu
- TSF (textured soy flour)
- TSP (textured soy protein)
- TVP (textured vegetable protein)
- Vitamin E (soy is an inexpensive compound from which you can extract tocopherol, the scientific name for vitamin E)

Grains

In Phase 1, the only grains we eliminated were the grains that contain toxic gluten: wheat, rye, and barley. In Phase 2, you're going to cut out all grains. A substantial portion of people with autoimmune diseases have sensitivities to different components of grains. Components of grains such as FODMAPs (which you'll learn about later in the chapter), nongluten proteins, and lectins in grains and legumes are common triggers to immune reactions.

What's more, single-ingredient processed foods, like grains, often contain toxic gluten because of contamination. They might be bred with gluten, they might be processed in a plant that also processes wheat, or they might be prepared in a factory or restaurant with added gluten. In one 2015 study published in the journal *Food Chemistry*, almost 24.7 percent of naturally gluten-free foods, like soy and oats, were contaminated with gluten.[2]

Some doctors believe that all gluten proteins are toxic. There are a number of research studies, including one from 2005 in the prominent scientific journal *Gut*, that show that patients with gluten sensitivity may react to the glutens in corn and rice.[3] More recently, there was a study done in 2012 that indicated that some of the protein structures in corn gluten can stimulate the exact same genetic receptor that we see in celiac patients.[4]

These grains need to be avoided in Phase 2 because they may contain different families of gluten or might be contaminated with toxic gluten:

- All gluten grains
- Amaranth
- Buckwheat
- Corn
- Millet
- Oats
- Quinoa
- Rice
- Sorghum
- Teff
- Wild rice

Each type of grain poses its own unique set of problems, some which I discuss below. This is why in Transition Phase 2 you will avoid all grains for 3 weeks and then reintroduce them one at a time, as long as they are clearly labeled as gluten-free.

Corn

According to the USDA, 88 percent of the corn grown in the United States is genetically modified. And 50 percent of people with celiac disease have a cross-reaction to corn because of molecular mimicry: The gluten proteins in corn look similar enough to gluten proteins in wheat, and the immune system can react to them.

Another problem with corn is the common mold that grows on it, called fumonisin, which the immune system will protect you from. Usually people at risk for fumonisin toxicity live in Third World countries, because their diet is primarily composed of corn. But if you follow a gluten-free diet, you may be compensating by eating a higher ratio of corn than the average American consumer, inadvertently exposing yourself to mold toxicity. Worse, one study found that toxic levels of fumonisin were found in 105 out of 118 foods labeled as gluten-free.[5] Consumption of these foods can keep your immune system highly vigilant.

Corn can also be found in:

- Baking powder
- Caramel
- Corn flour
- Corn malt
- Cornmeal
- Corn on the cob
- Cornstarch
- Corn tortillas
- Dextrin
- Dextrose
- Food starch
- Frozen corn
- Grits
- High fructose corn syrup
- Hominy
- Maltodextrin
- Masa
- Polenta
- Sorbitol
- Vegetable gum
- Vegetable protein
- Vegetable starch
- Xanthan gum

GLUTEN-CONTENT OF VARIOUS GRAINS

Food	Total protein	Giladins (% of total protein)	Glutenins (% of total protein)
Wheat	10–15	40–50	30–40
Rye	9–14	30–50	30–50
Oats	8–14	10–15	~5
Corn	7–13	50–55	30–45
Rice	8–10	1–5	85–90
Sorghum	9–13	>60	
Millet	7–16	57	30
Buckwheat			High

Reprinted by permission from *Alternative Medicine Review*, vol. 10, no. 3, 2005:174.

Rice

In restaurants, rice dishes are sometimes prepared with flour, believe it or not. Three of the last seven Japanese restaurants I've gone in have served rice that was prepared with wheat flour. I always ask the wait-staff to ask the sushi chef how rice is prepared and if the chef added flour to make it stickier.

While it's rare that the rice you cook at home is contaminated with gluten, it does contain some gluten and some lectins, which we are avoiding in Phase 2.

Quinoa

Quinoa is actually not a grain but a grass that comes from Peru. It is one of the healthiest options because it is naturally high in protein. Now that it has become so popular among the food conscious, it is also culti-vated in the United States. Farmers have been able to grow it here because they created a new strain that was crossbred with other grasses, like wheat. In one 2012 study published in the *American Journal of Clinical Nutrition*, 4 out of 15 quinoa strains contained toxic levels of gluten where the gluten occurred in the plant itself, not through cross-contamination during the manufacturing process.[6]

Nightshade Vegetables

Nightshade vegetables are a plant family that includes eggplant, peppers, potatoes, tomatoes, and a host of other flowering plants we use as herbs. The term *nightshade* may have been coined because some of these plants prefer to grow in shady areas, and some flower at night. All contain chemicals called saponins that can increase intestinal permeability and inflammation. During Phase 2, you should avoid the following, and then, afterward, add each back into your diet one at a time to see if any trigger inflammation for you.

- Ashwagandha (an herb)
- Cayenne pepper
- Chili powder
- Chipotle chili powder
- Curry powder
- Eggplant
- Goji berries
- Golden berries
- Hot sauce
- Ketchup
- Mexican seasoning
- Peppers (sweet and hot)
- Potatoes
- Taco seasoning
- Tomatillos
- Tomatoes
- Tomato sauce/paste

FODMAPs

FODMAPs are a family of carbohydrates (sugars) found in wheat as well as many other foods. The acronym FODMAP stands for fermentable oligo-di-monosaccharides and polyols. FODMAPs are osmotic (means they pull water into the intestinal tract), may not be digested or absorbed well, and could be fermented upon by bacteria in the intestinal tract when eaten in excess or if you have an imbalanced microbiome. The excess fermentation can cause bloating, gas, abdominal pain, diarrhea, and sometimes constipation. If you have a sensitivity to FODMAPs, you're likely to have some or many of these abdominal complaints. If you currently suffer from abdominal complaints, you should consider removing FODMAPs during Transition Phase 2. This may be more challenging, but it may make a host of difference in the way you feel. If you don't have abdominal complaints, you can enjoy the nongluten FODMAP foods from the list below.

FODMAP Fruits

- Apples
- Apricots
- Avocados
- Blackberries
- Boysenberries
- Cherries
- Figs
- Grapefruit
- Mangoes
- Nectarines
- Peaches
- Pears
- Persimmons
- Plums
- Pomegranates
- Watermelon

FODMAP Dried Fruits

- Cranberries, dried
- Currants
- Dates
- Prunes
- Raisins

FODMAP Nuts and Seeds

- Almond flour
- Almonds
- Cashews
- Pistachios

FODMAP Vegetables

- Artichoke, globe
- Artichoke hearts
- Artichoke, Jerusalem
- Asparagus
- Beans
- Beets
- Butternut squash (½ cup or more)
- Cabbage, Savoy
- Cauliflower
- Celery
- Frozen peas
- Garlic
- Leeks
- Mushrooms

- Onions and shallots
- Sugar pie pumpkin

- Sugar snap peas
- Sweet potato and yams

THE IMPORTANCE OF A CAREFULLY WORDED TITLE

In 2013, a group of researchers in Australia tried to determine if people with self-reported gluten sensitivity actually had a FODMAP sensitivity causing their symptoms. Their findings were published in an article in the journal *Gastroenterology* titled "No Effects of Gluten in Patients with Self-Reported Non-Celiac Gluten Sensitivity after Dietary Reduction of Fermentable, Poorly Absorbed, Short-Chain Carbohydrates."[7] What the study said was that there are other components of wheat besides gluten that cause problems for people. For some people, the culprits are the FODMAPs in wheat and other foods. To focus their research, and because they were looking for other possible causes or problems, the scientists excluded people with celiac or non-celiac gluten sensitivity identified by elevated antibodies to gluten. Even with that type of filtering, 8 percent of the people in the study still had a response to gluten proteins. The title of the study, "No Effects of Gluten . . . ," was just a poor choice of words. The title should have been "Minor Effects of Gluten . . ." Regardless, this paper is important because it was one of the first to say there are other parts of wheat besides gluten proteins that cause food-related symptoms: The FODMAPs can be the problem.

Because the article title was misleading, one blogger in Great Britain looked at the title and started reporting that gluten sensitivity must be a fad because science was saying that "there were no effects of gluten." Other bloggers picked up on this momentum by writing blog posts and magazine articles. Unfortunately, the bloggers didn't read the study but reacted to the title and created a backlash against gluten-free diets, which set back the public's perception on real scientific research. Their writings, in which they tried to prove that eating gluten-free is a fad and has no health benefits, were just not true. It was sensational journalism: writing copy without doing your homework to cause attention. Throughout this book, I've provided dozens of the latest findings. Read any one of them, and they will show clearly that for some people, gluten sensitivity without celiac disease is a real and dangerous problem.

FOODS THAT INFLUENCE YOUR HEALTH

Just as FODMAPs are associated with abdominal complaints, they also may cause common food sensitivities and specific symptoms. Here's a short list.

- If you have joint pain, it's likely that you have antibodies for nightshade vegetables and need to eliminate these from your diet.
- If you suffer migraines, you should consider lectin sensitivity and stay away from legumes.
- If you experience skin problems, cut out melons.
- If you have trouble with acne, eliminate trans fats.
- If you experience any number of symptoms of brain dysfunction (all the way from brain fog to autism), avoid glutamates (like MSG), which are notorious culprits behind neurological dysfunction.

OTHER LIKELY SUSPECTS

If you're still not feeling well after 6 weeks (finishing both Phase 1 and Phase 2), and you've done everything possible with food, and the focused attention you've applied has had no impact whatsoever, there is a hidden trigger that will require a thorough "investigative doctoring" approach. At this point, I would suggest finding a certified functional medicine practitioner. You might find that your inflammation is related to a microbiome so far out of balance that more than just a change of foods is necessary. You may have a toxic mold exposure or candida growth or a viral infection or Lyme disease. My Web site (theDr.com) has information about these common, non-food-related triggers.

For example, you could be living in a house or working in an office with a toxic mold problem that is making you sick. Mold sensitivity can be a minor inconvenience or a major immobilizing disruption to your life.

Here's one good way to validate a suspicion of a mold exposure problem: When you return to your home or workspace after leaving it for a few days, do you feel the need to open the windows to air the room

THE TRANSITION PROTOCOL CHEAT SHEET: PHASE 2

	Allowed	Not Allowed
Fruits/ Vegetables	All fresh fruits and vegetables Fermented vegetables that are not FODMAPs	Canned or dried fruits and vegetables Nightshade vegetables FODMAP fruits and vegetables if you suffer from abdominal complaints All soy products
Grains	Arrowroot flour Coconut flour	All grains: Amaranth Rice Barley Rye Buckwheat Sorghum Corn Teff Millet Wheat Oats Wild rice Quinoa
Proteins	Breakfast ham, bacon, or sausage, organic and gluten-free Fresh meats and poultry Legumes, unless you are sensitive to lectin Low-mercury fish and shellfish	All nuts and seeds, even if they are labeled as gluten-free Eggs Lunchmeats Self-basted or cured meat products
Condiments	Coconut, olive, avocado oils Honey Salt Vinegar	Flavored and malt vinegars Generic "vegetable" oil
Beverages	Kombucha Tea, coffee (unsweetened, no milk added) Unsweetened coconut milk Unsweetened fruit juices that are not FODMAPs Water	All sodas, including diet sodas Cow's, goat's, or soy milk Sweetened milk substitutes Sweetened fruit juices Sports drinks Unsweetened hemp, almond, or rice milk Unsweetened fruit juices that are FODMAPs if you suffer from abdominal complaints

out? If you do, it's likely because there's mold, and the concentrations are high enough that you recognize the smell, whereas before, when you were used to the smell, you might not have noticed it. Like food, exposure to mold can be constant and pervasive.

Mold sensitivity can be determined with a blood test or urinalysis of high concentration of mold metabolites. I've also found that people with mold allergies or sensitivities often have a pasty shine to their skin.

Samantha's Story, Part 6

By 2012, Samantha's health was beginning to turn around. She completed Phase 1 and Phase 2 of the Transition Protocol and was very careful about her diet. One day, she came into my office and we reviewed the foods she was eating. She told me that she was still off sugar. "Every time I eat it, I get a bladder infection or a yeast infection. I'm not talking about just sugar, Doc, I'm talking about fruit, too. I just know I can't eat fruit. I want to be healthy, and I want to be able to function and go to work and contribute to the planet."

Samantha had done the exactly right thing. What was the point of eating something that she knew would make her sick? I asked her if she had a similar reaction to wine. She told me, "I don't do that anymore, either. I pay for it every time, ending up on antibiotics."

I suggested that she keep going on the protocol, and she agreed. In 2013, she came back with a huge smile on her face. "You are not going to believe this," she said, "but after a year on the program, I can actually eat fruit again. I'm still off sugar, but that's not a problem because I never enjoyed it that much. Once in a while, at work, we'd have cupcakes that were gluten-free and dairy-free, but I would always pay for a transgression usually 2 or 3 days later, which is normal for my immune response. But now that I've cleaned up my gut, I did go back and try some fruit, and most of them aren't a problem. I went slow and reintroduced berries, and I'm sticking with that for a while."

Samantha's experience is not uncommon: When she restored her gut health and lowered her overall inflammation, she was able to go back to some of the foods she used to enjoy without a problem.

10

THE TRANSITION PROTOCOL RECIPES

One of the essential goals of the recipes I am sharing with you is that they be easy to prepare and family oriented. This means that whether you are a mother of five or a bachelor cooking for someone special, the recipes are user friendly. For example, the Hearty Beef and Mushroom Stew (page 252) is a tasty, nourishing meal that produces comments ranging from "Wow, this is really good, Mom!" to "If this man can cook like this, there's substance and depth to him!"

Most of the recipes can be prepared in advance, so that you don't have to scramble for a meal or panic that you won't have the right foods to support your transition. Each recipe indicates which Transition Phase it can be used for. We've also included some brands of products that we are most comfortable with, but feel free to source your own packaged goods as long as they meet the criteria I've laid out in this book.

Smoothies

GUT-HEALING SMOOTHIE

Phases 1 & 2

Yield: 2 servings

Blueberries not only have antioxidant properties that are remarkable at protecting your brain (consuming 1 cup of blueberries per day for 3 years gets your brain working as well as it did 11 years earlier[1]), but they also contain compounds that increase beneficial bacteria in the gut. Bananas are high in pectin, which helps to normalize movements of the large intestine.

Look for gelatin powders from pastured animals, such as those by Great Lakes Gelatin Company or Vital Proteins.

1–1½   cups water
½   cup coconut milk
2   frozen bananas
1   cup frozen blueberries
2   tablespoons ground flaxseeds
1   tablespoon unflavored gelatin powder
1   tablespoon high-quality fish oil
1   teaspoon ground cinnamon
1–2   scoops L-glutamine powder (optional)

In a blender, combine the water, coconut milk, bananas, blueberries, flaxseeds, gelatin powder, fish oil, cinnamon, and L-glutamine powder (if using). Blend until smooth. Add more water for a thinner smoothie, if desired. Serve immediately or pour into ice-pop molds and freeze for a sweet treat later on.

SUPER-ANTIOXIDANT GREEN SMOOTHIE

Yield: 2 servings

This smoothie is packed with anti-inflammatory antioxidants. You can vary the fruits and vegetables. Try wild blueberries in place of the raspberries; chopped fresh pears in place of the pineapple; or a whole, peeled orange in place of the cranberries. Use any type of greens—collards, bok choy, kale, dandelion greens, fresh spring nettles, or spinach. Stay away from FODMAP fruits and vegetables if you have abdominal complaints.

If you don't own a high-powdered blender—such as a Vitamix or Blentec—then be sure to use young, tender baby greens so they will blend well in the smoothie.

2 frozen bananas

1 cup chopped pineapple (fresh or frozen)

1 cup raspberries (fresh or frozen)

¼ cup frozen cranberries

2 cups water

2–3 cups firmly packed greens (baby kale, spinach, and bok choy)

In a blender, combine the bananas, pineapple, raspberries, cranberries, and water. Blend until smooth. Add the greens and blend again until very smooth. Serve immediately or store in a glass jar in the refrigerator for up to 1 day.

GLUTEN-FREE SANDWICH BREAD

Phase
I

Yield: 1 loaf

This delicious gluten-free bread loaf is perfect for making sandwiches or for breakfast toast. The dough can be separated into smaller portions to make individual dinner rolls.

2 cups warm water (105°–110°F)

2¼ teaspoons (1 package) active dry yeast

1 tablespoon pure maple syrup

1 tablespoon extra-virgin olive oil or avocado oil

⅓ cup whole psyllium husks (see Note)

2¼ cups brown rice flour

¾ cup tapioca flour

½ cup blanched almond flour

¾ cup potato starch

1½ teaspoons sea salt

1. In a 4-cup glass measuring cup, whisk together the warm water, yeast, and maple syrup. Let rest for 3 to 5 minutes, or until foamy and bubbly. Whisk in the oil and psyllium husks. Let rest for no more than 1 to 2 minutes.

2. While the yeast is proofing, in a large mixing bowl, whisk together the flours, potato starch, and salt. Pour the yeast mixture into the flour mixture and stir with a wooden spoon to incorporate. Continue incorporating the ingredients by kneading the dough with your hands in the mixing bowl or on a floured surface until well mixed together.

3. Grease an 8½" × 4½" glass bread pan with olive oil or coconut oil. Form the dough into a log shape and place in the pan. Cover with a damp cloth or a piece of parchment paper. Set in a warm spot or place the bread pan in a larger (such as a 13" × 9") pan of hot water. Let the bread rise for about 60 minutes.

4. Preheat the oven to 400°F. Bake the bread for 50 to 55 minutes, or until a wooden pick inserted in the center comes out clean. Let cool in the pan on a rack for a few minutes, then gently release the bread from the pan and cool on the rack. Slice as needed.

NOTE: You can buy psyllium husks on the Internet or at a local health food store.

Breakfast

COCONUT-RASPBERRY PANCAKES

Phase I

Yield: 5 small pancakes

This grain-free recipe uses a mixture of coconut flour and arrowroot to replace traditional flour. The pancakes are easy to make and very flavorful.

¼ cup coconut flour

¼ cup arrowroot powder or tapioca flour

1 teaspoon gluten-free baking powder

⅛ teaspoon sea salt

3 large organic eggs

2–3 tablespoons organic coconut milk

2–3 teaspoons pure maple syrup

⅓ cup raspberries, lightly mashed (fresh is preferred)

Coconut oil, for cooking

1. Heat a 10" cast-iron skillet over medium-low heat.

2. In a small mixing bowl, whisk together the coconut flour, arrowroot powder or tapioca flour, baking powder, and salt. In a separate bowl, whisk together the eggs, coconut milk, maple syrup, and raspberries. Pour the egg mixture into the flour mixture and whisk together. The mixture will seem thin at first. Let rest for a minute to thicken.

3. Add a few teaspoons of coconut oil to the preheated skillet. Drop the batter into the hot skillet by the quarter cup. Cook for about 90 seconds on each side.

GARDEN VEGETABLE FRITTATA

Phase
I

Yield: 4 servings

Eating a hearty, high-protein breakfast rich in vegetables will help curb sugar cravings later in the day. You can easily reheat a piece of frittata by placing it in a small skillet with a few tablespoons of water, or you can enjoy eating it cold or at room temperature. I suggest topping each slice with a spoonful of organic salsa. Serve with a small green salad or a few spoonfuls of Pickled Vegetables (page 278).

1 tablespoon extra-virgin olive oil

½ cup finely chopped onion

½ teaspoon sea salt

2 cups chopped broccoli florets

1 cup finely chopped red bell pepper

2 cups finely chopped kale

¼ cup finely chopped fresh basil

6 large pastured eggs, whisked

Freshly ground black pepper

1. Preheat the oven to 375°F.

2. Heat a deep 10" cast-iron skillet over medium heat. Add the oil, onion, and salt and cook for 5 minutes. Add the broccoli and bell pepper and cook for 5 to 7 minutes. Stir in the kale and basil, then pour in the eggs. Season with black pepper.

3. Place the skillet in the oven and bake for 20 minutes, or until the frittata is lightly browned. Slice into wedges and serve. Store leftover frittata in a covered glass container in the refrigerator for up to a week.

ITALIAN CHICKEN BREAKFAST SAUSAGES

Yield: 8 patties

These delicious sausage patties are packed with nutrients such as vitamin A, vitamin D, zinc, iron, and B vitamins. Serve with sautéed kale or the Super-Antioxidant Green Smoothie (page 243) for an energizing breakfast.

1½ **pounds organic boneless, skinless chicken thighs**

¼–½ **cup organic raw chicken livers**

¼ **cup chopped fresh chives or scallions**

2 **tablespoons chopped fresh sage leaves**

1 **tablespoon Italian seasoning**

2 **teaspoons fennel seeds**

1 **teaspoon garlic powder**

1 **teaspoon sea salt**

2–3 **tablespoons olive oil**

1. In a food processor fitted with the standard *S* blade, combine the chicken thighs, livers, chives or scallions, sage, Italian seasoning, fennel seeds, garlic powder, and salt. Process until the mixture is ground and begins to form a ball.

2. Lightly oil a large plate. With oiled hands, form the mixture into 8 equal-size patties and place on the prepared plate.

3. Preheat a 10" cast-iron skillet over medium-low heat for a few minutes. Add about 1 tablespoon of the oil and carefully place 3 or 4 patties into the pan. Cook for 3 to 5 minutes on each side, or until no longer pink. Repeat with the remaining patties. Uncooked patties can be stored between pieces of parchment paper in a container in the freezer for up to 6 months. Cooked patties can be stored in the refrigerator for up to 5 days.

KALE BREAKFAST HASH

Yield: 2 servings

If I make baked potatoes for dinner one night, I cook an additional one or two so I can prepare this quick-and-easy breakfast hash. If you are accustomed to eating a carb-rich breakfast such as bread or cereal in the morning, then this is a great replacement.

If you do not like eggs, substitute some leftover cooked salmon in place of the eggs.

2 tablespoons extra-virgin olive oil

1 medium whole baked potato, chopped into large pieces

Sea salt and freshly ground black pepper

2 scallions, thinly sliced

2–3 cups finely chopped kale

3 large pastured eggs, whisked

1. Heat a 12" cast-iron skillet over medium heat. Add the oil, then the potato. Season to taste with salt and pepper. Cook for a few minutes, until the potato pieces brown on all sides, then add the scallions and kale. Cook for a few minutes longer, until the kale is tender.

2. Move the mixture to one side of the pan. Pour the eggs into the other side of the pan and scramble. Once the eggs are cooked, mix them with the potato mixture. Taste and add more salt and pepper, if needed.

Soups

SLOW-COOKER CHICKEN STOCK

Phases
1 & 2

Yield: 2 quarts

Save the bones and skin from a roasted chicken (see the recipe on page 268) to make a rich, healing stock. There is just no comparison—the flavor of home-made stock is far superior to anything you could buy in a store. Using a slow cooker makes it incredibly easy to prepare homemade stock for soups, stews, or sauce recipes.

1	chicken carcass
1	small onion, chopped
2	carrots, chopped
2	ribs celery, chopped
1	bay leaf
	Few sprigs thyme
	Few sprigs rosemary
1–2	teaspoons sea salt
2	tablespoons raw apple cider vinegar
8–10	cups water

1. In a 4-quart slow cooker, combine the chicken, onion, carrots, celery, bay leaf, thyme, rosemary, salt, vinegar, and water. Cover and cook on low for 10 to 24 hours.

2. Place a colander over a large bowl and pour the stock through to strain. Discard the solids. Use the rich, flavorful stock immediately or pour into glass containers or widemouthed quart jars and freeze for later use.

CHICKEN, SQUASH, AND LEEK SOUP

Yield: 4 to 6 servings

If you like a rich, flavorful soup, then begin with a rich, flavorful homemade stock. I suggest using the Slow-Cooker Chicken Stock (page 249) in this recipe over anything store-bought.

Look for peeled and chopped butternut squash in the freezer section of your local supermarket or health food store. A 10-ounce bag of frozen squash equals about 2 cups. For a fresher flavor, purchase a small butternut squash with a long neck, and peel and chop it yourself—it's really quite simple!

2 tablespoons extra-virgin olive oil

1 medium leek, chopped

2 cloves garlic, crushed

4 cups chicken stock

2 cups peeled and chopped butternut squash

2 cups cooked, chopped chicken

1–2 teaspoons dried thyme

3–4 cups finely chopped kale

Sea salt and freshly ground black pepper

1. Heat the oil in a 4- or 6-quart pot over medium heat. Add the leek and garlic and cook for 4 to 5 minutes, or until the leek softens. Reduce the heat to low if the leek begins to brown. Stir in the stock, squash, chicken, and thyme. Cover and simmer for about 10 minutes, or until the squash is tender.

2. Turn off the heat and stir in the kale. Season to taste with salt and pepper.

CREAMY CARROT-FENNEL SOUP

Yield: 6 servings

Use the Slow-Cooker Chicken Stock (page 249) as the base for this soup. When using a fennel bulb in a recipe, simply cut off the green stalks and feathery leaves and use only the white bulb.

1 tablespoon extra-virgin olive oil

½ cup chopped onions

6 cups chopped carrots (2 pounds)

4 cups chopped fennel bulb (1 large bulb)

6 cups chicken stock

1 teaspoon dried thyme

½ cup chopped fresh chives

½ cup chopped fresh dill or parsley

Sea salt

1. Heat a 6-quart pot over medium heat. Add the oil and onions and cook for 5 minutes. Stir in the carrots, fennel, stock, and thyme. Cover and simmer for 30 to 35 minutes. Use an immersion blender to puree the soup in the pot, or pour it into a blender and puree in batches, covering the blender top with a towel in case the hot liquid splatters.

2. Return the soup to the pot and stir in the chives and dill or parsley. Add salt to taste. Serve immediately. Store leftover soup in a glass jar in your refrigerator for up to 1 week.

HEARTY BEEF AND MUSHROOM STEW

Phases
1 & 2

Yield: 6 servings

Serve this beef stew over cooked white or brown rice (Phase 1 only), and top it with a few spoonfuls of sauerkraut. The Transition Protocol allows cooked alcohol only. When you cook with wine, the alcohol evaporates and you are left with an acid that adds good flavor. For more information about alcohol consumption and a leaky gut, check out this online link: thepaleomom.com/2012/11/the-whys -behind-the-autoimmune-protocol-alcohol.html.

2 pounds grass-fed, organic beef stew meat

1 medium onion, chopped

2 cups chopped carrots

2 cups chopped and peeled rutabagas

3 cups chopped button mushrooms

1 tablespoon dried thyme

2 teaspoons sea salt

1½ cups water or Vital Choice organic beef bone broth

¾ cup organic red wine

3 tablespoons arrowroot powder

1–2 cups chopped kale

½ cup chopped fresh parsley

1. In a slow cooker, combine the stew meat, onion, carrots, rutabagas, mushrooms, thyme, and salt. In a small bowl, whisk together the water or broth, wine, and arrowroot powder and add to the slow cooker.

2. Cook on low for 8 hours or on high for 4 to 5 hours. Stir in the kale and parsley and cook for a few minutes. Taste and adjust the salt and seasonings, if desired. Store leftover stew in a covered glass container for up to a week or freeze in portion-size containers for up to 6 months.

HEARTY GARDEN VEGETABLE AND BEAN SOUP

Phase
1

Yield: 6 servings

The fiber found in vegetables and beans helps to feed beneficial bacteria in your gut. Serve this soup with a large green salad to boost healing. If you'd like to try this soup in Phase 2, omit the tomatoes and potatoes—as well as the beans if you have abdominal complaints.

Any type of cooked white bean will work in this recipe—try great Northern beans, navy, or cannellini. I've also used cooked chickpeas with great results. If you do not want to soak and cook your own beans, then substitute canned organic beans. Look for purveyors like Eden Foods who do not use BPA in their can linings.

2	tablespoons extra-virgin olive oil
1	small onion, finely chopped
2	cloves garlic, crushed
2	cups finely chopped yellow or red potatoes
1½	cups finely chopped celery
1½	cups chopped green beans
1–1½	cups diced roma tomatoes
1½	cups cooked white beans
4–6	cups chicken stock
1	teaspoon dried thyme
1	teaspoon dried oregano
2	cups chopped kale
½	cup chopped fresh parsley
½	cup chopped fresh basil
	Sea salt and freshly ground black pepper

1. Heat the oil in a 4- or 6-quart pot over medium heat. Add the onion and garlic and cook for 5 minutes, or until softened. Stir in the potatoes, celery, green beans, tomatoes, white beans, chicken stock, thyme, and oregano. Cover and cook for 10 to 15 minutes, or until the vegetables are tender.

2. Stir in the kale, parsley, and basil and simmer for a few minutes longer. Season to taste with salt and pepper. Serve immediately. Store leftover soup in glass quart jars and reheat as needed. Soup will last up to a week in the refrigerator.

THAI COCONUT FISH SOUP

Phases 1 & 2

Yield: 4 servings

Serve this warming and nourishing soup with a scoop of cooked white or brown rice and a few spoonfuls of fermented veggies such as kimchi. I like to use a mild-tasting Pacific-caught white fish such as halibut, black cod, or rockfish. Ask your fishmonger to skin the fillets when you purchase them at the market.

Gold Mine is an excellent brand of naturally fermented raw kimchi and sauerkraut.

1 tablespoon virgin coconut oil

½ medium onion, sliced

2 cloves garlic, crushed

1 red bell pepper, cut into matchsticks

2–3 carrots, cut into matchsticks

1 can (13.5 ounces) organic coconut milk

1 cup chicken stock

1–2 tablespoons sugar-free, gluten-free fish sauce

1–1½ pounds wild mild-flavored fish, pin bones removed, skinned, and chopped

¼ cup chopped fresh holy or sweet basil

¼ cup finely chopped fresh cilantro

1 tablespoon freshly squeezed lime juice

Sea salt

1–2 Thai chiles, finely chopped, wear plastic gloves when handling (optional)

1. Heat the oil in a 4-quart pot over medium heat. Add the onion and cook for 5 minutes, or until soft. Stir in the garlic, bell pepper, carrots, coconut milk, stock, and fish sauce. Cover and cook for 5 minutes. Add the fish and cook for 5 minutes, or until the fish is cooked through. Turn off the heat and add the basil, cilantro, lime juice, and salt to taste.

2. Serve over rice. Add Thai chiles to each bowl for extra spice, if desired. Store leftover soup in a tightly sealed glass jar for up to 5 days.

Salads and Vegetables

BAKED DELICATA SQUASH WITH CINNAMON

Phases 1 & 2

Yield: 4 servings

Delicata squash are a variety of winter squash. They are very sweet and mild flavored—perfect for baking. You can usually find them from September through March at grocery stores or farmers' markets. Serve this recipe with a big salad for lunch or with roasted chicken or fish and a salad for dinner.

2 **medium delicata squash**

2 **tablespoons extra-virgin olive oil**

½ **teaspoon ground cinnamon**

¼ **teaspoon sea salt**

1. Preheat the oven to 400°F. Cut the stem end off each squash, then cut each in half lengthwise. Use a spoon to scrape out the seeds.

2. Place the 4 squash halves skin side down in a glass baking dish. Drizzle the oil evenly over the flesh. Evenly sprinkle on the cinnamon and sea salt.

3. Bake for 40 minutes, or until tender. Scoop out the flesh and mash until smooth. Serve immediately, or store in the refrigerator for up to a week.

CHIPOTLE CABBAGE SLAW

Yield: 6 servings

Serve this colorful, antioxidant-rich slaw as a side dish with the Slow-Cooker Barbecued Chicken (page 270), or enjoy it alone as a snack.

½ **small head red cabbage, thinly sliced**

½ **small head green cabbage, thinly sliced**

3–4 **carrots, grated**

½ **bunch scallions, cut into thin rounds**

1 **recipe Creamy Chipotle-Lime Dressing (page 267)**

In a large bowl, toss together the cabbages, carrots, and scallions. If you plan to eat the entire salad at one meal, then pour the dressing over the salad, toss together, and serve. If you plan on eating only a small portion, then simply dress a serving-size portion and store the remaining salad in a loosely covered glass bowl in the refrigerator. Store the dressing separately in a glass jar.

FENNEL AND CABBAGE SALAD

Yield: 6 servings

Phases
1 & 2

You can prep this salad and keep it in your refrigerator all week, then take out serving-size portions as needed and add the dressing of your choice. This way, you can easily incorporate more vegetables into your daily routine without a lot of prep time.

1 **large fennel bulb**

½ **large head red or green cabbage**

1 **cup chopped fresh parsley**

½ **cup thinly sliced scallions or chives**

1 **recipe Citrus-Garlic Dressing (page 266)**

Set up a food processor with the slicing disk. Cut the fennel and cabbage into pieces small enough to fit into the feed tube, then process or thinly slice. Transfer to a large glass bowl and add the parsley and scallions or chives. Toss together. Pour the dressing over the salad and toss again. Store any leftover salad in a large glass container in the refrigerator for up to a week.

LEMON-CURRY ROASTED CAULIFLOWER

Yield: 4 servings

If you've never had roasted cauliflower before, then you're in for a real treat! My children fight over it, down to the last piece. On movie nights, try roasting a pan full of cauliflower and serving it in a bowl in lieu of popcorn—a much healthier alternative!

1 **medium head cauliflower, chopped**

1 **teaspoon mild curry powder**

1 **teaspoon finely grated lemon peel**

¼ **teaspoon sea salt**

1 **tablespoon freshly squeezed lemon juice**

2 **tablespoons extra-virgin olive oil or avocado oil**

1. Preheat the oven to 400°F.

2. On a large rimmed stainless steel baking sheet, toss together the cauliflower, curry powder, lemon peel, salt, lemon juice, and oil. Roast for 25 to 30 minutes, or until tender. Serve immediately.

ROSEMARY ROASTED FALL VEGETABLES

Yield: 4 to 6 servings

Serve roasted vegetables with baked fish and a large salad, or store them in your refrigerator and use them to top mixed greens. They pair well with leftover salmon and the Citrus-Garlic Dressing (page 266).

½ medium red onion, chopped into large pieces

3 medium carrots, cut into ½" rounds

1 pound Brussels sprouts, halved

2 small beets, peeled and chopped

1 small rutabaga, peeled and chopped

2 tablespoons extra-virgin olive oil or avocado oil

2 tablespoons chopped fresh rosemary

¼ teaspoon sea salt

1. Preheat the oven to 400°F.

2. On a large rimmed stainless steel baking sheet or in a glass baking dish, toss the onion, carrots, Brussels sprouts, beets, and rutabaga with the oil, rosemary, and salt. Spread the vegetables evenly so they are in a single layer.

3. Roast for 25 minutes, or until tender. Serve immediately.

SAUTÉED GREENS WITH GARLIC

Yield: 4 servings

Serve these tasty greens along with baked salmon, roasted lamb, or baked chicken for lunch or dinner or with fried eggs for a filling breakfast. Change the flavor by adding your favorite seasonings. I like to add a few dashes of raw apple cider vinegar and sea salt.

1 tablespoon extra-virgin olive oil or virgin coconut oil

1 bunch kale, rinsed and chopped

1 bunch collard greens, rinsed and chopped

1 bunch Swiss chard, rinsed and chopped

4–6 cloves garlic, crushed

¼–½ cup water

Heat the oil in a 6- or 8-quart pot over medium heat. Add the kale, collard greens, chard, and garlic and cook for a few minutes. Add the water, cover, and cook for 3 to 5 minutes, or until tender. Serve with your choice of optional seasonings to taste.

OPTIONAL SEASONINGS

Brown rice vinegar

Coconut vinegar

Ume plum vinegar

Freshly squeezed lemon juice

Coconut aminos

Wheat-free tamari

Sea salt

Toasted sesame seeds

Raw apple cider vinegar

BAKED SWEET POTATO FRIES

Phases
I & 2

Yield: 4 servings

For the perfect weeknight meal, serve these tasty baked fries with grass-fed burgers wrapped in lettuce leaves along with a few spoonfuls of Pickled Vegetables (page 278) on the side. I prefer to use white-fleshed sweet potatoes for this recipe rather than the orange variety; they have a little less moisture and work better as fries.

2½	**pounds white sweet potatoes, peeled**
½	**teaspoon freshly ground black pepper**
½	**teaspoon turmeric powder**
½	**teaspoon garlic powder**
½	**teaspoon sea salt**
3–4	**tablespoons extra-virgin olive oil or avocado oil**

1. Preheat the oven to 400°F.

2. Cut the sweet potatoes into ½"-thick strips that are about 4" long. Place on a large rimmed stainless steel baking sheet. In a small bowl, mix together the pepper, turmeric, garlic powder, and salt. Sprinkle evenly over the potatoes. Add the oil and toss to coat.

3. Bake for 25 to 30 minutes, or until tender. Serve immediately.

SPRING DETOX SALAD

Yield: 4 servings

This is my go-to salad for the week. I prepare it on the weekend and keep it in my refrigerator so I can use it as the base for salads throughout the week. Top it with leftovers like baked salmon or roasted chicken. Add some finely chopped avocado and walnuts for a heartier salad. Pour your favorite dressing into a small jar and dress your salad just before serving. I like to use the Raspberry-Lemon Vinaigrette (page 265), but any of the dressings in this chapter would be delicious.

6 cups mixed organic baby greens	In a large bowl, toss together the baby greens, arugula, dandelion, radishes, peas, pea shoots, and chives. Serve with your favorite dressing. Extra salad can be stored in a loosely covered container in the refrigerator for up to 5 days.
2 cups baby arugula	
1 cup chopped dandelion greens	
1 bunch radishes, chopped	
½ pound sugar snap peas, chopped	
1 cup pea shoots	
½ cup snipped fresh chives	

WARM QUINOA, KALE, AND CHICKEN SALAD

Phase I

Yield: 4 servings

Pack this comforting warm grain salad in a thermos for your lunch. Quinoa is an ancient pseudo-grain—a seed related to spinach and beets that resembles a grain—originating in the Andes of South America. You can find it at your local health food store.

1½ cups dry quinoa

2½ cups water or chicken stock

3 tablespoons extra-virgin olive oil

1 cup finely chopped onion

½ teaspoon sea salt

2–3 teaspoons mild curry powder

4 cups finely chopped kale

2–3 cups cooked, chopped chicken

¼ cup currants (see Note)

1–2 tablespoons freshly squeezed lemon juice

1. Rinse the quinoa well under warm water in a fine-mesh strainer. Place it in a 2-quart stainless steel pot and add the water or stock and a pinch of salt. Cover and bring to a boil, then reduce the heat to low and cook for 20 minutes.

2. Heat the oil in a 6-quart pot or a deep 11" skillet over medium heat. Add the onion and salt and cook for 7 minutes, or until soft. Stir in the curry powder. Add the cooked quinoa, kale, chicken, currants, and lemon juice. Stir together and cook for a few minutes, or until the kale has softened. Taste and adjust the salt and seasonings, if desired.

NOTE: Include the currants if FODMAPs are okay with your digestion; otherwise omit.

Salad Dressings

CREAMY ORANGE-GINGER DRESSING

Yield: about 1½ cups

Use this creamy orange-flavored dressing to top just about any salad. I like it tossed with chopped napa cabbage, scallions, and mung bean sprouts.

1 medium orange, peeled and seeded

2–3 teaspoons chopped fresh ginger

¼ cup creamy almond butter

3 tablespoons organic brown rice vinegar

1 teaspoon raw honey

¼ teaspoon sea salt

6 tablespoons extra-virgin olive oil

In a blender, combine the orange, ginger, almond butter, vinegar, honey, and salt. Blend on high speed until smooth. Slowly add the oil while the blender is running on low speed. Pour into a glass jar and store in the refrigerator for up to 10 days.

RASPBERRY-LEMON VINAIGRETTE

Phases
1 & 2

Yield: about ¾ cup

This vinaigrette recipe works well as a marinade for chicken. It also serves wonderfully as a dressing for a quinoa-vegetable salad or any green salad.

6 tablespoons extra-virgin olive oil

¼ cup mashed raspberries

2 tablespoons freshly squeezed lemon juice

2 tablespoons champagne vinegar

1 teaspoon raw honey

¼ teaspoon sea salt

In a glass jar, combine the oil, raspberries, lemon juice, vinegar, honey, and salt. Cover tightly with a lid and shake to combine. Store in the refrigerator for up to 10 days. Place the jar in a dish of hot water to thin the oil before serving.

CITRUS-GARLIC DRESSING

Phases 1 & 2

Yield: about 1 cup

Top your favorite salad with this dressing high in vitamin C. It pairs well with spicy greens such as arugula.

- **6 tablespoons extra-virgin olive oil**
- **¼ cup freshly squeezed orange juice**
- **2 tablespoons freshly squeezed lemon juice**
- **2 tablespoons freshly squeezed lime juice**
- **1 clove garlic, crushed**
- **2 teaspoons finely grated orange peel**
- **½ teaspoon finely grated lemon peel**
- **½ teaspoon finely grated lime peel**
- **½ teaspoon sea salt**

In a glass jar, combine the oil, citrus juices, garlic, citrus peels, and salt. Cover tightly with a lid and shake to combine. Store in the refrigerator for up to 10 days. Place the jar in a dish of hot water to thin the oil before serving.

TIP: Use a Microplane grater to finely grate the citrus peel before you squeeze the juice out.

CREAMY CHIPOTLE-LIME DRESSING

Phase I

Yield: about 1 cup

Serve this dressing over a salad of crunchy romaine lettuce, avocado, black beans, and toasted pumpkin seeds. I also like to serve it tossed with shredded cabbage, such as the Chipotle Cabbage Slaw (page 256).

½ cup raw cashews

½ cup water

1–2 tablespoons freshly squeezed lime juice

¼ cup extra-virgin olive oil

1 clove garlic, peeled

¼–½ teaspoon chipotle chili powder

½–1 teaspoon sea salt

Small handful of fresh parsley or cilantro

1. In a high-powered blender, combine the cashews, water, lime juice, oil, garlic, chili powder, and salt. Blend until smooth and creamy. Add the parsley or cilantro and blend on low speed to mince and combine. If you don't own a high-powered blender, soak the cashews in water in a small bowl for about 3 hours. Then drain and follow the instructions above, using a standard blender.

2. Pour into a glass jar and serve or store in the refrigerator for up to a week.

Main Dishes

BASIC ROASTED CHICKEN

Phases
1 & 2

Yield: 4 servings

Consider preparing this basic recipe over the weekend so you have precooked chicken in your refrigerator for quick meals and salads throughout the week. The cooked chicken can be used as a main dish or to top salads, or in recipes such as Warm Quinoa, Kale, and Chicken Salad (page 263); Chicken, Squash, and Leek Soup (page 250); and Chicken Salad Lettuce Wraps (page 269).

1 **whole organic chicken (3–4 pounds) separated into parts, or 2 organic bone-in chicken legs and 2 organic bone-in chicken breasts**

2–3 **tablespoons extra-virgin olive oil**

¼–½ **teaspoon sea salt**

¼ **teaspoon garlic powder**

Freshly ground black pepper

1. Preheat the oven to 375°F. Place the chicken pieces in a 13" × 9" glass baking dish. Drizzle with the oil, then evenly sprinkle on the salt, garlic powder, and a few pinches of pepper.

2. Roast, uncovered, for 60 minutes, or until a thermometer inserted into the thickest portion registers 170°F and the juices run clear. Use in recipes as desired. Cooked chicken can be stored in a covered glass container in the refrigerator for up to a week. Save the bones and skin for the Slow-Cooker Chicken Stock recipe on page 249.

CHICKEN SALAD LETTUCE WRAPS

Yield: 2 servings

For the chicken in this recipe, I like to use a leftover chicken breast from a whole organic chicken I have previously roasted. Be sure to use naturally fermented pickles, which have only a few ingredients: cucumbers, pickling spice, salt, and water—no vinegar!

Bubbies is the brand of pickles we like to use. We also highly recommend Primal Kitchen Mayo.

1½ cups cooked, chopped chicken breast

½ cup finely chopped celery

½ cup finely chopped pickles

¼ cup finely chopped carrots

¼ cup finely chopped fresh parsley

1–2 scallions, sliced into thin rounds

¼ cup mayonnaise

Sea salt and freshly ground black pepper

Butter lettuce leaves, rinsed and patted dry

In a large bowl, combine the chicken, celery, pickles, carrots, parsley, scallions, and mayonnaise. Mix well. Season to taste with salt and pepper. Place a scoop of the chicken salad onto a lettuce leaf and serve. Store leftover salad in the refrigerator for up to 3 days.

SLOW-COOKER BARBECUED CHICKEN

Phase
I

Yield: about 6 servings

This recipe can be assembled in a snap before you head to work in the morning. When you get home, bake some sweet potatoes and toss together a salad—you'll have a beautiful, nourishing meal. I like to scoop the shredded barbecued chicken into a sweet potato for serving.

1 small onion, sliced

1 jar (7 ounces) tomato paste (about ¾ cup)

1 cup water

2 tablespoons raw honey or pure maple syrup

2 tablespoons raw apple cider vinegar

2–3 teaspoons blackstrap molasses

2–3 cloves garlic, crushed

1 tablespoon smoked paprika

½ teaspoon chipotle chili powder

1–2 teaspoons sea salt

3 pounds pasture-raised boneless, skinless chicken breasts

In a 4-quart slow cooker, combine the onion, tomato paste, water, honey or maple syrup, vinegar, molasses, garlic, paprika, chili powder, and salt. Mix well. Add the chicken. Cover and cook on low for 8 hours. Using 2 forks, gently shred the chicken. Cook the shredded chicken for 30 minutes. Serve with baked sweet potatoes. Leftover barbecued chicken can be frozen in small containers for future use or refrigerated for up to 5 days.

COCONUT-CRUSTED FISH STICKS

Phases
1 & 2

Yield: 4 to 6 servings

Serve fish sticks with one of the salad recipes in this book and a baked sweet potato. When you purchase the fish at the market, have the fishmonger remove the skin.

Herbamare is an organic seasoning made from fresh herbs and vegetables and blended with natural sea salt.

1½–2 pounds halibut, skin removed

½ cup arrowroot powder

4–6 tablespoons water

1 teaspoon Herbamare or sea salt

½ teaspoon freshly ground black pepper

1 teaspoon dried thyme

2 cups unsweetened shredded coconut

3–4 tablespoons coconut oil

1. Rinse the halibut, then cut into "sticks" about ½" wide and 3" long.

2. In a bowl, whisk together the arrowroot, water, Herbamare or salt, pepper, and thyme. Place the coconut in a separate bowl.

3. Begin heating an 11" or 12" skillet over medium-high heat. While the skillet is heating, dip the fish sticks into the arrowroot mixture and coat evenly. Then dip the fish in the coconut, using your hands to press the coconut into the fish to ensure an even coating.

4. Add 2 tablespoons of the oil to the hot skillet. (The pan is hot enough when the oil spreads out quickly.) Add the fish sticks in batches so they don't overcrowd the pan. Cook for 4 to 6 minutes, turning once with tongs, or until the fish flakes easily. Timing may differ depending on the thickness of the fish. The fish will continue to cook once removed from the pan. Check doneness by breaking apart the thickest piece with a fork. Add the remaining oil as needed to the skillet and cook the remaining fish sticks.

ITALIAN MEATBALLS AND SPAGHETTI SQUASH NOODLES

Phases 1 & 2

Yield: 6 servings

This recipe is a spin on a traditional favorite, but without the tomatoes and wheat noodles. It's important to use a good-quality homemade stock in this recipe, as most of the store-bought varieties of beef stock—even the organic brands—use caramel coloring, which can contain gluten.

MEATBALLS

- 2 pounds grass-fed organic ground beef
- 1 cup grated carrots (firmly packed)
- ½ cup finely chopped scallions
- ½ cup finely chopped fresh parsley
- 2 large organic eggs, whisked
- 1 tablespoon Italian seasoning
- 1 teaspoon sea salt
- ½ teaspoon freshly ground black pepper
- ½ teaspoon garlic powder
- 2–3 teaspoons extra-virgin olive oil

SAUCE

- 3 cups Slow-Cooker Chicken Stock (page 249)
- 3 tablespoons arrowroot powder
- 1–2 teaspoons dried thyme
  Sea salt and freshly ground black pepper
- 1 medium spaghetti squash (about 3 pounds), cut in half lengthwise and seeded

1. Preheat the oven to 400°F.

2. *To make the meatballs:* In a large bowl, combine the beef, carrots, scallions, parsley, eggs, Italian seasoning, salt, pepper, and garlic powder. Mix well using your hands or a large spoon. With oiled hands, form the mixture into 2" meatballs and place on 2 plates. You should have 12 to 18 meatballs.

3. Heat a large cast-iron skillet over medium heat. Add 1 to 2 teaspoons of the oil to the pan. Cook the meatballs in batches for a few minutes on all sides, then transfer to a 13" × 9" glass baking dish (they won't be cooked through at this point). Repeat with the remaining oil and meatballs.

4. *To prepare the sauce:* In a large bowl, whisk together the stock, arrowroot, thyme, and salt and pepper to taste. Pour the sauce into the hot skillet used to cook the meatballs, return the skillet to the stove top, and whisk over medium heat until clear and thickened. Pour the sauce over the meatballs and bake, uncovered, for 40 to 45 minutes, or until no longer pink.

5. Place the spaghetti squash cut side down in another glass baking dish. Add a little water to the bottom of the dish and bake, uncovered, for 45 to 50 minutes. Scoop out the squash "noodles" with a spoon. Spaghetti squash naturally separates into noodles. Serve the meatballs and sauce over the noodles. Leftover meatballs, sauce, and squash can be frozen in individual serving-size containers for later use.

LEMON-GINGER SALMON

Yield: 6 servings

When shopping for salmon, be sure to purchase wild-caught fish. Farmed salmon often contains high levels of PCBs, which can increase the risk for diabetes, obesity, and insulin resistance. Serve salmon with some sautéed zucchini and a large green salad dressed with Citrus-Garlic Dressing (page 266).

2 **pounds wild salmon fillets**

3 **tablespoons freshly squeezed lemon juice**

1 **tablespoon raw honey**

1 **tablespoon toasted sesame oil**

1 **tablespoon arrowroot powder**

1 **clove garlic, crushed**

1–2 **teaspoons finely grated fresh ginger**

½ **teaspoon finely grated lemon peel**

½ **teaspoon sea salt**

1. Rinse the salmon fillets and place them skin side up in a small glass baking dish. In a small bowl, whisk together the lemon juice, honey, oil, arrowroot, garlic, ginger, lemon peel, and salt. Pour over the salmon. Cover and marinate at room temperature for 30 minutes or refrigerate and marinate for up to 2 hours. Drain off most of the marinade and flip the salmon fillets over so they are skin side down.

2. Preheat the oven to 400°F. Bake the salmon for 10 minutes per inch of thickness, or until the fish is opaque. A thin fillet such as coho might need 10 minutes, while a thick king salmon fillet might need 20 minutes. Fish will continue to cook after it comes out of the oven, so be careful not to overcook.

ROASTED CHICKEN
WITH SWEET POTATOES AND FIGS

Yield: 4 to 6 servings

Add ½ cup of organic white wine to the bottom of the pan when you add the water for even more flavor. If you don't use all of the pan juices, save them and add to your homemade Slow-Cooker Chicken Stock (page 249) with the bones. Serve this chicken with a large green salad tossed with Raspberry-Lemon Vinaigrette (page 265).

1 whole organic chicken
(3½–4-pounds)

2½ pounds sweet potatoes,
peeled and cut into
large pieces (see Note)

½–1 cup dried black Mission
figs (see Note)

3 tablespoons extra-virgin
olive oil, divided

1 teaspoon dried thyme

1 teaspoon dried
marjoram

1 teaspoon dried
rosemary

½–1 teaspoon sea salt
Freshly ground black
pepper

½ cup finely chopped
onion

1 cup water

1. Preheat the oven to 425°F.

2. Place the chicken in the center of a 13" × 9" glass baking dish. In a bowl, toss together the sweet potatoes, figs, and 2 tablespoons of the oil. Add to the pan around the chicken. Drizzle the remaining 1 tablespoon oil over the chicken. Sprinkle the thyme, marjoram, rosemary, salt, and pepper to taste over the chicken and sweet potatoes.

3. Place the chopped onion into the cavity of the chicken. Add the water to the pan.

4. Roast, uncovered, for 25 minutes, then reduce the heat to 325°F and roast for 1 hour, or until a thermometer inserted in a breast registers 180°F and the juices run clear. Let stand for 10 minutes before carving.

5. Transfer the sweet potatoes and figs to a serving bowl. Place the chicken on a carving board and slice. Pour the pan juices into a gravy boat and serve alongside the meat and vegetables.

NOTE: Include the sweet potatoes and figs if FODMAPs are okay with your digestion; otherwise omit.

Healthy Treats

NO-COOK CHOCOLATE CUSTARD

Yield: 6 servings

This recipe is perfect for the days when you are craving something rich, creamy, and chocolatey.

1   **can (13.5 ounces) organic coconut milk**

1   **tablespoon unflavored pastured gelatin powder**

¼   **cup organic raw cacao powder**

2–3   **tablespoons pure maple syrup**

2   **teaspoons pure vanilla extract**

    Fresh organic raspberries or strawberries, for garnish

1. In a blender, combine the coconut milk, gelatin powder, cacao, maple syrup, and vanilla. Blend to combine, then let the mixture rest in the blender for 5 minutes to soften the gelatin. Blend again on high speed for at least a minute, or until ultra-smooth.

2. Pour into 6 ramekins or small bowls and refrigerate for at least 30 minutes to set. Serve garnished with fresh berries. Cover any uneaten custard bowls and store in the refrigerator for up to a week.

CHEWY SPICE COOKIES

Phase
I

Yield: 10 to 12 cookies

This recipe uses an alternative baking flour called TigerNut flour—it's grain- and nut-free, making it the perfect flour to use in gluten-free treats. TigerNut flour is made from small tubers that are high in resistant starch—a type of prebiotic fiber that feeds the beneficial bacteria in our guts. You can buy this flour on the Internet or at a local health food store.

8   pitted medjool dates (about ½ cup firmly packed)
¼   cup virgin coconut oil
1   large egg
1   teaspoon pure vanilla extract
1   cup TigerNut flour (firmly packed)
1½   teaspoons ground cinnamon
½   teaspoon ground ginger
½   teaspoon baking soda
¼   teaspoon sea salt

1. Preheat the oven to 350°F. Line a baking sheet with unbleached parchment paper.

2. In a food processor fitted with the standard S blade, combine the dates, oil, egg, and vanilla. Process until the mixture is very smooth and pureed. Add the flour, cinnamon, ginger, baking soda, and salt and process again to combine.

3. Drop the dough by heaping tablespoonfuls onto the baking sheet. You should have 10 to 12 cookies. Using wet hands, gently flatten each one.

4. Bake for 10 minutes, or until the edges are crispy. Let cool for 5 to 10 minutes on the baking sheet before transferring to a plate to cool completely.

CHOCOLATE ALMOND APRICOT BARS

Yield: About 20 bars

Before you begin Phase 1, make a batch of these bars and stash them in your freezer. When you feel a craving coming on for sugar or chocolate, one of these bars will satiate your desire. Instead of "empty calorie" chocolate candy, this recipe offers healthy fats and protein from the almonds, healthy fiber from the dried apricots that feeds beneficial bacteria in your gut, and an array of powerful antioxidants in the organic bittersweet chocolate. I think of these as superfood bars. They can be enjoyed on Phase 2, as long as you are able to eat FODMAPs.

1 **cup raw almonds**

1 **cup dried apricots (unsulfured)**

3 **ounces organic bittersweet chocolate**

2 **tablespoons virgin coconut oil**

2 **tablespoons raw honey**

1 **teaspoon raw vanilla powder**

Pinch of sea salt

1. Line a 9" × 5" glass bread pan with unbleached parchment paper.

2. Place the almonds in a food processor fitted with the standard S blade and process until coarsely ground. Add the apricots and process until both are finely ground.

3. In a small saucepan, melt the chocolate and oil over very low heat. Pour over the almond mixture in the food processor, using a silicone spatula to scrape every last bit of chocolate goodness out of the pan. Add the honey, vanilla powder, and salt to the food processor. Process again to combine the ingredients.

4. Transfer the mixture to the prepared pan. Firmly and evenly press it into the pan. Freeze for 1 hour, or until the mixture is hard to the touch. Remove from the pan, peel off the parchment, and cut into bars with a large, sharp knife. Store in a stainless steel container in the freezer for up to 6 months.

TIP: Many chocolate companies process their chocolate on equipment that also processes gluten. Be sure to buy an organic bittersweet chocolate bar from a gluten-free company. We like to use Dagoba bars in this recipe. They are also divided into 1-ounce portions, making it easy to cut the amount you need from the bar.

Fermented Foods

PICKLED VEGETABLES

Yield: 1 quart

To make this recipe, you'll need a widemouthed quart jar with a lid or a 1-liter latch-lid jar.

3–4 **cloves garlic, chopped**

1½–2 **teaspoons whole black peppercorns**

Handful of fresh dill

1 **cup finely chopped carrots**

1 **cup finely chopped radishes**

1 **cup finely chopped green beans**

1 **tablespoon sea salt**

2 **cups filtered water**

1 **green cabbage leaf**

1. Place the garlic and peppercorns in the bottom of a widemouthed quart jar or a 1-liter latch-lid jar. Place the dill on top of that. Add the carrots, radishes, and beans, packing them down as you go, until they are ½" to 1" from the top of the jar.

2. In a small bowl, whisk together the salt and water until dissolved. Pour the brine solution over the vegetables until they are completely submerged. Fold up the cabbage leaf and press it into the vegetables so it fits under the lip of the jar. This will help keep the vegetables submerged, which is essential for proper fermentation. You could alternatively use a glass weight or boiled rock.

3. Cover the jar tightly with the lid and store in a location away from direct sunlight. "Burp" the jar every day once bubbles start forming, usually by day 2. Do this by slightly unscrewing the lid (or unlatching it) to release the gases and then screwing it back down. Fermentation should take 5 to 10 days, depending on the temperature of your house. The warmer it is, the shorter the fermentation time. Check the vegetables after 5 days. They should be sour and crispy.

4. Once the vegetables have fermented to your liking, place the jar in the refrigerator and store for up to 6 months. They will keep fermenting while in the refrigerator, but at a much slower rate.

HOMEMADE RAW SAUERKRAUT

Yield: 1 quart

Making your own sauerkraut is surprisingly easy. All you need is a widemouthed quart Mason jar, a wooden kraut pounder, cabbage, and some good sea salt. You may want to make a double or triple batch—once the sauerkraut is fermented, it will keep in the refrigerator for quite some time. When preparing this recipe, it's important to maintain the right cabbage-to-salt ratio. If you are doubling the recipe, use 5 pounds of cabbage and 3 tablespoons of sea salt.

2½ pounds cabbage
1½ tablespoons sea salt

1. Remove the outer 2 leaves from the cabbage and reserve 1 leaf. Cut the core out of the bottom of the cabbage and discard. Then cut the cabbage into pieces. Use a food processor fitted with the slicing blade to quickly and easily slice the cabbage. If you don't have a food processor, use a sharp knife to thinly slice the cabbage.

2. Place the sliced cabbage in a large bowl and sprinkle with the salt. Toss together, then let stand for 10 minutes. Use a wooden kraut pounder or meat hammer to pound the cabbage for 5 to 10 minutes, or until the juices have released. Using clean hands, place the cabbage in a widemouthed quart jar, firmly pressing down with the kraut pounder so there are no air bubbles. This recipe should fill 1 quart jar to the top. Press the cabbage down so the juices rise to the top of the jar. If there are not enough juices to completely cover the cabbage, whisk together ½ cup purified water with ½ teaspoon sea salt and pour over the cabbage. Press the reserved cabbage leaf into the cabbage. Screw on the lid and place the jar on a towel or in a pie plate to catch juices that may leak out.

3. Keep the jar on your kitchen counter away from direct sunlight. Let it ferment for 5 to 10 days, then place in the refrigerator, where it will keep for up to 6 months.

COCONUT-CHERRY PROBIOTIC SODA

Yield: 3¾ cups

This recipe is an excellent way to consume gut-healing probiotics in a tasty drink. Kids love it! If you can't find the Body Ecology kefir starter in your local health food store, you can order it online at bodyecology.com.

3 cups coconut water

¾ cup organic tart cherry juice

1 packet Body Ecology kefir starter

1. In a small saucepan, warm the coconut water and cherry juice over low heat until it nearly reaches 92°F. If it gets any hotter, the bacteria in the starter will die. The liquid should feel neutral to the touch—not too cold or hot. Pour it into a glass quart jar, add the kefir starter, and screw on the jar lid. Gently shake to combine.

2. Set the jar in a warm spot in your kitchen, ideally around 70°F, to ferment for 24 to 48 hours. It will ferment faster in a very warm kitchen, but in a cool kitchen (in the middle of winter), it may take longer than 48 hours. The beverage is done when it becomes less sweet and slightly bubbly. For a very bubbly "soda," you can pour it into a latch-lid bottle and let it sit on your counter for an additional day or two. Be careful when opening the lid, as pressure from the fermentation gases can build up.

SAMPLE MEAL PLANS

The following suggestions provide you with a week's worth of healthy food options for each phase of the Transition Protocol. Some of the suggestions incorporate the recipes from above; others rely on easy-to-find gluten-free, dairy-free, sugar-free options that are simple to prepare. I've also suggested where you can add fermented foods into your day.

Use the meal plan as a template for the first week, and then make adjustments based on your personal preferences and individual sensitivities going forward.

Transition Phase 1 Meal Plan

No gluten, dairy, sugar. Focus on whole, organic foods and fermented foods to replenish your microbiome.

DAY 1

Breakfast: 1 slice Gluten-Free Sandwich Bread (page 244) toasted and topped with ½ mashed avocado, a handful of arugula, 1 poached organic egg, and freshly ground black pepper

Lunch: Bowl of Hearty Garden Vegetable and Bean Soup (page 253)

Dinner: Grass-fed beef burgers wrapped in lettuce leaves, served with Baked Sweet Potato Fries (page 261), and naturally fermented pickles

Snack: No-Cook Chocolate Custard (page 275) and seasonal organic berries

DAY 2

Breakfast: Breakfast tacos (1 warmed gluten-free organic corn or brown rice tortilla, gluten-free organic refried beans, salsa, avocado, and scrambled organic eggs)

Lunch: Large salad made with organic mixed baby greens, chopped carrots, scallions, cooked quinoa, and leftover cooked chicken or salmon; topped with one of the salad dressings (pages 264–267)

Dinner: Slow-Cooker Barbecued Chicken (page 270), baked sweet potatoes, and sauerkraut

Snack: Gut-Healing Smoothie (page 242)

DAY 3

Breakfast: 2 slices Gluten-Free Sandwich Bread (page 244), toasted and topped with organic peanut butter or almond butter, plus 1 banana

Lunch: Warm Quinoa, Kale, and Chicken Salad (page 263)

Dinner: Grass-fed steak or leftover Slow-Cooker Barbecued Chicken, baked potato, steamed broccoli, and Pickled Vegetables (page 278)

Snack: Super-Antioxidant Green Smoothie (page 243)

DAY 4

Breakfast: Baked potato and Kale Breakfast Hash (page 248)

Lunch: Large salad made with organic baby mixed greens, chopped carrots, scallions, parsley, and leftover steak, cooked beans, or organic deli turkey slices; topped with one of the salad dressings (pages 264–267)

Dinner: Lemon-Ginger Salmon (page 273), cooked organic white or brown rice, and Fennel and Cabbage Salad (page 257)

Snack: Seasonal fruits and a Coconut-Cherry Probiotic Soda (page 280)

DAY 5

Breakfast: Gut-Healing Smoothie (page 242) and 1 poached organic egg

Lunch: Large salad made with organic baby mixed greens, leftover Fennel and Cabbage Salad, leftover cooked salmon, and a scoop of leftover cooked rice; topped with Citrus-Garlic Dressing (page 266)

Dinner: Chicken Salad Lettuce Wraps (page 269), Baked Delicata Squash with Cinnamon (page 255), and kimchi

Snack: Celery sticks and organic peanut butter or almond butter

DAY 6

Breakfast: Garden Vegetable Frittata (page 246)

Lunch: Sandwich made with 2 slices Gluten-Free Sandwich Bread (page 244), organic turkey slices, avocado, thinly sliced red onion, and mayo or mustard; served with a scoop of Homemade Raw Sauerkraut (page 279) or naturally fermented pickles

Dinner: Thai Coconut Fish Soup (page 254), cooked organic white basmati rice, and Lemon-Curry Roasted Cauliflower (page 258)

Snack: Chocolate Almond Apricot Bars (page 277)

DAY 7

Breakfast: Quinoa flakes hot cereal, topped with fresh or frozen blueberries, coconut milk, and chopped almonds

Lunch: Leftover Thai Coconut Fish Soup, plus Spring Detox Salad (page 262)

Dinner: Cooked brown rice spaghetti noodles topped with grass-fed beef and tomato pasta sauce (cook 1 pound ground beef and add 1 jar gluten-free, sugar-free organic pasta sauce), plus a large green salad

Snack: Seasonal fruits and a Coconut-Cherry Probiotic Soda (page 280)

Transition Phase 2 Meal Plan

No gluten, dairy, sugar, grains, or nightshades. Focus on whole, organic foods and fermented foods to replenish your microbiome.

DAY 1

Breakfast: Super-Antioxidant Green Smoothie (page 243) and fresh fruit

Lunch: Bowl of Chicken, Squash, and Leek Soup (page 250)

Dinner: Steak, baked winter squash, and Homemade Raw Sauerkraut (page 279)

Snack: Hummus and celery sticks

DAY 2

Breakfast: Italian Chicken Breakfast Sausages (page 248) and Pickled Vegetables (page 278)

Lunch: Large green salad made with mixed organic baby greens, bacon, and chopped cucumber; topped with one of the Phase 2 salad dressings (pages 264–266)

Dinner: Creamy Carrot-Fennel Soup (page 251) and Sautéed Greens with Garlic (page 260)

Snack: Hummus with sliced carrots and cucumbers

DAY 3

Breakfast: 1 slice Gluten-Free Sandwich Bread (page 244), toasted, and Pickled Vegetables (page 278)

Lunch: Leftover Creamy Carrot-Fennel Soup and half an avocado topped with Pickled Vegetables (page 278)

Dinner: Hearty Beef and Mushroom Stew (page 252) and a green salad

Snack: Fresh berries, and Coconut-Cherry Probiotic Soda (page 280)

DAY 4

Breakfast: Gut-Healing Smoothie (page 242)

Lunch: Leftover Hearty Beef and Mushroom Stew and Coconut-Cherry Probiotic Soda

Dinner: Grilled salmon, baked sweet potatoes, and a large baby greens salad

Snack: No-Cook Chocolate Custard (page 275)

DAY 5

Breakfast: Italian Chicken Breakfast Sausages (page 247) and Pickled Vegetables (page 278)

Lunch: Large salad made with organic mixed baby greens, chopped apples, leftover baked sweet potatoes, topped with one of the Phase 2 salad dressings (pages 264–266)

Dinner: Low-mercury tuna salad, 2 slices Gluten-Free Sandwich Bread (page 244), and Sautéed Greens with Garlic (page 260)

Snack: Super-Antioxidant Green Smoothie (page 243)

DAY 6

Breakfast: Fresh fruit salad with apples, blueberries, and 1 organic banana

Lunch: Spring Detox Salad (page 262), bacon, and kimchi

Dinner: Hearty Beef stew and Mushroom stew (page 252)

Snack: Celery sticks and hummus

DAY 7

Breakfast: Super-Antioxidant Green Smoothie (page 243)

Lunch: Large green salad made with mixed organic baby greens, chopped red cabbage, scallions, cucumbers, finely chopped fresh mango or apples; topped with one of the Phase 2 salad dressings (pages 264–266)

Dinner: Grass-fed beef burgers wrapped in lettuce leaves, served with Rosemary Roasted Fall Vegetables (page 259) or baked winter squash; served with a Coconut-Cherry Probiotic Soda (page 280)

Snack: No-Cook Chocolate Custard (page 275) and 1 organic banana

The Transition Meal Plan Shopping List (for Both Phase 1 and Phase 2)

Active dry yeast

Almond butter

Almond flour (blanched)

Almonds

Apples

Apricots (dried)

Arrowroot powder

Arugula

Avocados

Avocado oil

Baby greens (mixed organic)

Baking powder (gluten-free)

Baking soda

Bananas

Basil

Bay leaf

Beef bone broth (organic)

Beef stew meat (organic)

Beets

Bittersweet chocolate (organic)

Black pepper

Black peppercorns (whole)

Blueberries

Body Ecology kefir starter

Bok choy

Broccoli

Brown rice flour

Brown rice spaghetti noodles

Brown rice tortilla (gluten-free)

Brown rice vinegar

Brussels sprouts

Butternut squash

Button mushrooms

Cabbage

Carrots

Cashews (raw)

Cauliflower

Celery

Champagne vinegar

Chicken (whole, organic)

Chicken breasts (boneless, skinless)

Chicken livers

Chicken stock

Chicken thighs (boneless, skinless)

Chipotle chili powder

Chives

Cilantro

Cinnamon

Coconut

Coconut aminos

Coconut flour

Coconut milk

Coconut oil

Coconut (unsweetened shredded)

Coconut vinegar

Coconut water

Collard greens

Corn tortilla (organic, gluten-free)

Cranberries (frozen)

Cucumbers

Currants

Curry powder

Dandelion greens

Delicata squash

Deli turkey slices (organic)

Dill

Eggs

Fennel

Fennel seeds

Figs

Fish oil

Fish sauce (sugar-free, gluten-free)

Flaxseeds (ground)

Garlic

Garlic powder

Gelatin powder (unflavored)

Ginger (fresh and ground)

Grass-fed beef

Green beans

Green cabbage

Halibut

Herbamare

Hummus (gluten-free)

Italian seasoning

Kale

Kimchi

Leeks

Lemons

Lettuce

L-glutamine powder

Limes

Marjoram (dried)

Maple syrup

Marjoram (dried)

Mayonnaise

Medjool dates

Molasses

Mushrooms

Mustard

Olive oil, extra-virgin

Onions

Oranges

Oregano (dried)

Paprika

Parsley

Pasta sauce (organic, gluten-free)

Peanut butter

Pea shoots

Pickles (naturally fermented)

Pineapple

Potatoes

Potato starch

Psyllium husks (whole)

Pumpkin seeds

Quinoa
Quinoa flakes hot cereal
Radishes
Raspberries
Raw apple cider vinegar
Raw cacao powder
Raw honey
Raw vanilla powder
Red bell pepper
Red cabbage
Red wine
Refried beans (organic, gluten-free)
Roma tomatoes
Rosemary
Rutabaga
Sage
Salmon
Salsa
Sauerkraut
Scallions
Sea salt
Sesame oil, toasted

Sesame seeds
Spaghetti squash
Spinach
Steak
Sugar snap peas
Sweet potatoes
Swiss chard
Tamari (wheat-free)
Tapioca flour
Tart cherry juice
Thai chiles
Thyme (dried)
TigerNut flour
Tomato paste
Turmeric
Ume plum vinegar
Vanilla extract (pure)
White basmati rice
White beans
White or brown rice
Winter squash

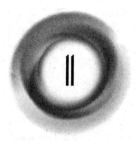

WEEK 7 AND BEYOND:

A LIFETIME OF BETTER HEALTH

By week 7, it's very likely that you'll be beginning to look and feel differently and know that you are solidly on the right track to better health. I hope that you are feeling less sick, fat, and tired after these 6 full weeks of going gluten-free, dairy-free, and sugar-free, as well as investigating the other most common foods that can cause sensitivities. You may notice that you are less bloated, that your skin has cleared up a bit, and that you have more energy. These are all signs that your body is winding down the inflammatory cascade and your immune system is returning to a more normal, balanced response.

If this is true, you can now transition to the maintenance part of the program. This is when you begin to expand your options by adding back one food at a time—the foods you've been avoiding—and determining how your body responds to each one. You'll begin by slowly reintroducing the foods removed during Phase 2 in Chapter 9, while still staying clear of gluten, dairy, and sugar.

HOW TO ADD FOODS BACK INTO YOUR DIET

Continue to eat as many of the approved foods that you learned to enjoy on the plan as you begin to reintroduce the foods you have been avoiding. Start with one food at a time, perhaps one of the nightshade vegetables, until you have reintroduced all the foods that you enjoy. For example, add a tomato to one meal for one day. The following day, have tomatoes twice, then three times on the third day. Given that nightshades are a food group that commonly triggers reactions, it's helpful to find out quickly if they can be tolerated.

Reintroducing foods requires patience, so go slowly. The process of reintroduction will take a few weeks, because we can reintroduce only one food at a time. The reason is that food reactions can occur anywhere from immediately after eating to within 72 hours. If you don't experience any change in the way you feel within 3 days of reintroducing tomatoes, for example, then it's likely that tomatoes do not cause an adverse reaction. Of course, if any food causes any kind of symptoms, that is a clear message from your body that you have a sensitivity to that particular food item. It may be your energy that suffers with the introduced food, or your ability to sleep, or your bowel activity. Use the chart on page 292 to remember which foods you are sensitive to so you can continue to avoid them in the future.

Many people feel different symptoms or even stronger symptoms than they experienced before trying the Transition Protocol. If this is the case for you, don't worry: This experience is completely normal. As you remove inflammation in one area of the body, you unmask symptoms that were occurring simultaneously but to a lesser extent in another area. This is a sign that you are getting stronger and healthier. Your body is recognizing toxins a little faster and sending you a little clearer message.

As you slowly reintroduce the foods eliminated during the last 3 weeks, you may be able to clearly see if any of these foods actually trigger a physical or mental reaction. In fact, having symptoms develop with the reintroduction of eliminated foods is a blessing. No one can argue with how you feel. You may choose to ignore the symptoms, but that's not why you bought this book. Then you can take the Medical Symptoms Quiz again in Chapter 4, which will let you know if you've made progress along the autoimmune spectrum. The most common changes you might experience are increases or decreases in any of the following:

- Digestion/bowel function
- Brain function, clarity of thinking

- Energy level
- Headache/head pressure
- Joint/muscle aches
- Kidney/bladder/skin function
- Nasal and chest congestion

On day 4, move to another nightshade vegetable (perhaps white potatoes), and try that food for 3 days using the same pattern. No reaction? Go on to another food on day 7, and so on. Once those are completely reintroduced, move to the organic gluten-free grains and repeat the process, continuing through all of the foods eliminated during Phase 2.

Next try reintroducing a little bit of sugar, but only if you want to. It is not mandatory to reintroduce the foods that you have eliminated. Your sweet tooth will have diminished so that you can stay away from toxic sugar as much as possible. Because of the excess amounts of sugar we have been exposed to throughout our lives, many researchers say the sugar-related disease of diabetes is the most pressing health problem today.[1] It's also important to note that more than 46 percent of the 386 million people worldwide with diabetes are undiagnosed. This alarming number suggests that sometimes how we "feel" with diabetes is not debilitating enough to see a doctor. Many undiagnosed diabetics feel fine. For this reason, I suggest waiting to reintroduce refined sugar for at least 6 months to a year. This will give your blood-sugar-regulating metabolic pathways a chance to rebuild a stronger tolerance to occasional sugar exposures.

When you think you can tolerate a bit of sugar, you can reintroduce alcoholic beverages. I advise my patients to begin with ones that are inherently gluten-free, like tequila or gluten-free hard cider made from apples or other fruits. If you wake up the next morning feeling groggy or with low energy after having just one gluten-free drink, it might be a sign that it's too early to introduce something even modestly high in sugar. You'll then know that you need to continue being vigilant avoiding sugar. If so, wait another 3 weeks and try again.

I suggest you reintroduce dairy last. As you've learned, dairy is such a common and potent trigger that it can set you back if you have a reaction. Because the protein molecules of dairy are eight times the size of human breast milk, dairy can cause a host of different reactions,

FOOD INTRODUCTION DELAYED RESPONSE CHART

Name:_____

Day	Food		Digestion/ bowel function	Brain function, clarity of thinking	Energy level
	time	food			

Day	Headache/ head pressure	Joint/muscle aches	Kidney/ bladder/skin function	Nasal and chest congestion

including excessive mucus production. Kids with recurrent ear infections, or adults with chronic sinus infections, develop a scenario where the head becomes a human petri dish full of mucus. Bacteria thrive within this nutrient-dense, dark, no-immune-system environment. There is no bloodflow through the accumulated mucus, thus no white blood cells can get in to kill off the bacteria.

THE ELEPHANT IN THE ROOM: THE DILEMMA OF THE ELIMINATION DIET

The concept of reintroducing foods into the diet is one I have had difficulty with for most of my career. The standard method everyone uses is as I've explained: to reintroduce one food at a time and then notice how you feel. This is referred to as an elimination diet. On the surface, the logic is sound. The problem is, as you have learned, that the spectrum of autoimmunity development is going on in your body for years without noticeable symptoms. When we have elevated antibodies to our brain, for example, we cannot "feel" the inflammation that is roaring inside until enough brain cells have been damaged and we develop symptoms. If you've eliminated the offending foods and taken the nutrition to support healing the gut and balancing your microbiome, your body is purring along like a finely tuned sports car. But when you reintroduce suspected foods into the diet, if a particular food is a problem and if you're lucky, you may have a noticeable symptom wherever the weak link is in your chain. While this works well for some people, there has never been a study looking at how many people do not have symptoms with food reintroduction, yet their bodies reactivate an immune response and, once again, elevate antibodies. And if you reactivate the immune cascade without noticeable symptoms, you reactivate the destruction of tissue cells from elevated antibodies wherever the weak link is in your chain. This is the conundrum with food reintroduction: Unless you try these foods, you'll never know if they affect you. Yet if you eat them and they cause problems, symptoms might not be noticeable for a very long time.

The only strategy I know to help protect you in the long term is a two-pronged approach: First, follow this elimination diet, reintroducing foods one at a time as I've just outlined. Second, 6 months after you've completed the reintroduction and you're feeling great, redo the blood tests discussed in Chapter 5 that identified the initial problems. If they show that the antibodies to the weak link in your chain are reactivated, now you have evidence that despite how you "feel," tissue damage has begun again and you are at high risk of eventually developing the disease associated with that specific tissue destruction. With my two-step approach, you are more assured of not unintentionally reactivating the tissue-destruction cascade.

Remember, the triad necessary for the development of autoimmune disease is genetics, environmental triggers, and intestinal permeability. There are many environmental triggers that we are testing during the reintroduction phase—not just gluten. Any food that you have an adverse reaction to will cause intestinal permeability and is a problem, irrespective of whether you "feel" the problem or not.[2]

HOW TO EAT AT RESTAURANTS

Since I travel so often for teaching, I find myself in restaurants all the time. This wouldn't be my preference: I know I'm much safer eating foods I prepare at home. Eating out is fraught with hazards. Often, many food service professionals—from the waitstaff to the restaurant managers and even the chefs—may not be fully aware of how to best assist people with food sensitivities. But thanks to the availability of supportive digestive enzymes discussed in Chapter 8, I feel an incredible sense of relief, and I feel safe outside of my own kitchen.

People who work in restaurants are usually service-oriented folks who want to deliver a pleasant experience for diners. Unfortunately, many of them have not been taught the significance of an inadvertent exposure. On top of that is the fact that in general, people are kind: We don't want to make a scene and might even think, *I don't want to be a bother*. But I have learned that maintaining your good health trumps politeness.

I am a strong advocate that whenever you are in a restaurant, you need to make your specific needs heard and then have the waitstaff follow through on them. Don't be afraid to be dramatic: You need to capture someone's attention. At restaurants, I make sure I look the waiter/waitress directly in the eye and say the following in a friendly but direct tone:

"Hello, I'm hoping you can help me. I have a gluten sensitivity. Can you help me ensure that all the food brought to our table is gluten-free?"

Most of the time, a good waitperson will understand your concerns and make sure everything coming to your table is safe. I have also found that when you engage the waitstaff (*"Can you help me ensure . . . "*), it gives you a little more protection because you have created an ally who hopefully will be your advocate in the kitchen, protecting your food along the dangerous journey from the cutting board to your plate. Gluten exposure can occur anywhere in the preparation stage. Besides hidden sources of gluten, dairy, or sugar in recipes, there are serious concerns about cross-contamination: when pots, pans, and cooking utensils are used repeatedly without being thoroughly cleaned. So even if there is no gluten in any of the ingredients, you can be exposed if the cook uses the same cutting board that bread was sliced on, stirs your gluten-free pasta with the same fork used for the regular pasta on the other burner, or deep-fries your French fries in the same oil that cooked breaded shrimp. Remember, it takes only $\frac{1}{8}$ of a thumbnail of gluten to activate your protective immune inflammatory response. Good waitstaff will remind the kitchen staff to use only the cleanest pots and pans when preparing food for someone with sensitivities.

If I do not have confidence in my waitperson, I ask for the owner or the manager. Don't feel like you are making staff go out of their way. Restaurants make these types of accommodations all the time. That's their job—to give you a wonderful experience so that you want to return. Help them help you have a great experience by letting them know what you need. I politely say to the boss, "I have a gluten sensitivity, so to avoid a 911 incident in your restaurant, could you please make sure that everything I order is completely gluten-free?"

I also select foods from the menu that I know can be simply prepared. I steer clear of sauces completely, and I ask for proteins or vegetables to be sautéed with just a little garlic and olive oil. I tend to go back to the restaurants where I've had good experiences, so that the people who work there know me and understand my needs. When I'm on the road, I look for chain restaurants that have a reputation of being amenable. My favorite chains include McCormick & Schmick's and the Oceanaire Seafood Room, although to be honest, an inadvertent contamination can occur anywhere. Once, my girlfriend and I were having dinner with my friend, a leading functional medicine gastroenterologist, in one of my favorite chain restaurants, and the staff served us a gluten-containing appetizer even though we were very clear about our needs.

My girlfriend is a sensitive celiac. It was sobering to see that even with clear communication from all three of us about the need for gluten-free dishes, mistakes can happen.

Two years later, I was at an upscale chain restaurant with my sister, and I told the waiter very clearly that we both have a gluten sensitivity. The waiter said confidently, "No problem. We can handle gluten sensitivity. Almost every entree on the menu can be made gluten-free."

We were thrilled to hear it. My sister and I both ordered a simply prepared piece of grilled salmon, with rice and green vegetables on the side. Just before the waiter left with our order, I said, "Please make sure to tell the chef everything needs to be gluten-free." I looked him directly in the eye as I spoke. His look back to me showed his annoyance, as if he were saying, "You idiot, I already said that we can do everything gluten-free," but he replied, "Yes, sir."

Yet when the food arrived, everything was swimming in an unidentifiable sauce. I immediately asked the waiter to find out what it was, and sure enough, it contained flour as a thickening agent. This time the waiter was embarrassed, took the food back to the kitchen, and put in a completely new order. I asked for the manager and told him that I was going to post our experience on my Facebook page—how clear we were with the waiter and the unfortunate result—and that tens of thousands of people were going to read about the mistake "your restaurant" made. The look of shock on his face was obvious. I then said, "And here's my card with my personal e-mail address. When you send me photos and an explanation of the additional training you have completed with your staff for accommodating gluten-free eating, I will post an update with the caption, 'They Blew It, and Now They're Going out of Their Way to Make It Right.'"

I've used this method a number of times over the years, and in most cases the manager gets back to me with the update on staff training. In the end, making a point is a win-win for everyone.

PUTTING IT ALL TOGETHER TO UNDERSTAND THE BIG PICTURE

In this book, you've learned how to identify where you are on the auto-immune spectrum and discovered how you got there in the first place. You've also learned how to stop throwing gasoline on the fire of inflammation by avoiding the foods that are making you sick. And you've learned how to heal and seal your gut so that you can rebuild the tissue that's been damaged and stop triggering the autoimmune cascade once and for all.

You may have noticed that within the discussion of experimenting with the foods you have been avoiding, I clearly left off gluten. This decision was deliberate because the only food that we know with certainty you cannot reintroduce is gluten. According to the research I have seen, gluten is the only food for which our bodies make memory B cells (remember General Measles?). That means once the sensitivity has begun and your immune system makes antibodies to gluten, you will have a lifelong sensitivity. It will never go away. General Gluten will always be vigilant. A number of clinical trials now in process are looking for a "cure" to gluten sensitivity, yet as of this writing, none has been confirmed.

In my office, we retest patients 6 to 12 months after they've started following a gluten-free diet. Unlike testing for other antibodies, the time frame is determined by the patients' age, their response to the Transition Protocol, and their overall health. The further along they may be in development of the autoimmune spectrum, the more time it takes before autoimmune and food antibodies come back down into normal range. We look to see if the immune system has calmed down, which is confirmed by the bloodwork.

If bloodwork confirms you no longer have elevated antibodies to gluten, there is a natural tendency to ask, "Is it okay now to go back to eating gluten, Doc?" Unfortunately, the answer is no. First, even when the right blood test comes back normal, it just means there have been no assaults in the last few months, and the armed forces are back on sentry duty instead of high alert. When the threat is reduced, the alert level drops down (reduced antibody levels). It takes 2 to 6 months to reduce the antibody levels after the threat is completely removed, so be patient.

The two most common culprits for keeping the immune system activated are cheating and inadvertent exposures. The story I shared about the nun in Chapter 7 tells the whole story: Just ⅛ of a thumbnail of gluten a week was keeping this woman sick. As soon as she was ordered by her bishop to stop eating that tiny bit, she returned to full vitality. So no matter where you are on the spectrum, you cannot go back to eating gluten, not even once in a while. As I have been telling doctors and the public for years, a gluten-related disorder—meaning celiac disease or non-celiac gluten sensitivity—requires a 100 percent gluten-free diet for life.

If you still don't believe me, listen carefully to the science. According to a 2009 study published in the journal *Alimentary Pharmacology and Therapeutics*, 65 percent of celiac patients still have inflammation in their intestines causing intestinal permeability *even when they are following a gluten-free diet for years.*[3] You read that correctly. The few who heal completely (only 8 percent) do so only because their intestinal shag carpeting (the microvilli) and tissue are given the chance to heal. Intestinal permeability remains for the majority of people for two reasons: Either there are inadvertent exposures that continue to fuel the fire, or because the intestines were so severely damaged, the fire cannot stop and the intestines cannot heal on their own.

So what does this mean? Well, in terms of long-term health, the studies are disheartening. If you have either celiac disease or a gluten sensitivity, your likelihood of dying early in life, which is known as the *standard mortality ratio* (SMR), is high compared to the general population because of ongoing intestinal permeability that is cascading into ongoing inflammation. Here is the exact language used in a 2001 landmark study: "Death was most significantly affected by diagnostic delay, pattern of presentation, and adherence to the gluten-free diet. . . . Non-adherence to the gluten-free diet, defined as eating gluten once-per-month, increased the relative risk of death sixfold."[4] Simply put, the SMR for someone with celiac is 2 to 1, which includes everyone regardless of whether or not they are following a gluten-free diet. That means if I'm 63 and I have celiac disease, and my brother is 62 and he does not have celiac disease, I am twice as likely to die at 63 of some disease—heart disease, cancer, Alzheimer's, diabetes, stroke, Parkinson's—than my brother is when he reaches 63. And if I already have another autoimmune disease, the likelihood increases. Add asthma, the SMR is 3 to 1; kidney disease, it's 6 to 1; with tuberculosis, it's 5 to 1; with Crohn's and colitis, it's 70.9 to 1; with Hashimoto's thyroid disease, it's 64.5 to 1. The reason is simple: Unless you allow the shags of your intestinal lining to completely heal, you are not addressing the inflammation. Without addressing the inflammation, the autoimmune cascade continues, and even though you are trying your best, you continue along the autoimmune spectrum. And in a shocking study in 2006, the mortality from gluten-sensitive individuals negative for celiac disease was shown to be even worse. Here's what the study authors said: "Overall mortality and mortality from malignant neoplasms were increased in patients who were gluten sensitive with a celiac test."[5]

However, there is good news. The research shows that for those who continue to follow a gluten-free diet (meaning they're working hard at it), their SMR was 0.5 to 1; the risk of dying early is half as often instead of twice as often, because they're really taking care of themselves.

My intention with this book has been to help you understand that gluten-free eating is not a 3-week or even a 6-week program. When you connect the dots from a gluten sensitivity to intestinal permeability to initiating the spectrum of autoimmune disease, you now realize this is a guiding principle for a lifetime, and vigilance is a small price to pay for the higher levels of health and vitality you will experience. Most important, remember that it doesn't matter how you feel. In fact, most autoimmune diseases are known as silent killers because you're going to feel fine even as these diseases progress. Osteoporosis, anemia, a vitamin B deficiency: You feel fine. Yet these are all malabsorption conditions linked directly to gut inflammation, where your body is not absorbing important nutrients like calcium, vitamin B, or magnesium. You don't feel symptoms with malabsorption until it gets so bad it becomes obvious. And you do not feel when you have elevated antibodies to your thyroid or your brain or your heart. The elevated antibodies destroying your tissue are the true "silent killers," slowly reducing your tissue and organ function until the function diminishes enough that you begin having symptoms. Then here comes the diagnosis: psoriasis, rheumatoid arthritis, Alzheimer's disease, and so on—conditions that affect your body and brain wherever your weak link is located.

This is why it's important to understand the world of predictive autoimmunity. If you can identify diseases before the earliest symptoms, and you learn how to stop throwing fuel on the fire, you can turn these SMR numbers around and achieve optimal healing. This is true not only for you but for your entire family. Genetics is part of the triad in the development of autoimmune disease. If you have a gluten sensitivity, it's likely that your family will suffer from one of the 300 different types of autoimmune conditions—whether they know it now or not.

Their health, as well as your own, is in your hands. Only you can control your destiny.

Remember, the series of base hits is what wins the ball game. In practically every lecture I have given over the last decade, whether to the public or to the most sophisticated health-care practitioners, I end my talk with the following quote from my mentor, Dr. Jeffrey Bland, because it sums up my message so well:

> *Throughout your life, the most profound influences on your health, vitality, and function are not the doctors you have visited or the drugs, surgery, or other therapies you have undertaken. The most profound influences are the cumulative effects of the decisions you make about your diet and lifestyle on the expression of your genes.*

Thank you, and God bless you.

ENDNOTES

INTRODUCTION

1   L. H. Sigal, "Basic Science for the Clinician 44. Atherosclerosis: An Immunologically Mediated (Autoimmune?) Disease," *Journal of Clinical Rheumatology* 13, no. 3 (Jun 2007): 160–68.
   Y. Sherer and Y. Shoenfeld, "Mechanisms of Disease: Atherosclerosis in Autoimmune Diseases," *Nature Clinical Practice: Rheumatology* 2, no. 2 (Feb 2006): 99–106.
   N. Rose and M. Afanasyeva, "Autoimmunity: Busting the Atherosclerotic Plaque," *Nature Medicine* 9, no. 6 (Jun 2003): 641–42.
   C. J. Binder et al., "The Role of Natural Antibodies in Atherogenesis," *Journal of Lipid Research* 46, no. 7 (Jul 2005): 1353–63.
   P. A. Gordon et al., "Atherosclerosis and Autoimmunity," *Lupus* 10, no. 4 (2001): 249–52.

2   V. G. Khurana et al., "Cell Phones and Brain Tumors: A Review Including the Long-Term Epidemiologic Data," *Surgical Neurology* 72, no. 3 (Sep 2009): 205–14; discussion 214–15. doi: 10.1016/j.surneu.2009.01.019.

3   Z. S. Morris, S. Wooding, and J. Grant, "The Answer Is 17 Years, What Is the Question: Understanding Time Lags in Translational Research," *Journal of the Royal Society of Medicine* 104, no. 12 (Dec 2011): 510–20.

CHAPTER 1

1   M. R. Arbuckle et al., "Development of Autoantibodies before the Clinical Onset of Systemic Lupus Erythematosus," *New England Journal of Medicine* 349, no. 16 (Oct 16, 2003): 1526–33.

2   G. Davies et al., "Effects of Metronidazole and Misoprostol on Indomethacin-Induced Changes in Intestinal Permeability," *Digestive Diseases and Sciences* 38, no. 3 (Mar 1993): 417–25.

3   J. S. Strauss et al., "Guidelines of Care for Acne Vulgaris Management," *Journal of the American Academy of Dermatology* 56, no. 4 (Apr 2007): 651–63.

4   G. Corrao et al., "Mortality in Patients with Coeliac Disease and Their Relatives: A Cohort Study," *Lancet* 358, no. 9279: 356–61.

5   S. Helms, "Celiac Disease and Gluten-Associated Diseases," *Alternative Medicine Review* 10, no. 3 (Sep 2005): 172–92.

6   ACCORD Study Group, "Long-Term Effects of Intensive Glucose Lowering on Cardiovascular Outcomes," *New England Journal of Medicine* 364, no. 9 (Mar 2011): 818–28. doi: 10.1056/NEJMoa1006524.

7   M. Gundestrup and H. H. Storm, "Radiation-Induced Acute Myeloid Leukemia and Other Cancers in Commercial Jet Cockpit Crew: A Population-Based Cohort Study," *Lancet* 354, no. 9195 (Dec 11, 1999): 2029–31.

8   O. H. Franco et al., "The Polymeal: A More Natural, Safer, and Probably Tastier (Than the Polypill) Strategy to Reduce Cardiovascular Disease by More Than 75%," *British Medical Journal* 329, no. 7480 (Dec 18, 2004): 1447–50.

9   NIH Autoimmune Diseases Coordinating Committee, *Autoimmune Diseases Research Plan*, 2006.

10   E. Lionetti et al., "Subclinic Cardiac Involvement in Paediatric Patients with Celiac Disease: A Novel Sign for a Case Finding Approach," *Journal of Biological Regulators and Homeostatic Agents* 26, Suppl. 1(Jan–Mar 2012): S63–68.

11   American Autoimmune Related Diseases Association, "List of Diseases: Autoimmune and Autoimmune-Related Diseases," http://www.aarda.org /autoimmune-information/list-of-diseases/.

12   J. F. Ludvigsson et al., "Small-Intestinal Histopathology and Mortality Risk in Celiac Disease," *Journal of the American Medical Association* 302, no. 11 (Sep 16, 2009): 1171–78.

13   A. Carroccio et al., "Non-Celiac Wheat Sensitivity Diagnosed by Double-Blind Placebo-Controlled Challenge: Exploring a New Clinical Entity," *American Journal of Gastroenterology* 107, no. 12 (Dec 2012): 1898–906.

14   A. Carroccio et al., "High Proportions of People with Nonceliac Wheat Sensitivity Have Autoimmune Disease or Antinuclear Antibodies," *Gastroenterology* 149, no. 3 (Sep 2015): 596–603.

15   Helms, "Celiac Disease and Gluten-Associated Diseases."

16   W. F. Stenson et al., "Increased Prevalence of Celiac Disease and Need for Routine Screening among Patients with Osteoporosis," *Archives of Internal Medicine* 165, no. 4 (Feb 28, 2005): 393–99.

CHAPTER 2

1   A. Fasano and T. Shea-Donohue, "Mechanisms of Disease: The Role of Intestinal Barrier Function in the Pathogenesis of Gastrointestinal Autoimmune Diseases," *Nature Clinical Practice: Gastroenterology and Hepatology* 2, no. 4 (Sep 2005): 416–22.

2   M. F. Cusick, J. E. Libbey, and R. S. Fujinami, "Molecular Mimicry as a Mechanism of Autoimmune Disease," *Clinical Reviews in Allergy and Immunology* 42, no. 1 (Feb 2012): 102–11. doi: 10.1007/s12016-011-8293-8.

3   Ahmed El-Sohemy, "Coffee, CYP1A2 Genotype and Risk of Myocardial Infarction," *Genes and Nutrition* 2, no. 1 (Oct 2007): 155–56.

4   C. Catassi et al., "Natural History of Celiac Disease Autoimmunity in a USA Cohort Followed since 1974," *Annals of Medicine* 42, no. 7 (Oct 2010): 530–38.

5   P. H. Green et al., "Mechanisms Underlying Celiac Disease and Its Neurologic Manifestations," *Cellular and Molecular Life Sciences* 62, no. 7–8 (Apr 2005): 791–99.

6   I. W. Davidson et al., "Antibodies to Maize in Patients with Crohn's Disease, Ulcerative Colitis and Coeliac Disease," *Clinical and Experimental Immunology* 35, no. 1 (Jan 1979): 147–48.

7   J. Hollon et al., "Effect of Gliadin on Permeability of Intestinal Biopsy Explants from Celiac Disease Patients and Patients with Non-Celiac Gluten Sensitivity," *Nutrients* 7, no. 3 (Feb 27, 2015): 1565–76. doi: 10.3390/nu7031565.

8   A. Sanchez et al., "Role of Sugars in Human Neutrophilic Phagocytosis," *American Journal of Clinical Nutrition* 26, no. 11 (Nov 1973): 1180–84. J. Bernstein et al., "Depression of Lymphocyte Transformation Following Oral Glucose Ingestion," *American Journal of Clinical Nutrition* 30, no. 4 (Apr 1977): 613. W. Ringsdorf Jr., E. Cheraskin, and

R. Ramsay Jr., "Sucrose, Neutrophilic Phagocytosis and Resistance to Disease," *Dental Survey* 52, no. 12 (Dec 1976): 46–48.

9   F. Couzy et al., "Nutritional Implications of the Interactions between Minerals," *Progressive Food and Nutrition Science* 17, no. 1 (Jan–Feb 1933): 65–87. A. Kozlovsky et al., "Effects of Diets High in Simple Sugars on Urinary Chromium Losses," *Metabolism* 35, no. 6 (June 1986): 515–18. M. Fields et al., "Effect of Copper Deficiency on Metabolism and Mortality in Rats Fed Sucrose or Starch Diets," *Journal of Nutrition* 113, no. 7 (July 1, 1983): 1335–45. J. Lemann, "Evidence That Glucose Ingestion Inhibits Net Renal Tubular Reabsorption of Calcium and Magnesium," *Journal of Clinical Nutrition* 70 (1976): 236–45.

10   E. Takahashi, Tohoku University School of Medicine, *Wholistic Health Digest* 41 (Oct 1982): 10. Patrick Quillin, "Cancer's Sweet Tooth," *Nutrition Science News* Apr 2000. M. Rothkopf, "Fuel Utilization in Neoplastic Disease: Implications for the Use of Nutritional Support in Cancer Patients," *Nutrition* 6, no. 4 (July–Aug 1990): 14S–16S. D. Michaud, "Dietary Sugar, Glycemic Load, and Pancreatic Cancer Risk in a Prospective Study," *Journal of the National Cancer Institute* 94, no. 17 (Sep 4, 2002): 1293–300.

11   J. Cornée et al., "A Case-Control Study of Gastric Cancer and Nutritional Factors in Marseille, France," *European Journal of Epidemiology* 11, no. 1 (Feb 1995): 55–65.

12   A. T. Lee and A. Cerami, "The Role of Glycation in Aging," *Annals of the New York Academy of Science* 663 (Nov 21, 1992): 63–70.

13   L. Darlington, N. W. Ramsey, and J. R. Mansfield, "Placebo-Controlled, Blind Study of Dietary Manipulation Therapy in Rheumatoid Arthritis," *Lancet* 1, no. 8475 (Feb 1, 1986): 236–38. J. Cheng et al., "Preliminary Clinical Study on the Correlation between Allergic Rhinitis and Food Factors," *Journal of Clinical Otorhinolaryngology* (China) 16, no. 8 (Aug 2002): 393–96.

14   S. Reiser et al., "Effects of Sugars on Indices on Glucose Tolerance in Humans," *American Journal of Clinical Nutrition* 43, no. 1 (Jan 1986): 151–59.

15   S. Ayres Jr and R. Mihan, "Is Vitamin E Involved in the Autoimmune Mechanism?" *Cutis* 21, no. 3 (Mar 1978): 321–25.

16   A. Furth and J. Harding, "Why Sugar Is Bad for You," *New Scientist* Sep 23, 1989, 44.

17   Nancy Appleton, *Lick the Sugar Habit* (New York: Avery Penguin Putnam, 1988).

18   Thomas Cleave, *The Saccharine Disease* (New Canaan, CT: Keats Publishing, 1974).

19   M. Tominaga et al., "Impaired Glucose Tolerance Is a Risk Factor for Cardiovascular Disease, but Not Impaired Fasting Glucose: The Funagata Diabetes Study," *Diabetes Care* 22, no. 6 (Jun 1999): 920–24.

20   A. T. Lee and A. Cerami, "Modifications of Proteins and Nucleic Acids by Reducing Sugars: Possible Role in Aging," *Handbook of the Biology of Aging* (New York: Academic Press, 1990).

21   V. M. Monnier, "Nonenzymatic Glycosylation, the Maillard Reaction and the Aging Process," *Journal of Gerontology* 45, no. 4 (Jul 1990): 105–10.

22   D. G. Dyer et al., "Accumulation of Maillard Reaction Products in Skin Collagen in Diabetes and Aging," *Journal of Clinical Investigation* 93, no. 6 (1993): 421–22.

23   Monnier, "Nonenzymatic Glycosylation."

24   Appleton, *Lick the Sugar Habit.*

25   W. Hellenbrand et al., "Diet and Parkinson's Disease II: A Possible Role for the Past Intake of Specific Nutrients; Results from a Self-Administered Food-Frequency Questionnaire in a Case-Control Study," *Neurology* 47, no. 3 (Sep 1996): 644–50.

26   N. J. Blacklock, "Sucrose and Idiopathic Renal Stone," *Nutrition and Health* 5, no. 1–2 (1987): 9–17. G. C. Curhan et al., "Beverage Use and Risk for Kidney Stones in Women," *Annals of Internal Medicine* 28, no. 7 (Apr 1, 1998): 534–40.

27   F. S. Goulart, "Are You Sugar Smart?" *American Fitness,* Mar–Apr 1991, 34–38.

28   E. Grand, "Food Allergies and Migraine," *Lancet* 1, no. 8123 (May 5, 1979): 955–59.

29   John Yudkin, *Sweet and Dangerous* (New York: Bantam Books, 1974), 129.

30   J. Frey, "Is There Sugar in the Alzheimer's Disease?" *Annales de biologie clinique* (Paris) 59, no. 3 (May–Jun 2001): 253–57.

31   A. Ceriello, "Oxidative Stress and Glycemic Regulation," *Metabolism* 49, no. 2 (Suppl 1; Feb 2000): 27–29.

32   Blacklock, "Sucrose and Idiopathic Renal Stone."

33   F. Lechin et al., "Effects of an Oral Glucose Load on Plasma Neurotransmitters in Humans," *Neuropsychobiology* 26, no. 1–2 (1992): 4–11.

34   M. Fields, "Nutritional Factors Adversely Influencing the Glucose/Insulin System," *Journal of the American College of Nutrition* 17, no. 4 (Aug 1998): 317–21.

35   Patricia Murphy, "The Role of Sugar in Epileptic Seizures," *Townsend Letter for Doctors and Patients*, May, 2001.

36   N. Stern and M. Tuck, *Pathogenesis of Hypertension in Diabetes Mellitus. Diabetes Mellitus, a Fundamental and Clinical Test,* 2nd ed. (Philadelphia: Lippincott Williams & Wilkins, 2000), 943–57.

37   D. Donnini et al., "Glucose May Induce Cell Death through a Free Radical-Mediated Mechanism," *Biochemical and Biophysical Research Communications* 219, no. 2 (Feb 15, 1996): 412–17.

38   W. Glinsmann, H. Irausquin, and Y. K. Park, "Evaluation of Health Aspects of Sugar Contained in Carbohydrate Sweeteners: Report of Sugars Task Force, 1986," *Journal of Nutrition* 116 (Suppl 11; Nov 1986): S1–216. J. Yudkin and O. Eisa, "Dietary Sucrose and Oestradiol Concentration in Young Men," *Annals of Nutrition and Metabolism* 32, no. 2 (1988): 53–55.

39   T. Feehley and C. R. Nagler, "Health: The Weighty Costs of Non-Caloric Sweeteners," *Nature* 514, no. 7521 (Oct 9, 2014): 176–77. doi: 10.1038/nature13752.

40   Nicholas A. Bokulich and Martin J. Blaser, "A Bitter Aftertaste: Unintended Effects of Artificial Sweeteners on the Gut Microbiome," *Cell Metabolism* 20, no. 5 (Nov 4, 2014): 701–3.

41   G. Kristjánsson, P. Venge , and R. Hällgren, "Mucosal Reactivity to Cow's Milk Protein in Coeliac Disease," *Clinical and Experimental Immunology* 147, no. 3 (Mar 2007): 449–55.

42   J. Wasilewska et al., "The Exogenous Opioid Peptides and DPPIV Serum Activity in Infants with Apnoea Expressed as Apparent Life Threatening Events (ALTE)," *Neuropeptides* 45, no. 3 (Jun 2011): 189–95. doi:10.1016/j.npep.2011.01.005.

43   M. Knip et al., "Dietary Intervention in Infancy and Later Signs of Beta-Cell Autoimmunity," *New England Journal of Medicine* 363, no. 20 (Nov 11, 2010): 1900–8. doi: 10.1056/NEJMoa1004809.

44   A. Ebringer and T. Rashid, "Rheumatoid Arthritis Is Caused by Proteus: The Molecular Mimicry Theory and Karl Popper," *Frontiers in Bioscience (elite edition)* 1 (Jun 1, 2009): 577–86.

45   Michael H. Silverman and Marc J. Ostro, *Bacterial Endotoxin in Human Disease* (Berkeley, CA: XOMA, 1999).

46   J. Hollon et al., "Effect of Gliadin on Permeability."

CHAPTER 3

1   J. Simon-Areces, "UCP2 Induced by Natural Birth Regulates Neuronal Differentiation of the Hippocampus and Related Adult Behavior," *PLoS One* 7, no. 8 (2012): e42911.

2   K. Kristensen and L. Henriksen, "Cesarean Section and Disease Associated with Immune Function," *Journal of Allergy and Clinical Immunology* 137, no. 2 (Feb 2016): 587–90.

3   J. R. Marchesi et al., "The Gut Microbiota and Host Health: A New Clinical Frontier," *Gut* 65, no. 2 (Feb 2016): 330–39.

4   H. J. Zapata and V. J. Quagliarello, "The Microbiota and Microbiome in Aging: Potential Implications in Health and Age-Related Diseases," *Journal of the American Geriatrics Society* 63, no. 4 (Apr 2015): 776–81.

5   J. L. Round and S. K. Mazmanian, "The Gut Microbiota Shapes Intestinal Immune Responses during Health and Disease," *Nature Reviews: Immunology* 9, no. 5 (May 2009): 313–23.

6   S. Bengmark, "Nutrition of the Critically Ill—A 21st-Century Perspective," *Nutrients* 5, no. 1 (2013): 162–207.

7   G. D. Hermes, E. G. Zoetendal, and H. Smidt, "Molecular Ecological Tools to Decipher the Role of Our Microbial Mass in Obesity," *Beneficial Microbes* 6, no. 1 (Mar 2015): 61–81.

8   C. De Filippo et al., "Impact of Diet in Shaping Gut Microbiota Revealed by a Comparative Study in Children from Europe and Rural Africa," *Proceedings of the National Academy of Sciences of the United States of America* 107, no. 33 (Aug 17, 2010): 14691–96.

9   C. Costelloe et al., "Effect of Antibiotic Prescribing in Primary Care on Antimicrobial Resistance in Individual Patients: Systematic Review and Meta-Analysis," *BMJ* 340 (May 18, 2010): c2096. doi: 10.1136/bmj.c2096.

10   T. J. Martin, J. E. Kerschner, and V. A. Flanary, "Fungal Causes of Otitis Externa and Tympanostomy Tube Otorrhea," *International Journal of Pediatric Otorhinolaryngology* 69, no. 11 (Nov 2005): 1503–8.

11   A. I. Petra et al., "Gut-Microbiota-Brain Axis and Its Effect on Neuropsychiatric Disorders with Suspected Immune Dysregulation," *Clinical Therapeutics* 37, no. 5 (May 1, 2015): 984–95. doi: 10.1016/j.clinthera.2015.04.002.

12   N. Sudo, "Role of Microbiome in Regulating the HPA Axis and Its Relevance to Allergy," *Chemical Immunology and Allergy* 98 (2012): 163–75. doi: 10.1159/000336510.

13   G. Ou et al., "Proximal Small Intestinal Microbiota and Identification of Rod-Shaped Bacteria Associated with Childhood Celiac Disease," *American Journal of Gastroenterology* 104, no. 12 (Dec 2009): 3058–67. doi: 10.1038/ajg.2009.524.

14   N. Hayek, "Chocolate, Gut Microbiota, and Human Health," *Frontiers in Pharmacology* 4 (Feb 7, 2013): 11. doi:10.3389/fphar.2013.00011.

15   A. Duda-Chodak, "The Inhibitory Effect of Polyphenols on Human Gut Microbiota," *Journal of Physiology and Pharmacology* 63, no. 5 (Oct 2012): 497–503.

16   O. H. Franco et al. "The Polymeal" (see chap. 1, n. 8).

17   M. I. Queipo-Ortuno et al., "Influence of Red Wine Polyphenols and Ethanol on the Gut Microbiota Ecology and Biochemical Biomarkers," *American Journal of Clinical Nutrition* 95, no. 6 (Jun 2012): 1323–34. doi:10.3945/ajcn.111.027847.

18   M. Massot-Cladera et al., "Cocoa Modulatory Effect on Rat Faecal Microbiota and Colonic Crosstalk," *Archives of Biochemistry and Biophysics* 527, no. 2 (Nov 15, 2012): 105–12. doi: 10.1016/j.abb.2012.05.015.

19   Mara Hvistendahl, "My Microbiome and Me," *Science* 336, no. 6086 (Jun 8, 2012): 1248–50.

20   M. Jackson et al., "Signatures of Early Frailty in the Gut Microbiota," *Genome Medicine* 8, no. 1 (Jan 29, 2016): 8.

21   J. Suez et al., "Artificial Sweeteners Induce Glucose Intolerance by Altering the Gut Microbiota," *Nature* 514, no. 7521 (Oct 9, 2014): 181–86.

22   I. R. Redovnikovic et al., "Polyphenolic Content and Composition and Antioxidative Activity of Different Cocoa Liquors," *Czech Journal of Food Sciences* 27, no. 5 (2009): 330–37.

CHAPTER 4

1   R. Valentino et al., "Markers of Potential Coeliac Disease in Patients with Hashimoto's Thyroiditis," *European Journal of Endocrinology* 146, no. 4 (Apr 2002): 479–83.

2   J. P. Bercz et al., "Mechanistic Aspects of Ingested Chlorine Dioxide on Thyroid Function: Impact of Oxidants on Iodide Metabolism," *Environmental Health Perspectives* 69 (Nov 1986): 249–54.

3   V. M. Darras, "Endocrine Disrupting Polyhalogenated Organic Pollutants Interfere with Thyroid Hormone Signalling in the Developing Brain," *Cerebellum* 7, no. 1 (2008): 26–37.

4   US Department of Health and Human Services, Office on Women's Health, "Hashimoto's Disease, Frequently Asked Questions," http://www.womenshealth.gov /publications/our-publications/fact-sheet/hashimoto-disease.pdf.

5   Jonas F. Ludvigsson et al., "Small-Intestinal Histopathology and Mortality Risk in Celiac Disease," *Journal of the American Medical Association* 302, no. 11 (Sep 16, 2009): 1171–78.

6   C. Zanchi et al., "Leonardo da Vinci Meets Celiac Disease," *Journal of Pediatric Gastroenterology and Nutrition* 56, no. 2 (Feb 2013): 206–10.

7   M. Finizio et al., "Large Forehead: A Novel Sign of Undiagnosed Coeliac Disease," *Digestive and Liver Disease* 37, no. 9 (Sep 2005): 659–64.

CHAPTER 5

1   M. R. Arbuckle et al., "Development of Autoantibodies" (see chap. 1, n. 1).

2   Y. Shoenfeld et al., "The Mosaic of Autoimmunity: Prediction, Autoantibodies, and Therapy in Autoimmune Disease—2008," *Israel Medical Association Journal* 10, no. 1 (Jan 2008): 13–19.

3   B. Lindberg et al., "Islet Autoantibodies in Cord Blood from Children Who Developed Type I (Insulin-Dependent) Diabetes Mellitus before 15 Years of Age," *Diabetologia* 42, no. 2 (Feb 1999): 181–87.

4   A. Lanzini et al., "Complete Recovery of Intestinal Mucosa Occurs Very Rarely in Adult Coeliac Patients despite Adherence to Gluten-Free Diet," *Alimentary Pharmacology and Therapeutics* 29, no. 12 (Jun 15, 2009): 1299–1308. doi: 10.1111/j.1365-2036.2009.03992.x.

5   A. Sugrue, A. Egan, and A. O'Regan, "A Woman with Macrocytic Anaemia and Confusion," *BMJ* 349 (Jul 8, 2014): g4388.

6   R. Shaoul and A. Lerner, "Associated Autoantibodies in Celiac Disease," *Autoimmunity Reviews* 6, no. 8 (Sep 2007): 559–65.

7   J. V. Wright, "The Unexpected Culprits behind Rheumatoid Arthritis," *Nutrition and Healing*, Dec. 18, 2008.

8   N. H. Shah et al., "Proton Pump Inhibitor Usage and the Risk of Myocardial Infarction in the General Population," *PLoS One* 10, no. 6 (Jun 10, 2015): e0124653.

9   D. E. Freedberg et al., "Use of Proton Pump Inhibitors Is Associated with Fractures in Young Adults: A Population-Based Study," *Osteoporosis International* 26, no. 10 (Oct 2015): 2501–7.

10   K. Tucker, "Are you Vitamin B$_{12}$ Deficient?" *Agricultural Research* 48, no. 8 (Aug 2000).

11   L. Viitasalo et al., "Early Microbial Markers of Celiac Disease," *Journal of Clinical Gastroenterology* 48, no. 7 (Aug 2014): 620–24.

12   B. Kaila, K. Orr, and C. N. Bernstein, "The Anti-*Saccharomyces Cerevisiae* Antibody Assay in a Province-Wide Practice: Accurate in Identifying Cases of Crohn's Disease and Predicting Inflammatory Disease," *Canadian Journal of Gastroenterology* 19, no. 12 (Dec 2005): 717–21.

13   E. Israeli et al., "Anti-*Saccharomyces Cerevisiae* and Antineutrophil Cytoplasmic Antibodies as Predictors of Inflammatory Bowel Disease," *Gut* 54, no. 9 (Sep 2005): 1232–36. doi:10.1136/gut.2004.060228.

14   K. M. Das et al., "Autoimmunity to Cytoskeletal Protein Tropomyosin: A Clue to the Pathogenetic Mechanism for Ulcerative Colitis," *Journal of Immunology* 150, no. 6 (Mar 15, 1993): 2487–93.

15   M. Hendricks and H. Weintraub, "Tropomyosin Is Decreased in Transformed Cells," *Proceedings of the National Academy of Sciences of the United States of America* 78, no. 9 (Sep 1981): 5633–37.

16   C. Betterle and R. Zanchetta, "Update on Autoimmune Polyendocrine Syndromes (APS)," *Acta Bio-Medica* 74, no. 1 (Apr 2003): 9–33.

17   L. H. Duntas, "Does Celiac Disease Trigger Autoimmune Thyroiditis?" *Nature Reviews: Endocrinology* 5, no. 4 (Apr 2009): 190–91.

18   C. Virili et al., "Atypical Celiac Disease as Cause of Increased Need for Thyroxine: A Systematic Study," *Journal of Clinical Endocrinology and Metabolism* 97, no. 3 (Mar 2012): E419–22.

19   C. J. Murray and J. Frenk, "Ranking 37th—Measuring the Performance of the US Health Care System," *New England Journal of Medicine* 362, no. 2 (Jan 14, 2010): 98–99. doi: 10.1056/NEJMp0910064. P. A. Muennig and S. A. Glied, "What Changes in Survival Rates Tell Us about US Health Care," *Health Affairs*. 29, no. 11 (Nov 2010): 2105–13. doi: 10.1377/hlthaff.2010.0073.

20   P. Lencel and D. Magne, "Inflammaging: The Driving Force in Osteoporosis?" *Medical Hypotheses* 76, no. 3 (Mar 2011): 317–21. doi: 10.1016/j.mehy.2010.09.023.

21   P. Jepsen, "Comorbidity in Cirrhosis," *World Journal of Gastroenterology* 20, no. 23 (Jun 21, 2014): 7223–30.

22   G. Gobbi et al., "Coeliac Disease, Epilepsy, and Cerebral Calcifications: The Italian Working Group on Coeliac Disease and Epilepsy," *Lancet* 340, no. 8817 (Aug 22, 1992): 439–43.

23   M. Hadjivassiliou, R. A. Grünewald, and G. A. Davies-Jones, "Gluten Sensitivity as a Neurological Illness," *Journal of Neurology, Neurosurgery, and Psychiatry* 72, no. 5 (May 2002): 560–63.

CHAPTER 6

1   P. J. Turnbaugh et al., "The Effect of Diet on the Human Gut Microbiome: A Metagenomic Analysis in Humanized Gnotobiotic Mice," *Science Translational Medicine* 1, no. 6 (Nov 11, 2009): 6ra14.

2   Environmental Working Group analysis of tests of 10 umbilical cord blood samples conducted by AXYS Analytical Services (Sydney, BC) and Flett Research Ltd. (Winnipeg, MB).

3   L. Geurts et al., "Gut Microbiota Controls Adipose Tissue Expansion, Gut Barrier and Glucose Metabolism: Novel Insights into Molecular Targets and Interventions Using Prebiotics," *Beneficial Microbes* 5, no. 1 (Mar 2014): 3–17.

4   L. O. Schulz et al., "Effects of Traditional and Western Environments on Prevalence of Type 2 Diabetes in Pima Indians in Mexico and the US," *Diabetes Care* 29, no. 8 (Aug 2006): 1866–71.

5   William Davis, *Wheat Belly: Lose the Wheat, Lose the Weight, and Find Your Path Back to Health* (Emmaus, PA: Rodale, 2011).

CHAPTER 7

1   USDA Economic Research Service, "Recent trends in GE Adoption," http://www.ers.usda.gov/data-products/adoption-of-genetically-engineered-crops-in-the-us/recent-trends-in-ge-adoption.aspx.

2   R. Mesnage et al., "Cytotoxicity on Human Cells of Cry1Ab and Cry1Ac Bt Insecticidal Toxins Alone or with a Glyphosate-Based Herbicide," *Journal of Applied Toxicology* 33, no. 7 (Jul 2013): 695–99.

3   Anthony Samsel and Stephanie Seneff, "Glyphosate's Suppression of Cytochrome P450 Enzymes and Amino Acid Biosynthesis by the Gut Microbiome: Pathways to Modern Diseases," *Entropy* 15, no. 4 (Apr 2013): 1416–63. doi:10.3390/e15041416.

4   R. A. Hites et al.,"Global Assessment of Organic Contaminants in Farmed Salmon," *Science* 303, no. 5655 (Jan 9, 2004): 226–29.

5   S. L. Seierstad et al., "Dietary Intake of Differently Fed Salmon: The Influence on Markers of Human Atherosclerosis," *European Journal of Clinical Investigation* 35, no. 1 (Jan 2005): 52–59.

6   J. Foran et al., "Quantitative Analysis of the Benefits and Risks of Consuming Farmed and Wild Salmon," *Journal of Nutrition* 135, no. 11 (Nov 2005): 2639–43.

7   National Resources Defense Council, "The Smart Seafood Buying Guide," August 25, 2015. https://www.nrdc.org/stories/smart-seafood-buying-guide.

8   T. Thompson, "Gluten Contamination of Commercial Oat Products in the United States," *New England Journal of Medicine* 351, no. 19 (Nov 4, 2004): 2021–22.

9   G. M. Sharma, M. Pereira, and K. M. Williams, "Gluten Detection in Foods Available in the United States—A Market Survey," *Food Chemistry* 169 (Feb 15, 2015): 120–26.

10   B. Bellioni-Businco et al., "Allergenicity of Goat's Milk in Children with Cow's Milk Allergy," *Journal of Allergy and Clinical Immunology* 103, no. 6 (Jun 1999): 1191–94.

11   J. Jenkins, H. Breiteneder, and E. N. Mills, "Evolutionary Distance from Human Homologs Reflects Allergenicity of Animal Food Proteins," *Journal of Allergy and Clinical Immunology* 120, no. 6 (Dec 2007): 1399–405.

12   P. Restani et al., "Cross-Reactivity between Milk Proteins from Different Animal Species," *Clinical and Experimental Allergy* 29, no. 7 (Jul 1999): 997–1004.

13   T. J. Suutari et al., "IgE Cross Reactivity between Reindeer and Bovine Milk Beta-Lactoglobulins in Cow's Milk Allergic Patients," *Journal of Investigational Allergology and Clinical Immunology* 16, no. 5 (2006): 296–302.

14   G. Iacono et al., "Use of Ass' Milk in Multiple Food Allergy," *Journal of Pediatric Gastroenterology and Nutrition* 14, no. 2 (Feb 1992): 177–81.

15   A. V. Finkel, J. A. Yerry, and J. D. Mann, "Dietary Considerations in Migraine Management: Does a Consistent Diet Improve Migraine?" *Current Pain and Headache Reports* 17, no. 11 (Nov 2013): 373. doi: 10.1007/s11916-013-0373-4.

16   B. M. Popkin and C. Hawkes, "Sweetening of the Global Diet, Particularly Beverages: Patterns, Trends, and Policy Responses," *Lancet Diabetes and Endocrinology* 4, no. 2 (Feb 2016): 174–86.

17   USDA, Profiling Food Consumption in America. http://www.usda.gov/factbook /chapter2.pdf.

18   A. Singh et al., "Phytochemical Profile of Sugarcane and Its Potential Health Aspects," *Pharmacognosy Reviews* 9, no. 17 (Jan–Jun 2015): 45–54.

19   Nicholas A. Bokulich and Martin J. Blaser, "A Bitter Aftertaste: Unintended Effects of Artificial Sweeteners on the Gut Microbiome," *Cell Metabolism* 20, no. 5 (Nov 4, 2014): 701–3.

20   J. James et al., "Preventing Childhood Obesity by Reducing Consumption of Carbonated Drinks: Cluster Randomised Controlled Trial," *BMJ* 328, no. 7450 (May 22, 2004): 1237. doi: 10.1136/bmj.38077.458438.EE.

21   F. Biagi et al., "A Milligram of Gluten a Day Keeps the Mucosal Recovery Away: A Case Report," *Nutrition Reviews* 62, no. 9 (Sep 2004): 360–63.

22   Chiara Dall'asta et al., "Dietary Exposure to Fumonisins and Evaluation of Nutrient Intake in a Group of Adult Celiac Patients on a Gluten-Free Diet," *Molecular Nutrition and Food Research* 56, no. 4 (Apr 2012): 632–40.

CHAPTER 8

1   A. Fasano and T. Shea-Donohue, "Mechanisms of Disease: The Role of Intestinal Barrier Function in the Pathogenesis of Gastrointestinal Autoimmune Diseases," *Nature Clinical Practices: Gastroenterology and Hepatology* 2, no. 9 (Sep 2005): 416–22.

2   J. L. Watson et al., "Green Tea Polyphenol (-)-Epigallocatechin Gallate Blocks Epithelial Barrier Dysfunction Provoked by IFN-Gamma but Not by IL-4," *American Journal of Physiology: Gastrointestinal and Liver Physiology* 287, no. 5 (Nov 2004): G954–61.

3   S. D. Hsu et al., "Green Tea Polyphenols Reduce Autoimmune Symptoms in a Murine Model for Human Sjogren's Syndrome and Protect Human Salivary Acinar Cells from TNF-Alpha-Induced Cytotoxicity," *Autoimmunity* 40, no. 2 (Mar 2007): 138–47.

4   Jeong-a Kim et al., "Epigallocatechin Gallate, a Green Tea Polyphenol, Mediates NO-Dependent Vasodilation Using Signaling Pathways in Vascular Endothelium Requiring Reactive Oxygen Species and Fyn," *Journal of Biological Chemistry* 282, no. 18 (May 4, 2007): 13736–45.

5   S. Kuriyama et al., "Green Tea Consumption and Cognitive Function: A Cross-Sectional Study from the Tsurugaya Project," *American Journal of Clinical Nutrition* 83, no. 2 (Feb 2006): 355–61.

6   Q. Collins et al., "Epigallocatechin-3-Gallate (EGCG), a Green Tea Polyphenol, Suppresses Hepatic Gluconeogenesis through 5-AMP-Activated Protein Kinase," *Journal of Biological Chemistry* 282, no. 41 (Oct 12, 2007): 30143–49.

7   S. Kuriyama et al., "Green Tea Consumption and Mortality due to Cardiovascular Disease, Cancer, and All Causes in Japan: The Ohsaki Study," *Journal of the American Medical Association* 296, no. 10 (Sep 13, 2006): 1255–65.

8   A. C. Bronstein et al., "Annual Report of the American Association of Poison Control Centers' National Poison Data System (NPDS): 28th Annual Report," *Clinical Toxicology* 49, no. 10 (Dec 2010): 910–41.

9   K. M. Adams, M. Kohlmeier, and S. H. Zeisel, "Nutrition Education in US Medical Schools: Latest Update of a National Survey," *Academic Medicine* 85, no. 9 (Sep 2010): 1537–42.

10   B. Diosdado et al., "Neutrophil Recruitment and Barrier Impairment in Celiac Disease: A Genomic Study," *Clinical Gastroenterology and Hepatology* 5, no. 5 (May 2007): 574–81.

11   B. Muehleisen and R. L. Gallo, "Vitamin D in Allergic Disease: Shedding Light on a Complex Problem," *Journal of Allergy and Clinical Immunology* 131, no. 2 (Feb 2013): 324–29. doi: 10.1016/j.jaci.2012.12.1562.

12   J. O. Clarke and G. E. Mullin, "A Review of Complementary and Alternative Approaches to Immunomodulation," *Nutrition in Clinical Practice* 23, no. 1 (Feb 2008): 49–62.

13   Y. Wang et al., "High Molecular Weight Barley β-Glucan Alters Gut Microbiota toward Reduced Cardiovascular Disease Risk," *Frontiers in Microbiology* 7 (Feb 10, 2016): 129.

14   A. Mahmood et al., "Zinc Carnosine, a Health Food Supplement That Stabilises Small Bowel Integrity and Stimulates Gut Repair Processes," *Gut* 56, no. 2 (Feb 2007): 168–75.

15   M. R. Griffin, "Epidemiology of Nonsteroidal Anti-Inflammatory Drug-Associated Gastroduodenal Injury," *American Journal of Medicine* 104, no. 3A (Mar 30, 1998) :23S–29S.

16   C. M. Wilcox et al., "Consensus Development Conference on the Use of Nonsteroidal Anti-Inflammatory Agents, including Cyclooxygenase-2 Enzyme Inhibitors and Aspirin," *Clinical Gastroenterology and Hepatology* 4, no. 9 (Sep 2006): 1082–89.

17   B. Cryer, "NSAID-Associated Deaths: The Rise and Fall of NSAID-Associated GI Mortality," *American Journal of Gastroenterology* 100, no. 8 (Aug 2005): 1694–95.

18   B. Cryer and M. Feldman, "Effects of Very Low Doses of Daily, Long-Term Aspirin Therapy on Gastric, Duodenal and Rectal Prostaglandins and on Mucosal Injury in Healthy Humans," *Gastroenterology* 117, no. 1 (Jul 1999): 17–25.

19   C.M. Wilcox, B. Cryer, and G. Triadafilopoulos, "Patterns of Use and Public Perception of Over-the-Counter Pain Relievers: Focus on Nonsteroidal Antiinflammatory Drugs," *Journal of Rheumatology* 32, no. 11 (Nov 2005): 2218–24.

20   Daniel A. Leffler et al., "A Randomized, Double-Blind Study of Larazotide Acetate to Prevent the Activation of Celiac Disease during Gluten Challenge," *American Journal of Gastroenterology* 107, no. 10 (Oct 2012): 1554–62.

21   Ilus Tuire et al., "Persistent Duodenal Intraepithelial Lymphocytosis despite a Long-Term Strict Gluten-Free Diet in Celiac Disease," *American Journal of Gastroenterology* 107, no. 10 (Oct 2012): 1563–69.

22   M. V. Tulstrup, "Antibiotic Treatment Affects Intestinal Permeability and Gut Microbial Composition in Wistar Rats Dependent on Antibiotic Class," *PLoS One* 10, no. 12 (Dec 21, 2015): e0144854.

23   F. C. Peedikayil, P. Sreenivasan, and A. Narayanan, "Effect of Coconut Oil in Plaque Related Gingivitis—A Preliminary Report," *Nigerian Medical Journal* 56, no. 2 (Mar–Apr 2015): 143–47.

24   K. Scherf et al., "Wheat-Dependent Exercise-Induced Anaphylaxis," *Clinical and Experimental Allergy* 46, no. 1 (Jan 2016): 10–20.

25   T. Thompson and T. Grace, "Gluten in Cosmetics: Is There a Reason for Concern?" *Journal of the Academy of Nutrition and Dietetics* 112, no. 23 (Sep 2012): 1316–23.

26   R. Teshima, "Food Allergen in Cosmetics," *Yakugaku Zasshi* 134, no. 1 (2014): 33–38.

27   K. Kwangmi, "Influences of Environmental Chemicals on Atopic Dermatitis," *Toxicological Research* 31, no. 2 (Jun 2015): 89–96.

28   A. R. Heurung, "Adverse Reactions to Sunscreen Agents: Epidemiology, Responsible Irritants and Allergens, Clinical Characteristics, and Management," *Dermatitis* 25, no. 6 (Nov–Dec 2014): 289–326.

CHAPTER 9

1   Margie Kelly, "Top 7 Genetically Modified Crops," *Huffpost Green* (blog), Oct 30, 2012, http://www.huffingtonpost.com/margie-kelly/genetically-modified-food_b _2039455.html.

2   G. M. Sharma, M. Pereira, and K. M. Williams, "Gluten Detection in Foods Available in the United States—A Market Survey," *Food Chemistry* 169 (Feb 15, 2015): 120–26.

3   G. Kristjánsson et al., "Gut Mucosal Granulocyte Activation Precedes Nitric Oxide Production: Studies in Coeliac Patients Challenged with Gluten and Corn," *Gut* 54, no. 6 (Jun 2005): 769–74. doi:10.1136/gut.2004.057174.

4   F. Cabrera-Chávez et al., "Maize Prolamins Resistant to Peptic-Tryptic Digestion Maintain Immune-Recognition by IgA from Some Celiac Disease Patients," *Plant Foods for Human Nutrition* 67, no. 1 (Mar 2012): 24, 30.

5   Chiara Dall'asta et al., "Dietary Exposure to Fumonisins and Evaluation of Nutrient Intake in a Group of Adult Celiac Patients on a Gluten-Free Diet," *Molecular Nutrition and Food Research* 56, no. 4 (Apr 2012): 632–40.

6   V. F. Zevallos et al., "Variable Activation of Immune Response by Quinoa (Chenopodium Quinoa Willd.) Prolamins in Celiac Disease," *American Journal of Clinical Nutrition* 96, no. 2 (Aug 2012): 337–44.

7   J. R. Biesiekierski et al., "No Effects of Gluten in Patients with Self-Reported Non-Celiac Gluten Sensitivity after Dietary Reduction of Fermentable, Poorly Absorbed, Short-Chain Carbohydrates," *Gastroenterology* 145, no. 2 (Aug 2013): 320–28.

CHAPTER 11

1   P. Tiwari, "Recent Trends in Therapeutic Approaches for Diabetes Management: A Comprehensive Update," *Journal of Diabetes Research* 2015 (2015): 340838.

2   M. T. Ventura et al., "Intestinal Permeability in Patients with Adverse Reactions to Food," *Digestive and Liver Disease* 38, no. 10 (Oct 2006): 732–36.

3   A. Lanzini et al., "Complete Recovery of Intestinal Mucosa Occurs Very Rarely in Adult Coeliac Patients despite Adherence to Gluten-Free Diet," *Alimentary Pharmacology and Therapeutics* 29, no. 12 (Jun 15, 2009): 1299–308.

4   G. Corrao et al., "Mortality in Patients with Coeliac Disease and Their Relatives: A Cohort Study," *Lancet* 358, no. 9279 (Aug 4, 2001): 356–61.

5   L. A. Anderson et al., "Malignancy and Mortality in a Population-Based Cohort of Patients with Coeliac Disease or 'Gluten Sensitivity,'" *World Journal of Gastroenterology* 13, no. 1 (Jan 7, 2007): 146–51.

INDEX

Underscored page references indicate boxed text. **Boldface** references indicate illustrations and photographs.

arthritic peptide, 127
artificial sweeteners, 50, 86, 159, 186–87
ASCA (anti-Saccharomyces cerevisiae
   antibodies), 122
asialoganglioside GM 1, 128–29
aspartame, 50, 159
atherosclerosis, 15–16, 127
atopic dermatitis, 219
ATPase, 118–21
autism spectrum disorder, 148–49
autoantibodies, 35–37
autoimmune diseases
   identifying, 20–21, 24–27
   organ-specific, 114
   primary pathway in development of,
      5
   systemic, 113
autoimmune spectrum
   allostasis, 7
   antibiotics and, 8
   autoimmune diseases, 20–21, 24–27
   benign autoimmunity, 4
   celiac disease, 27–32
   common symptoms of gluten-related
      disorders, 107–9
   comparing traditional and functional
      medicine approaches, 91–92
   creating timeline, 102–4
   determining place on, 91
   diagnosing celiac disease and gluten
      sensitivity, 105–7
   early pathogenic autoimmunity, 5–7
   elevated antibodies, 11–15
   gluten sensitivity, 27–32
   inflammation, 15–20
   lifestyle perspective to health, 93–94
   Medical Symptoms Quiz, 100–102
   normal immunity, 4
   NSAIDs and, 7–8
   overview, 3–4, 9–11
   pathogenic autoimmunity, 4
   Ready-to-Change Quiz, 96–98
   stages of lifestyle change, 95–96
   starting Transition Protocol, 109–10
autoimmunity. See also autoimmune
      spectrum; predictive
      autoimmunity
   benign, 4
   early pathogenic, 5–7
   pathogenic, 4

B

Bacillus subtilis bacteria, 209
bacteria. *See also* microbiome
   Bacillus subtilis , 209
   Bacteroidetes, 66
   Bifidobacterium , 209
   Firmicutes, 66, 70

Lactobacillus , 209
Porphyromonas gingivalis, 216
Prevotella, 67
Saccharomyces boulardii , 209
Saccharomyces cervisae, 113
superbugs, 11
survival, 152
bacteriocidins, 82
Bacteroidetes bacteria, 66
baking flours, 172–73
bananas, 163
beans, biological value of, 167
beef
   biological value of, 167
   grass-fed, 86, 166
benign autoimmunity, 4, 35
benzodiazepines, 30
Bifidobacterium bacteria, 209
biofilms, 76
biological value (BV), 167
biomarkers, 112, **116**
biomarker testing, 112
Bland, Jeffrey, 19, 20, 40–41
body burden, 147–49, **148–49**, 151
body-care products, 218–23
body composition analysis, 16
body fat
   adipose fat, 16, 48
   retention of, 153–54
   white fat, 153
brain
   microbiota-gut-brain axis, 80–81
   multiple autoimmune reactivity screen
      asialoganglioside GM 1, 128–29
      cerebellar, 129–30
      glutamic-acid decarboxylase, 128
      myelin basic protein, 128–29
      synapsin, 129–30
      tubulin, 129
butyrate (butyric acid), 72, 88, 163
BV (biological value), 167

C

caffeine, 193–94
Campbell-McBride, Natasha, 229
carbohydrates
   alcoholic beverages, 187
   choosing good carbohydrates, 86
   complex, 186
   FODMAPs, 30, 234–36
   fructan, 162
   glycemic index and, 51
   refined, 186, 190
casein
   biological value of, 167
   in colostrum, 210
   defined, 55
   dysbiosis and, 71

in nondairy products, 183–84
Samantha's story, **63**
casomorphins, 55, 189
catabolism, 144
celiac disease
    cranial facial morphology of patients
        with, <u>108</u>, 108–9, <u>109</u>
    diagnosing, 105–7
    genetic testing for, **135**
    microvilli, 27, **28**
    overview, 27–32
cerebellar antibodies test, 129–30
CFUs (colony-forming units), 87, 90
change, stages of, 95–96
cheat sheet
    Phase 1 of Transition Protocol, **197**
    Phase 2 of Transition Protocol, **238**
chicken, biological value of, 167
chicory root, 162
children
    fish consumption, 169
    following Transition Protocol, 196
    sweetened beverages and, 187
chlorine, 93, 124–25
chocolate, 85, **85**
coconut butter, 172
coconut cream, 172
coconut milk, 172, 183
coconut oil, 172, 218
coffee
    factors in determining health benefits/
        risks, 39–40
    gluten-free, 193–94
collagen complex, 127
collateral damage, 36
colony-forming units (CFUs), 87, 90
colostrum, 209–10
common symptoms, defined, 7
comorbidity, 17
conditions, defined, 20
contemplation stage of change, 95–96
cooking oils, 172
corn
    as GMO crop, 158–59
    maltodextrin, 211
    Phase 2 of Transition Protocol, 232
cosmetics, 218–23
cow's milk
    biological value of, 167
    casein, 55
    infants at risk for type 1 diabetes and, 55,
        128
    protein structure, 183
cranial facial morphology (of patients with
    celiac disease), <u>108</u>, 108–9, <u>109</u>
cross-reactivity, 55
curcumin, 201
cytochrome P450 hepatocyte, 127–28
cytokines, 10, 199

D

dairy
    casein, 55
    eliminating during Phase 1 of Transition
        Protocol, 183–85
    homogenization, 54
    lactose intolerance, 54–55
    pasteurization, 54
dark rings under eyes (allergic shiners), 153
Davis, William, 51, 189–90
Dennie's lines, 153
Dennis, Melinda, 174
dermatitis, 219
determination stage of change, 96
detox diet, **150**
DHA (in fish), 207
diabetes
    cow's milk and infants at risk for, 55, 128
    glyphosate and, <u>160</u>
    sugar and, 47–48
    type 1, 47–48
    type 2, 48
    type 3, 48
dietary fat
    healthy fats, 86, 172
    lipid raft transcytosis, 56
differential (repeat stool analysis), 142–43
digestive enzyme supplements
    E3 Advanced Plus, 216
    overview, 215–16
disease process (pathogenic autoimmunity),
    4
dysbiosis
    antibiotics and, 75–76, **77**
    defined, 60
    general discussion, 71–74
    stress and, 76, 78–82
    symptoms of, 74–75

E

early pathogenic autoimmunity, 5–7
edema (fluid retention), 153
EGCG (epigallocatechin gallate)
    antioxidant, 201
elevated antibodies. *See also* antibodies
    lupus, 6
    overview, 11–15
endorphins, **85**, 189
endoscopy report, 105
endotoxins, 56
enkephalins, **85**, 189
environmental exposures
    dairy, 54–56
    gluten, 43–46
    lipopolysaccharides, 56–57, **58**
    overview, 41–42
    sugar, 46–54

EPA (in fish), 207
epigallocatechin gallate (EGCG)
    antioxidant, 201
epigenetics, 39–41, 69–70, 143
epithelial intestinal lining, 59
epithelium cells, 206
erythrocyte sedimentation rate (ESR), 142
euthyroidism, 124

F

fad diets, 31
Fasano, Alessio, 44, 59, 60, 68
fat (body)
    adipose fat, 16, 48
    retention of, 153–54
    white fat, 153
fat (dietary)
    healthy, 86, 172
    lipid raft transcytosis, 56
fermentable oligo-di-monosaccharides and
        polyols. *See* FODMAPs
fermented foods
    introducing to diet, 87
    overview, 173
    probiotics from, 208–9
    recipes, 278–80
    Samantha's story, **89**
fibulin, 127
"fight, flight, or fright" response, 78–79
Firmicutes bacteria
    defined, 66
    Pima Indians, 70
fish
    biological value of, 167
    highest mercury content, 171
    high mercury content, 170
    low-mercury content, 170
    moderate mercury content, 170
    overview, 169
fish oils, 207–8
flours (baking), 172–73
fluid retention (edema), 153
FODMAPs (fermentable oligo-di-
        monosaccharides and polyols)
    defined, 30
    Phase 2 of Transition Protocol, 234–36
food allergies, 42
food sensitivities. *See also* gluten sensitivity
    food allergies versus, 42
    non-celiac wheat sensitivity, 30–31
    Samantha's story, **62–63**
Ford, Rodney, 196
free radicals
    defined, 18
    from hot oils, 172
    oxidative stress and, 19
fresh foods
    animal proteins, 166–68
    fruits, 163–64

nuts and seeds, 164–65
    overview, 161–63
    vegetables, 165–66
fruits
    FODMAP, 235
    Phase 1 of Transition Protocol, 163–64
    polyphenols, 84
fumonisin, 232
functional medicine approach, 91–92

G

gastrointestinal system
    gastrointestinal tract, 9
    multiple autoimmune reactivity screen
        ANCA antibodies, 122
        ASCA antibodies, 122
        ATPase, 118–21
        intrinsic factor, 121–22
        parietal cells, 118–21
        tropomyosin, 122–23
general adaptation syndrome, 79
genetics
    epigenetics, 39–41
    genetic testing for celiac disease, **135**
    molecular mimicry, 35–37
    overview, 37–38
Glass cleaner formula, 225
glia cells, 9
glucocorticoids, 80
glutamic-acid decarboxylase, 128
glutamine, 206–7
gluten
    classification of gluten proteins, **43**
    common symptoms of gluten-related
        disorders, 107–9
    diagnosing celiac disease and gluten
        sensitivity, 105–7
    digestibility, 44
    eliminating during Phase 1 of Transition
        Protocol, 173–76
    ingredients that may contain, **179–82**
    intestinal permeability and, 61
    Kaposi's sarcoma and, <u>45</u>
    thyroid function and, 93
gluten ataxia, 30
gluten sensitivity
    diagnosing, 105–7
    medications that worsen, **200**
    osteoporosis and, <u>32</u>
    overview, 27–32
    Samantha's story, **62–63**
Gluten Sensitivity Support Packs, 205
gluteomorphin, 189
glycemic index
    bananas, 163
    overview, 51–53
    vegetables, 165
glyphosate, 159, <u>160</u>
GMOs, 158–61

goat's milk, 183
grains
  genetically modified, 158–61
  increased gluten content of, 46
  Phase 1 of Transition Protocol, 173–74
  Phase 2 of Transition Protocol, 231–34
  Triticeae family of, 43
grass-fed beef, 86, 166
green tea, 202–3, <u>203</u>

H

Hadjivassiliou, Marios, 30
Hashimoto's thyroid disease, 30
HCl (hydrochloric acid)
  defined, 118
  hypochlorhydria, 119
  supplements, 120–21
  symptoms of deficiency, 119–20
"heal and repair" state, 142
healthy fats, 86, 172
heart
  multiple autoimmune reactivity screen
    alpha-myosin, 125
    myocardial peptide, 125
    phospholipid, 125–27
    platelet glycoprotein, 125–27
    predictive autoimmunity, **117**
hemoglobin A1C, 17–18
high-sensitivity C-reactive protein test, 142
homeostasis model assessment (HOMA), 54
homogenization, 54
household products
  All-purpose cleaner formula, 224
  All-purpose disinfectant formula, 225
  All-purpose scouring powder formula, 224
  Glass cleaner formula, 225
  Porcelain polish formula, 225
  toxic food exposures in, 224, **226–27**
  Wood cabinet cleaner formula, 225
  Wood floor cleaner formula, 225
Houston, Mark, 10, 115
hunger, managing, 194–95
hydrochloric acid. *See* HCl

I

IBD (inflammatory bowel disease), <u>160</u>
IBS (Irritable bowel syndrome), 29
IgA antibody, 11–12
IgD antibody, 11–12
IgE antibody, 11–12
IgG antibody, 11–12
IgM antibody, 11–12
immune system
  adaptive, 10–11
  antibodies, 10
  antigens, 11
  cytokines, 10

elevated antibodies, 11–15
  inflammation, 15–20
    overview, 15–16
    oxidative stress and, 18–20
    weak link and, 17–18
  innate, 10, 14, 28–29
  types of, 9
inadvertent food exposures, avoiding, 213–16
inflammation
  genetic weak link and, 17–18
  overview, 15–16
  oxidative stress and, 18–20
  systemic inflammatory cascade, **58**
inflammatory bowel disease (IBD), <u>160</u>
innate immune system
  elevated antibodies, 14
  gluten sensitivity, 28–29
  overview, 10
insulin
  insulin resistance, 48
  multiple autoimmune reactivity screen, 128
intestinal antigenic permeability screen, 135, 136
intestinal permeability
  general discussion, 59–61
  reversibility of, 64
  Samantha's story, **63**
intrinsic factor, 121–22
inulin, 162
investigative doctoring approach, 237, 239
iodine 131, 93–94
Irritable bowel syndrome (IBS), 29
islet cell antigen antibodies, 128

K

Kaposi's sarcoma, <u>45</u>
Kasuli, Erica, 187, 194–95
Keech, Andrew, 210
kefir, 87
KeVita, 87
kimchi, 87
kombucha, 87
Kupffer cells, 9

L

Lactobacillus bacteria, 209
lactose intolerance, 54–55
leaky gut syndrome
  general discussion, 59–61
  reversibility of, 64
  Samantha's story, **63**
lectins, 30
lifestyle perspective to health, 93–94
lipid raft transcytosis, 56
lipopolysaccharides. *See* LPS
Lipski, Liz, 186

Wood cabinet cleaner formula, 225
Wood floor cleaner formula, 225
normal immunity, 4
NSAIDs (nonsteroidal anti-inflammatory
    drugs)
    autoimmune spectrum and, 7–8
    zinc carnosine and, 209
nut milks, 183
nutrients supporting Transition Protocol
    colostrum, 209–10
    fish oils, 207–8
    glutamine, 206–7
    Gluten Sensitivity Support Packs, 205
    green tea, 202–3, <u>203</u>
    pleiotropic approach, 202–3
    Polymeal approach, 203
    polyphenol, 201–2
    probiotics, 208–9
    vitamin D, 205–6
    zinc carnosine, 209
nuts and seeds, 164–65

O

oats, 174
oil pulling, 218
oils (cooking), 172
omega-3 fatty acids, 207–8
oral (mouth) hygiene, 216, 218
osteocyte, 127
osteoporosis
    gluten sensitivity and, <u>32</u>
    proton-pump inhibitors and, 120
ovaries, testing, 127
oxidative stress, 18–20

P

Paleo diet
    coconut products, 172
    compared to Transition Protocol, 191
pancreas, testing, 128
parasympathetic dominance (adrenal
    glands), 80
parasympathetic nervous system, 78
pareve labeling, 183, **184**
parietal cells, 118–21
pasteurization, 54
pathogenic autoimmunity (disease process), 4
pathogenic intestinal permeability, 64, 206
Phase 1 (Transition Protocol)
    baking flours, 172–73
    cheat sheet, **197**
    eliminating dairy, 183–85
    eliminating gluten, 173–76
    eliminating sugar, 186–91
    FAQs, 191–96
    fermented foods, 173
    fish, 169–71
        highest mercury content, 171
        high mercury content, 170

low-mercury content, 170
        moderate mercury content, 170
        overview, 169
    fresh foods, 161–68
        animal proteins, 166–68
        fruits, 163–64
        nuts and seeds, 164–65
        overview, 161–63
        vegetables, 165–66
    GMOs and, 158–61
    healthy fats, 172
    ingredients that may contain gluten,
        179–82
    overview, 157–58
    reviewing ingredients, 176–79
    wheatgrass juice, **179**
Phase 2 (Transition Protocol)
    cheat sheet, **238**
    foods to avoid, 229–36
        corn, 232
        FODMAPs, 234–36
        grains, 231–34
        nightshade vegetables, 234
        overview, 229–30
        quinoa, 233–34
        rice, 233
        soy, 230–31
    investigative doctoring approach, 237,
        239
    overview, 228–29
    Samantha's story, **240**
phospholipid, 125–27
Pima Indians
    Firmicutes bacteria, 70–71
    US Pima Indian diet versus Mexican
        Pima Indian diet, 152–53
platelet glycoprotein, 125–27
pleiotropic approach, 202–3
Polymeal approach, 84–85, 203
polyphenols, 84–85, 201–2
Porcelain polish formula, 225
Porphyromonas gingivalis bacteria, 216
positive predictive value (PPV), 112–13,
        113–14
PPIs (proton-pump inhibitors), 120
prebiotics, 84, <u>85</u>, 90, 216
precontemplation stage of change, 95
predictive autoimmunity
    genetic weak link and, 114–16
    intestinal antigenic permeability screen,
        135, 136
    multiple autoimmune reactivity screen
        adrenal glands, 125
        brain, 128–30
        gastrointestinal system, 118–23
        heart, 125–27
        liver, 127–28
        musculoskeletal health, 127
        overview, 116, 118
        pancreas, 128